This is the first book to focus on injury in the aging, an area of increasing concern given the rapid rise in the elderly population. Because of this demographic increase and the burgeoning costs of health care, it is crucial to understand the nature of, and responses to, injuries in older people. Trauma and injury in this group present unique clinical problems. Even in those who survive, recovery may not be complete and the associated loss of independence has an enormous impact on society. This volume is a pioneering attempt to distil and summarise our state of knowledge, and to identify those areas where new medical research might help to alleviate or overcome this problem. The contributors span a comprehensive range of clinical and scientific issues pertinent to improving the care of injured elderly patients.

INJURY IN THE AGING

INJURY IN THE AGING

Edited by

M. A. HORAN AND R. A. LITTLE

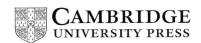

CAMBRIDGE
UNIVERSITY PRESS

PUBLISHED BY THE PRESS SYNDICATE OF THE UNIVERSITY OF CAMBRIDGE
The Pitt Building, Trumpington Street, Cambridge CB2 1RP, United Kingdom

CAMBRIDGE UNIVERSITY PRESS
The Edinburgh Building, Cambridge CB2 2RU, United Kingdom
40 West 20th Street, New York, NY 10011-4211, USA
10 Stamford Road, Oakleigh, Melbourne 3166, Australia

First published 1998

Printed in the United Kingdom at the University Press, Cambridge

Typeset in 10/13 pt Times [VN]

A catalogue record for this book is available from the British Library

Every effort has been made in preparing this book to provide accurate and
up-to-date information which is in accord with accepted standards and practice
at the time of publication. Nevertheless, the authors, editors and publisher can
make no warranties that the information herein is totally free from error, not
least because clinical standards are constantly changing through research and
regulation. The authors, editors and publisher therefore disclaim all liability for
direct or consequential damages resulting from the use of the material contained
in this book. The reader is strongly advised to pay careful attention to
information provided by the manufacturer of any drugs or equipment that they
plan to use.

ISBN 0 521 62160 7 hardback

Contents

Contributors

S. P. Allison
Department of Medicine Ward C54, University Hospital, Nottingham NG7 2UH, UK

G. S. Ashcroft
School of Biological Sciences and Department of Geriatric Medicine, University of Manchester, Manchester M13 9PT, UK

R. N. Barton
North Western Injury Research Centre, University of Manchester, Manchester M13 9PT, UK

M. R. Bliss
London E9 7DP, UK

F. Carli
McGill Department of Anesthesia, Royal Victoria Hospital, Montreal, Quebec H3A 1A1, Canada

B. Clift
Department of Orthopaedics, Dundee Royal Infirmary, Dundee DD1 9ND, UK

W. J. K. Cumming
Neuroscience Unit, Alexandra Hospital, Cheadle SK8 2PX, UK

C. T. Currie
Department of Medicine, Geriatric Medicine Unit, University of Edinburgh, City Hospital, Edinburgh EH10 5SB, UK

H. T. Davenport
Northwood HA6 2UZ, UK

J. H. Downton
St Thomas' Hospital, Stockport SK3 8BL, UK

J. Duggan
James Connelly Memorial Hospital, Blanchardstown, Co Dublin, Ireland

J. D. Edwards
Intensive Care Unit, University Hospital of South Manchester, Manchester M20 8LR, UK

M. W. J. Ferguson
School of Biological Sciences, University of Manchester, Manchester M13 9PT, UK

R. M. Francis
Musculoskeletal Unit, Freeman Hospital, Newcastle upon Tyne NE7 7DN, UK

L. Gormally
The Linacre Centre, London NW8 9NH, UK

J. Grimley Evans
Nuffield Department of Clinical Medicine, Geriatric Medicine Division, Radcliffe Infirmary, Oxford OX2 6HE, UK

M. A. Horan
Department of Geriatric Medicine, Hope Hospital, Salford M6 8HD, UK

R. A. Little
North Western Injury Research Centre, University of Manchester, Manchester M13 9PT, UK

W. J. MacLennan
Geriatric Medicine Unit, Department of Medicine, University of Edinburgh, City Hospital, Edinburgh EH10 5SB, UK

J. McClure
Diagnostic Cytology, Christie Hospital, Manchester M20 9BX, UK

P. A. O'Neill
Department of Geriatric Medicine, Hope Hospital, Salford M6 8HD, UK

S. G. Parker
University of Leicester, Leicester, UK

N. J. Rothwell
University of Manchester, Manchester M13 9PT, UK

D. I. Rowley
The University of Dundee, Department of Orthopaedic and Trauma Surgery, Royal Infirmary, Dundee DD1 9ND, UK

P. J. L. M. Strijbos
Department of Pharmacology, Wellcome Research Laboratories, Beckenham BR3 3BS, UK

A. M. Sutcliffe
Musculoskeletal Unit, Freeman Hospital, Newcastle upon Tyne NE7 7DN, UK

G. M. Watkins
Department of Surgery, Easton Hospital, Easton, PA 18042, USA

J. Wattis
Leeds Community and Mental Health Services, Meanwood Park Hospital, Leeds LS6 4QB, UK

1

An overview of injury

M. A. HORAN and R. A. LITTLE

The nature of injury

For the purpose of this volume, injury may be defined as physical damage to tissue caused by, for example, the dissipation of energy on contact with an external object (e.g. motor vehicle) or agent (heat) and the whole body (systemic) responses elicited by such a localised injury. We will not consider directly 'injuries' such as vascular occlusion although many of the local and general responses that are discussed will be relevant to such situations as the host has only a limited number of homoeostatic mechanisms to recruit.

Why should injury, especially to the elderly, be considered worthy of discussion? It is accepted, perhaps begrudgingly, by those responsible for resourcing health care that injury is now a major problem. Thus injury has been described as the last major plague of the young, with road traffic accidents already posing a global threat while penetrating injuries from bullets and knives which are an epidemic in the USA are following the advance of civilisation/westernisation through the rest of the world. Although attracting most publicity, deaths are only part (and perhaps the least important part) of the problems posed to society by injury. For every death there are at least 100 injured patients who require admission to hospital, often for long periods. Recovery and rehabilitation may not be complete and many survivors suffer permanent disability/handicap, especially after head injuries (see below).

While most attention has been focused on the problems of injury in the young and its cost to society in terms of loss of productive life (Baker *et al.*, 1985) the present volume will, we hope, draw attention to the increasing and largely unrecognised situation with the elderly. The population of all developed countries is aging and although cancer and cardiovascular diseases remain the main causes of death, injury, both accidental and premeditated (surgery), is increasing. For example, although improvements in health care enable the elderly to be more active, they live in an environment which exposes them to many dangers. Thus falls in or close to home and

1

the resultant injuries such as a fractured neck of femur are associated with an excess mortality of about 35% at 1 year after the accident. Many of the survivors fail to regain their independence, even after long periods of hospitalisation, and thereby pose great strains on the providers of health care.

Measurement of injury

It is to be expected that advances in treatment will come from a better understanding of both the epidemiology of, and the biological responses to, injury. If such studies are to be put on a scientific base then it is essential that there are scoring systems to grade the severity of such injuries and the responses to them. Thus most scales are based on either the extent of anatomical injury or the physiological disturbance induced by an injury. Anatomical scores are most accurate when confirmed by post-mortem examination and are, therefore, of limited use in the initial assessment of the patient. The most robust anatomical scores are those based on the Abbreviated Injury Scale first introduced in 1956 by Baker and colleagues (Baker *et al.*, 1974). This system provides lists of injuries divided by body region and graded according to severity by scores from 1 to 5. From such scores a total Injury Severity Score (ISS) can be calculated and this has been validated in numerous studies against mortality (Bull, 1975) and against metabolic/endocrine responses (Stoner *et al.*, 1979).

Although the ISS is a discontinuous scale regression techniques can be used and it has also been subjected to probit analysis which has shown the importance of age in determining mortality (Bull, 1975). Thus it has been demonstrated that the LD_{50} ISS fell from 40 in young adults (age approximately 25 years) to 20 in the elderly (age approximately 75 years). Also the slope of the relation between ISS and mortality was steeper in the elderly, indicating that a given increase in injury severity had a greater influence on mortality in this age group. While this finding of the increased susceptibility of the elderly to injury has been accepted without question, recent studies have cast doubt on what might have been too simplistic an analysis. It is now recognised that the prevalence of significant pre-existing medical conditions which might influence the acute metabolic and cardiovascular responses to injury increases in the elderly. Indeed if the compounding influence of such conditions is taken into account then the effect of age *per se* on mortality after injury is not very marked (D. W. Yates, personal communication).

The importance of intercurrent diseases in determining outcome after injury is recognised in the scales used to assess the physiological responses to injury. For example, the Acute Physiology and Chronic Health Evaluation (APACHE) scale first introduced in 1983 showed, with a multivariate logistic regression analysis of data obtained within 24 hours of intensive care unit (ICU) admission, that the severity of illness and age were significantly related to survival (Wagner *et al.*, 1983). In its original form, APACHE included 33 variables (selected and weighted by clinical consensus to reflect the degree of derangement of seven physiological systems: neurological, cardiovascular, respiratory, gastrointestinal, renal, metabolic, haematological) and age. It was soon simplified to 12 physiological variables, including the Glasgow Coma Score, plus age and chronic health evaluation (Knaus *et al.*, 1985). A similar exercise resulted in the Simplified Acute Physiological Score (SAPS II; Le Gall *et al.*, 1993). The latter scale has been shown to be a better predictor of outcome after injury than, for example, ISS (Maurette *et al.*, 1986). SAPS is also a good predictor of short (1 month) and long-term mortality in the elderly (more than 70 years of age) intensive care patient (Mahul *et al.*, 1991). This study also provides data to guide the debate about the use of intensive care facilities for the care of the elderly. Of 295 patients admitted 103 (35%) were alive at 1 year and 88% had returned to home and 82% had the same or improved functional status. The factors influencing mortality in critical illness have been divided into intrinsic (e.g. age, severity of acute illness, previous health status) and extrinsic (e.g. those related to the medical environment such as the quality of health care factors) (Maurette & Valentine, 1990). It is to be expected that a greater awareness and recognition of such problems will improve the care of the injured elderly patient – hence the present volume.

Measuring recovery

Although scales for scoring the severity of injury have been widely accepted as tools for population studies it has to be emphasised that their value in predicting outcome in individual patients is very limited, a caveat that may be of even greater significance in the elderly (Lonner & Koval, 1995). While most outcome studies are focused on survival very little attention has been paid to the quality of that survival. This may reflect the fact that rehabilitation is not usually considered an integral part of trauma services.

To study recovery requires the ability to measure function, disability and handicap and their rates of change. All the available scales that have been used so far may exhibit 'floor' and/or 'ceiling' effects at either end of the spectrum of function and, because they are ordinal in nature, are not good measures of the rate of change when the patients start at different baselines. Despite these difficulties, Mackenzie *et al.* (1988), who recruited 479 patients from two North American Trauma Centres and followed functional improvement over a year, found that at one year, 27% had quite marked limitations and 16% had more modest limitations. Those who survived injuries to the thorax or abdomen usually had a good functional outcome with only 5% still convalescing at 1 year. Patients with minor injuries to the head and spine also had good functional recovery; however, moderate to severe brain, spine and limb injuries were associated with persistent impairments. Interestingly, even minor injuries to the limbs were associated with substantial morbidity at 1 year. Another study (Jurkovich *et al.*, 1995) using the Sickness Impact Profile (SIP) to evaluate function in a group of patients with lower limb fracture reported that about half had some detectable disability a year later and about half of these rated the disability as moderate to severe. Interestingly, the domain most markedly affected was 'psychosocial'.

Emhoff *et al.* (1991) have reported the use of the Functional Independence Measure (FIM) to study 109 consecutive trauma patients, all with multiple injuries and fully independent before injury. They showed that those with the most marked impairments on admission were the most likely to present discharge problems and require rehabilitation. Furthermore, those with the slowest rates of improvement soon after admission presented similar discharge problems. Recently, a series of weighting factors has been described for the FIM which the authors claim to transfer the scale to behave as if it were interval in nature and this transformed scale appears to be robust in practice (Kidd *et al.*, 1995). Similarly, the recently described London Handicap Scale is also claimed to behave as an interval measure; neither of these scales has yet been applied in the setting of traumatic injury.

The factors that determine the quality of survival or recovery after injury are poorly understood. For example, it is not known how the well-characterised disturbances in homoeostatic reflexes and neuroendocrine and metabolic control associated with the ebb and flow phase of the response to injury resolve or how they influence outcome. The only aspect of the whole-body response to have been studied extensively beyond the flow phase is postoperative fatigue which may last beyond 2 months in about a third of patients (Christensen & Kehlet, 1993). There is some evidence that in the elderly muscle is more resistant to fatigue despite being weaker (Narici *et al.*, 1991). Mild muscle weakness and reduced exercise capacity have been reported in patients with postoperative fatigue. Although fatigue is related to the magnitude of the surgical procedure the relative roles of under-nutrition, protein catabolism, inactivity and physiological deconditioning have yet to be resolved. While psychological factors are not thought to play a major role in postoperative fatigue the contribution of sleep disorders which form part of the response to injury and critical illness is not known.

In addition to considering the 'biological' factors that might influence outcome, the roles of psychological and social factors should not be overlooked (Johnston, 1996). Thus, the effects of initial cognitive status, nature of coping strategies, incidence of depression, residual accessibility of main life interests, level of care and social support and other factors affecting quality of life have to be taken into account. The complexity of the situation is illustrated by the demonstration that psychosocial stress can affect immune functions and thereby possibly limit host-defence responses (Khansari *et al.*, 1990).

Injuries at specific sites

Head injuries

As the brain ages, its dura becomes tightly adherent to the skull which makes epidural haematomas uncommon. A progressive loss of brain volume leads to an increase in the space around the brain that is thought to protect it against contusions, but makes subdural haematomas more likely. Intraparenchymal haemorrhage is also commoner in the elderly. The epidemiology of head injuries has been reviewed recently (Jennett, 1996). Two aspects are particularly worthy of note. First, there is a modest increase in incidence rates after the age of about 60 years and, second, head injuries are commoner in men than in women, even in extreme old age. Thus, crude figures, unadjusted for sex, may underestimate the importance of head injuries among older people owing to the preponderance of women in older age groups.

Head injuries in older people can be devastating. Severe injuries (Glasgow Coma Scale (GCS) less than 8) have a fatality rate of about 90% (Bybee, 1987). Those who survive the initial injury have long hospital stays and more severe residual neurological deficits. In a study comparing 33 younger patients with acute subdural haematomas with 34 older patients with similar lesions, none of the older patients with a GCS less than 13 made a functional recovery (Howard *et al.*, 1989). Similarly, of 76 patients aged over 70 years admitted to three major neurosurgical centres (Newcastle and Glasgow in the UK and San Diego in the USA) only three lived to recover to an independent existence and only one of these made a good recovery as assessed using the Glasgow Outcome Scale (GOS; A. D. Mendelow, personal communication). It is widely believed that the aged also have poorer outcomes after minor head injuries (GCS 13 on presentation) but there is little published evidence to support this conclusion.

It is not entirely clear why the old have such poor outcomes after head injuries but it is likely that co-morbid factors, suboptimal management and a predisposition to systemic complications play important roles. In addition, a recent study suggests that there is a reduced capacity of the aging brain to recover from injuries (Vollmer *et al.*, 1991).

Thoracic trauma

Older people with isolated chest injuries have a two to three times greater risk of death than similarly injured younger people (Kulshrestha & Iyer, 1988; Shorr *et al.*, 1989). Rib fractures often complicate even mild blunt trauma to the chest in old people. Similarly, insignificant falls or blows to the chest may cause occult pneumothorax or haemothorax and pulmonary contusions often accompany even mild thoracic injuries. Prompt mechanical ventilation is warranted in older patients showing signs of respiratory distress in any of these circumstances. A history of rapid deceleration should alert us to the possibility of traumatic rupture of the aorta in all older patients (Camp *et al.*, 1994). Mediastinal widening or an ill-defined aortic knob are characteristic radiographic appearances. Although more than 80% of those with this complication die at the accident scene, the remainder may be haemodynamically stable on presentation.

Abdominal trauma

The death rate in old patients with visceral injuries is about 80% (Finelli *et al.*, 1989). The principles of management of abdominal injuries change little with age; however, it should be borne in mind that the old are intolerant of both shock and unnecessary laparotomy and their management demands a sense of urgency and a high degree of clinical acumen. Those with a history of previous significant abdominal surgery should have either a computed tomography (CT) scan or ultrasound scan rather than diagnostic peritoneal lavage.

Fall-related fractures

The nature of the fall dictates the nature of the fracture. Fractures of the wrist and proximal humerus are classically associated with falls on an outstretched arm, implying that the person was moving reasonably fast at the time of the fall. Falls from a stationary position or during slow locomotion will most likely result in proximal femoral fractures and it is these that account for most of the old-age peak in trauma deaths (Tubbs, 1976). Falls also account for the majority of cervical spine fractures in older people (Lieberman & Webb, 1994). Frail older people may sustain long bone fractures without a clear history of injury or falls (Kane *et al.*, 1995). These have been termed 'minimal trauma fractures' and the only precipitating factor clearly identified is severely impaired mobility.

Multiple injuries

Visceral injuries in the absence of fractures are very rare in older trauma victims (Naam & Brown, 1983; Schmidt & Moore, 1993). The bony injuries that present the most immediate threats to life are skull fractures (with underlying brain injury) and fractures of the pelvis. The main problem with pelvic fractures is massive bleeding from lacerations to the pelvic venous plexus, but this can generally be controlled by external fixators. About 15% of older people with closed pelvic fractures die whereas for open fractures the death rate is around 80% (Martin & Teberian, 1990).

Long bone fractures, especially the tibia, are common and must be stabilised early to control blood loss, to reduce the risk of fat embolism and to enable early mobilisation.

Older people do not tolerate well delays before surgical stabilisation (Riska & Myllynen, 1982).

Conclusion

Blunt trauma is an important cause of death and disability for older people. There is also quite a large literature on injuries in the aging, although it is to be found in disparate sources. One of the reasons for this book is to try to draw together this literature so that we may better see where we are and, therefore, where we might go most appropriately. In this brief overview, we have sought to define injuries and to describe how their severity might be measured and related to outcomes. Death is the easiest outcome to which injury severity might be related but we do not consider it to be the most important outcome. The extent of recovery is much more important, and for this reason we have tried to highlight how it might be measured. Finally, to illustrate some of the peculiarities and problems of injuries in the aging, we have given brief descriptions of injuries affecting different body regions and how old age modifies their clinical features and/or management.

References

Baker, S. P., O'Neill, B., Haddon, W., Jr & Long, W. B. (1974). The Injury Severity Score: a method for describing patients with multiple injuries and evaluating emergency care. *J Trauma*, **14**, 187–96.

Baker, S. P., O'Neill, B. & Karpf, R. S. (1985). *The Injury Fact Book*. Lexington: Lexington Books, DC Health & Company.

Bull, J. P. (1975). The Injury Severity Score of road traffic casualties in relation to mortality, time of death, hospital treatment time and disability. *Accid Anal Prev*, **7**, 249–55.

Bybee, D. E. (1987). Toleration of head injury by the elderly. *Neurosurgery*, **20**, 954–8.

Camp, P. C., Rogers, F. B., Shackford, S. R., Leavitt, B. J., Cobean, R. A. & Clark, D. E. (1994). Blunt traumatic aortic lacerations in the elderly. *J Trauma*, **37**, 418–25.

Christensen, T. & Kehlet, H. (1993). Postoperative fatigue. *World J Surg*, **17**, 220–5.

Emhoff, T. A., McCarthy, M., Cushman, M., Garb, J. L. & Valenziano, C. (1991). Functional scoring of multi-trauma patients: who ends up where? *J Trauma*, **31**, 1227–32.

Finelli, F., Jonsson, J., Champion, H., Monelli, S. & Fouty, W. J. (1989). A case control study for major trauma in geriatric patients. *J Trauma*, **29**, 541–8.

Howard, M. A., Gross, A. S., Dacey, R. G. & Winn, H. R. (1989). Acute subdural haematomas: an independent clinical entity. *J Neurosurg*, **71**, 858–63.

Jennett, B. (1996). Epidemiology of head injury. *J Neurol Neurosurg Psychiatry*, **60**, 362–9.

Johnston, M. (1996). Psychological factors in recovery from illness and from surgery. *Proc R Coll Phys Edinb*, **26**, 451–60.

Jurkovich, G., Mock, C., MacKenzie, E., Burgess, A., Cushing, B., deLateur, B., McAndrew, M., Morris, J. & Swiontkowski, M. (1995). The sickness impact profile as a tool to evaluate functional outcome in trauma patients. *J Trauma*, **39**, 625–31.

Kane, R. S., Burns, E. A. & Goodwin, J. S. (1995). Minimal trauma fractures in older nursing home residents: the interaction of functional status, trauma, and site of fracture. *J Am Geriatr Soc*, **43**, 156–9.

Khansari, D. N., Murgo, A. J. & Faith, R. E. (1990). Effects of stress on the immune system. *Immunol Today*, **11**, 170–5.

Kidd, D., Stewart, G., Baldry, J., Johnson, J., Rossiter, D., Petruckevitch, A. & Thompson, A. J. (1995). The Functional Independence Measure: a comparative validity and reliability study. *Disabil Rehab*, **17**, 10–14.

Knaus, W.A., Draper, E. A., Wagner, D. P. & Zimmerman, J. E. (1985). APACHE II: a severity of disease classification system. *Crit Care Med*, **13**, 818–29.

Kulshrestha, P. & Iyer, K. S. (1988). Chest injuries: a clinical and autopsy profile. *J Trauma*, **28**, 844–7.

Le Gall, J. R., Lemeshow, S. & Saulnier, F. (1993). A new Simplified Acute Physiology Score (SAPS II) based on a European/North American multicenter study. *JAMA*, **270**, 2957–63.

Lieberman, J. H. & Webb, J. K. (1994). Cervical spine injuries in the elderly. *J Bone Joint Surg (Br)*, **76–B**, 877–81.

Lonner, J. H. & Koval, K. J. (1995). Polytrauma in the elderly. *Clin Orthop*, **318**, 136–43.

MacKenzie, E. J., Siegel, J. H., Shapiro, S., Moody, M. & Smith, R. T. (1988). Functional recovery and medical costs of trauma: an analysis by type and severity of injury. *J Trauma*, **28**, 281–97.

Mahul, P., Perrot, D., Tempelhoff, G., Gaussorgues, P., Jospe, R., Ducreux, J. C., Dumont, A., Motin, J., Auboyer, C. & Robert, D. (1991). Short- and long-term prognosis, functional outcome following ICU for elderly. *Intensive Care Med*, **17**, 7–10.

Martin, R. E. & Teberian, G. (1990). Multiple trauma and the elderly patient. *Emerg Med Clin North Am*, **8**, 411–20.

Maurette, P., Dabadie, P., Chochard, J. F., Erny, P. & Salamon, R. (1986). Measuring severity in trauma resuscitation. *Ann Fr Anesth Reanim*, **5**, 367–71.

Maurette, P. & Valentine, M. L. (1990). Resuscitation in the elderly: prognostic factors. *Ann Fr Anesth Reanim*, **9**, 245–8.

Naam, N. H. & Brown, W. H. (1983). Major pelvic fracture. *Arch Surg*, **16**, 610–15.

Narici, M. V., Bordini, M. & Cerretelli, P. (1991). Effect of aging on human adductor pollicis muscle function. *J Appl Physiol*, **71**, 1277–81.

Riska, E. B. & Myllynen, P. (1982). Fat embolism in patients with multiple injuries. *J Trauma*, **22**, 891–4.

Schmidt, J. & Moore, G. P. (1993). Management of multiple trauma. *Emerg Med Clin North Am*, **11**, 29–51.

Shorr, R. M., Rodriguez, A., Indeck, M. C., Crittenden, M. D., Hartunian, S. & Cowley, R. A. (1989). Blunt chest trauma in the elderly. *J Trauma*, **29**, 234–7.

Stoner, H. B., Frayn, K. N., Barton, R. N., Threlfall, C. J. & Little, R. A. (1979). The relationships between plasma substrates and hormones and the severity of injury in 277 recently injured patients. *Clin Sci*, **56**, 563–73.

Tubbs, N. (1976). A comparison of deaths from injury: 1947–56 compared with 1962–71. *Injury*, **7**, 233–41.

Vollmer, D. G., Torner, J. C., Jane, J. A., Sadovnic, B., Charlebois, D., Eisenberg, H. M., Foulkes, M. A., Marmarou, A. & Marshall, L. F. (1991). Age and outcome following traumatic coma: why do older patients fare worse? *J Neurosurg*, **75**, S37–S49.

Wagner, D. P., Knaus, W. A. & Draper, D. A. (1983). Statistical validation of a severity of illness measure. *AJPH*, **73**, 878–84.

2

The attributes of old age

M. A. HORAN

The old and their injuries

Few readers will be unaware of the demographic changes that have taken place in developed, industrialised nations with both a relative and absolute increase in the number of old people. This change has been brought about by two important factors: increased life expectancy and reduced birth rate. While the rate of increase of the elderly population in these developed countries has slowed, similar increases can now be seen in the developing world. It is estimated that the world population of those over 60 years of age will have risen from 8.5% in 1980 to 9.6% in 2000 and 12.5% by 2020 (Macfadyen, 1990). These demographic changes are often referred to as population aging, or sometimes as the greying of nations.

Even though injuries are much commoner in younger people, old people who sustain injuries are more likely to die as a result of them, regardless of injury severity (Tubbs, 1976; Oreskovich et al., 1984; Gustilo et al., 1985; Fife, 1987; Evans, 1988a; Osler et al., 1988; Champion et al., 1989; Finelli et al., 1989; McCoy et al., 1989; Sklar et al., 1989). Accidental injuries are the tenth commonest cause of death in old age. Figures from the USA for 1986 report that 38% of hospital bed-days for all patients in which injury was the primary cause of admission were accounted for by those over the age of 65 years (Champion et al., 1989). Using 1986 average daily costs in hospital ($500) and in intensive units ($1200–2000), their hospital expenses exceeded $4.4 billion. Despite the considerable proportion of trauma care resources consumed by the oldest people, research has tended to be directed towards the needs of younger ones.

Do older trauma victims differ from their younger counterparts? The first and most obvious difference is that accidental injuries in older people are largely a problem for women while in younger age groups, they are much commoner in men. In our population, old women greatly outnumber old men and, moreover, their thinner bones are more likely to fracture on impact. Another important difference from trauma in the young is the occurrence of 'late deaths'. The peak death rate for upper femur fractures occurs about a month after the injury (Tubbs, 1976) but continues at an increased level for a considerable time, reported as 12 months by one group (Holmberg et al., 1986) and 20 months by another (Jensen & Tøndevold, 1979). A more recent study looking at survival times of fatally injured pedestrians stratified for injury severity (Injury Severity Score, ISS) showed that older patients had a higher proportion of their total mortality late after the injury (Fife, 1987).

Scoring systems to measure trauma severity and predict outcome have become essential tools in trauma research and management. Many such scales exist; some are based on anatomical indices and some on physiological ones, while others (e.g. TRISS – used in the Major Trauma Outcome Study, MTOS) are hybrids. Until comparatively recently, the only outcome to have been considered is survival. There is now increasing interest in disability as an equally important outcome measure.

The MTOS is a retrospective study of over 120000 patients treated at US trauma centres, of whom about 10% were elderly (Champion et al., 1990). The purpose of the study was to set national norms of trauma care and survival probability. As might be expected, old people had an increased likelihood of death; however, this study also showed that the aged were over-represented among the unexpected deaths, over 50% of which had significant head, neck and thoracic injuries. This suggests the TRISS system fails accurately to measure severity or predict survival for these types of injury, particularly in the old.

One prevalent medical response to the high death rate seen in the aged trauma victim is to assume that a poor outcome is an inevitable characteristic of advanced age and to treat less actively and, in the extreme, to use age as a criterion to ration medical care. It is now clear that such an attitude is inappropriate as it is based on a false premise, as is clearly demonstrated by the recent study of Knaus et al. (1991 a,b). The objective of their researches was to refine the APACHE (Acute Physiology, Age, Chronic Health Evaluation) methodology to predict more accurately hospital mortality risk for critically ill hospitalised adults. Using the APACHE III system, chronological age alone accounted for only 3% of the variation in outcome; acute physiological abnormalities accounted for 86%. Indeed, this conclusion is emphasised in a study reported by Osler et al. (1988); when Injury Severity Score (ISS), Trauma Score (TS) and Glasgow Coma Scale (GCS) had been corrected for, the presence of shock emerged as an enormously potent predictive factor of outcome. Likewise, Scalea et al. (1990) reached a similar conclusion and reported that the appropriate response was early invasive monitoring as a means to improve survival.

It seems reasonable to conclude that it is not age per se that accounts for the poor outcome of older trauma victims but factors that are strongly age related. Intrinsic factors such as co-existing disease, undernutrition and age-related changes in organs and physiological systems may contribute to outcome directly by limiting protective responses or indirectly by confronting the medical attendants' diagnostic efforts.

Extrinsic factors such as medication and the doctors' attitudes may have similarly important adverse effects.

The nature of aging

What constitutes an old person?

I have already used terms such as old people and the elderly, but who are they? There is no precise answer to this question and many research publications seem conveniently flexible about which individuals should be included in the 'old' age group and are often equally flexible about which ones should be assigned to the 'young' group. This can often lead to problems when comparing the results of different studies. Most people who reach retirement age are likely to enjoy good health and the functional impairments generally associated with 'aging' do not become particularly prevalent until after the age of about 75 years and become increasingly common thereafter. Hence, the more recent literature has started to adopt terms used for census purposes in the USA (US Bureau of the Census, 1989): young-old (age 65–74 years), old (age 75–84 years) and oldest-old (age 85+ years).

What constitutes aging?

All multicellular organisms pass through stages of development, sexual maturity and 'aging', although the characteristic senescent changes observed in mammals do not necessarily represent those seen in lower order animals (Goss, 1994). There is overwhelming evidence that the longevity of a species is genetically determined (Rose, 1991), although the precise mechanisms involved are not clear. Despite numerous theories about how an organism ages, it is now widely accepted that no single mechanism can account for the varied manifestations of the aged phenotype and the singular expression 'biological aging' is being replaced by terms such as 'aging mechanisms' and 'aging processes'. This trend is consistent with the considerable variation in rates of decline in systems, both between and within individuals. Such declines probably represent the summation of intrinsic processes, environmental factors, nutrition, lifestyle and disease. Perhaps we have been in error by trying to distinguish 'aging' from these other factors and might have been wiser to view 'aging' as the effect of these changes, and not the cause.

These 'aging changes' are seen at all levels: social, psychological, morphological, systemic, cellular and molecular. The most relevant of these for a discussion about injury are the systemic physiological changes that arise during aging and how responses to medications change with age.

Physiological changes

Many of these changes can be observed to commence long before old age, some even before middle age (Curb *et al.*, 1990). I have already stated that no all-encompassing description of aging at any level is possible but at least four patterns of change can be identified:

1. Total loss of function, e.g. reproductive capacity in women or the ability to hear sounds above a certain frequency.
2. Diminished function associated with loss of anatomical units but with surviving units retaining more or less normal function, e.g. loss of nephrons or muscle fibres.
3. Little or no loss of functional units but with a generalised decline in the function of those units, e.g. reduced nerve conduction velocity.
4. Secondary and adaptive changes, e.g. increased plasma gonadotrophic hormone concentrations caused by loss of feedback inhibition from gonadal steroids or the reliance on stroke volume to maintain cardiac output (the Starling mechanism) secondary to an inability to raise heart rate sufficiently because of changes in cardiovascular adrenergic receptors.

Even though increasing age is strongly linked to deteriorating average functional performances (Table 2.1), not all functions decline at the same rate or to the same extent and this is the case both within individuals and between individuals. Functions that require very precise regulation because they are essential for life (e.g. body fluid pH, PaO_2, body temperature, resting heart rate) change hardly at all. Organisms could not sustain major deviations in these parameters and would die. On the other hand, quite large changes may be seen in systems possessed of a large reserve capacity (Table 2.1).

The interindividual variation in the age-related decline of numerous body systems has led some investigators to attempt a distinction between 'chronological age' and 'biological age'; those with the greater declines in particular functions are regarded as biologically older (Mooradian, 1990). Combinations of physiological measures have been used in theoretical models to calculate a 'biological age' for individuals that is distinct from their 'chronological age' (Ruiz-Torres *et al.*, 1990). Although interesting, and despite considerable effort, this approach has not identified any convincing biomarkers for aging. Furthermore, this approach has only tangential relevance for the practice of medicine in old age. Of much greater importance is the identification of those factors that predispose to medical problems and determine poor outcomes, regardless of whether they represent some intrinsic process, environmental influences or disease. It is only then that we will be able to target interventions to the needs of the individual. Regrettably, too little effort has yet been expended on this approach.

As the individual progresses through the life span, the functional declines mentioned

Table 2.1. *Average decline in some selected physiological variables between the ages of* 30 *and* 80 *years*

Variable	Reduction (%)
Resting cardiac output	30
Vital capacity	50
Renal blood flow	50
Maximum breathing capacity	60
Maximum oxygen uptake	70

Source: Shock (1983).

above will proceed towards some theoretical threshold, which, if exceeded, would result in decompensation of the relevant system. Furthermore, this progressive erosion of reserve capacity will limit the ability to respond to an increased demand or stress. This is most likely to be of clinical importance for cardiopulmonary, renal and cognitive functions. Furthermore, changes in discrete systems interact and one highly characteristic feature is the disruption of the many regulatory processes that provide functional integration between cells and organs (Shock, 1983). The resulting impairment of the ability to coordinate the various functions needed to defend the internal environment probably also contributes to the increased vulnerability of the aged organism to both internal and external stresses (Shock, 1983). Thus old age can be regarded in terms of reductions in reserve capacities together with alterations in the integration of the control mechanisms that regulate functional activities within and between cells, tissues and organs rather than simply to the diminished capacity of one or other organ system. These various impairments might well interact so that the overall effect is greater than the sum of individual impairments, although decompensation in a single system may become critical in some circumstances. This line of reasoning is entirely consistent with the observation that although there is a gradual, linear decline in individual functions, the probability of dying increases approximately exponentially with increasing age (Timiras, 1972).

Pharmacological aspects of aging

Medicines commonly cause problems for old people and are strongly implicated in many hospital admissions. Many drugs cause hypotension and confusion in the elderly, thus predisposing to falls and possible injury. The reasons for such problems (usually called adverse drug reactions or ADRs) may be changes in the host that predispose to drug toxicity, or the co-administration of several drugs with the potential for interactions. The more drugs a person is taking, the higher the risk of ADRs and when nine or more drugs are being taken, drug-related problems are virtually inevitable (Denham, 1990).

Many changes occur with aging that alter the handling of a drug or responsiveness to it and the likely behaviour of a drug in an elderly recipient can seldom be inferred from its behaviour in younger ones. Although many age-related changes have been described in the gastrointestinal tract, they mostly have little effect on drug absorption. Age-related changes in body composition such as a reduced body size, reduced lean body mass and reduced total body water together with increased fat mass mean that the volume of distribution for lipid-soluble drugs tends to increase in old age while that of water-soluble ones diminishes. This means, for example, that highly water-soluble drugs like digoxin will achieve therapeutic concentrations with a lower dose. Furthermore, many of these water-soluble drugs are excreted by the kidneys and age-related declines in glomerular filtration will prolong the elimination of such drugs.

Many drugs bind to plasma proteins, particularly albumin, although it is generally only unbound drug that is active. Healthy aging is not associated with significant changes in albumin concentration but sick old people often have hypoalbuminaemia. Drugs that bind extensively to albumin (e.g. warfarin, tolbutamide) will have much higher concentrations of free drug in hypoalbuminaemic people and there will be considerable potential for toxicity.

Many drugs are metabolised in the liver, either by phase 1 reactions (mainly oxidation, reduction, demethylation and hydrolysis) or by phase 2 reactions (mainly acetylation, glucuronide formation and sulphation). Impairments of all kinds of reactions have been described in old people but there is considerable variation from drug to drug and from person to person. Much more consistent and larger impairments are associated with illness, frailty and co-administration of other drugs (Woodhouse & James, 1990).

As well as the pharmacokinetic changes just described, pharmacodynamic changes are also common in old age. These changes represent altered responsiveness to a drug and might occur because of age-related changes in homoeostatic mechanisms such as cardiovascular reflexes or from receptor and postreceptor events. The former changes predispose to hypotension caused by many drugs and the latter changes are associated with the increased sensitivity to benzodiazepines, drugs with anticholinergic properties and many anaesthetic agents.

The nature of disease

Basic concepts

At the turn of the century, concepts of disease were firmly rooted in pathology as notions of disease arose from systematic clinical descriptions that were related to autopsy findings and, later, to changes at the microscopic level. Infectious diseases were the great killers and, as microbiology advanced, disease came to be seen in terms of specific aetiology. In this perspective, diseases were seen as attributable to a single, necessary and sufficient cause (e.g. typhoid fever was caused by *Salmonella typhi*). Within a few decades, this view had to be modified because not all individuals exposed to 'necessary causes' developed the disease. From such observations came the concept of differential susceptibility.

Improved hygiene, immunisation programmes and effective drugs tamed the great infectious diseases and altered the pattern of medical practice so that chronic diseases became increasingly important. This changing pattern of disease brought changes in the understanding of the nature of disease; in particular, there was an increased emphasis on multiple predisposing factors. Unlike the acute conditions that fit the classical model of disease, the distinction between these chronic conditions and 'aging' is much less clear. Much debate has been stimulated in trying to make a distinction between them (Blumenthal, 1993). That this debate cannot yet (and perhaps will never) be resolved has been succinctly summarised by Evans (1988b) who wrote: 'To draw a distinction between disease and normal aging is to separate the undefined from the undefinable'.

Disease presentation in old age

The traditional model for the practice of medicine comes mainly from disease presentation in younger people. In this model it is usually possible to account for all abnormal findings with a single diagnosis. A particular pattern of symptoms and signs characterises a disease or pathophysiological state (e.g. heart failure). Deviations from this model are common in older people.

The most overt deviation from this traditional model is that multiple diseases often co-exist in old people (co-morbidity) (Wilson *et al.*, 1962; Abrams, 1985) and the symptoms and signs that have been recorded may be attributable to more than one disease. Furthermore, a patient may have multiple complaints without any one of them dominating the clinical picture or even a major complaint that cannot be explained by the most overt or most serious underlying problem. As a result of the age-related erosion of functional reserve in many systems and organs, impaired adaptation to challenges and co-morbidity, a disease in one organ (e.g. respiratory infection) may precipitate decompensation in another (e.g. heart failure or confusion). This is often referred to as the atypical presentation of disease.

Underlying senescent changes and co-morbidity may also contribute to late or even silent presentations when disease at one site limits the symptoms of disease at another (e.g. mobility problems limiting activity so that dyspnoea does not occur until heart failure is very advanced). The tendency for disease to present in an advanced state in old people is well documented. Patients may have a low expectation for health and may misinterpret symptoms as manifestations of aging. The doctor may share his patients' views about old age and, wrongly attributing treatable conditions to aging, deny patients the benefits of effective treatment. Furthermore, doctors may misinterpret the significance of certain changes and commence treatment for a condition that the patient does not have. For example, ankle swelling is often caused by local mechanical factors rather than signifying fluid overload. Diuretic treatment under these circumstances will usually be inappropriate and may be harmful by depleting circulating blood volume or causing electrolyte disturbances.

Even the diagnosis of hip fracture may be delayed. Eastwood (1987) reported reasons for late diagnosis in 33 patients from a group of 374 consecutive admissions to a trauma unit over a 1 year period. Eight patients presented late, confirmation of the diagnosis of hip fracture was difficult in five and the diagnosis was simply missed in 20. Missed diagnoses were particularly likely in patients who were confused, dependent or prone to repeated falls.

Co-morbidity and disability

I have already emphasised the importance of chronic disease in modern medical practice. The numbers of older people with chronic conditions is high (Table 2.2). Owing to their high prevalence in old age, it is common for several of them to co-exist within an individual, sometimes in association with more acute conditions. It is this phenomenon that is often referred to as co-morbidity. For example, Guralnik *et al.* (1989) reported that 49% of community dwelling people aged over 60 years had two or more of nine chronic conditions surveyed, 23% had three or more and 8% had four or more. For those aged over 80 years, 70% of women and 53% of men had two or more chronic conditions. Thus, it would be anticipated that elderly victims of trauma will have other conditions that might alter management or influence outcome.

The most comprehensive information is available for hip fracture patients. For example, one study reported that 90% of hip fracture patients had co-existing disorders that would have benefited from the help of a physician (Campbell, 1976). Furthermore, these co-existing problems were associated with a difficult peri- and postoperative course, prolonged and difficult rehabilitation, institutionalisation and death (Miller, 1978; Magaziner *et al.*, 1989).

Just as the prevalence of chronic conditions increases with age, so does the prevalence of disability (Table 2.3), often to a degree that threatens independence (Schneider & Guralnik, 1990). Hip fractures contribute markedly to disability. One study of these fractures in a community dwelling population of old people showed a decline in

Table 2.2. *Prevalence of some chronic diseases in the USA noninstitutionalised population*

Condition	Age group (years)			
	18–44	45–64	65–74	≥75
Arthritis	52.1	268.5	459.3	494.7
Heart disease	40.1	129.0	276.8	349.1
Hearing impairment	49.8	159.0	261.9	346.9
Visual impairment	32.8	43.7	76.4	128.8
Cerebrovascular disease	1.0	17.9	54.0	72.6

Note: Prevalence per 1000 persons.
Source: Data from Seeman *et al.* (1989).

Table 2.3. *Definition of impairment, disability and handicap*

Impairment	Any loss or abnormality of psychological, physiological or anatomical structure or function
Disability	Any restriction or lack (resulting from an impairment) of ability to perform an activity in the manner, or within the range, considered normal for a human being
Handicap	A disadvantage for a given individual, resulting from an impairment or a disability, that limits or prevents the fulfilment of a role that is normal (depending on age, sex and social and cultural factors) for that individual

function at 6 weeks after fracture with little improvement when reassessed at 6 months (Marottoli *et al.*, 1992). In another study of functional outcome, this time in an institutionalised population, Folman *et al.* (1994) reported that only 17% regained their pre-injury level of overall function and only 13% regained their pre-injury level of mobility. Interestingly, functional improvement was better in the oldest-old than in the young-old.

The concept of frailty

It is common to hear old people described as frail but the term, like aging, has no precise meaning. It implies vulnerability and feebleness, as might occur with marked erosion of functional reserves and a very limited ability to resist stressful stimuli. This is probably what some authors mean by the term 'unsuccessful aging'. Speechley & Tinetti (1991) have attempted to define frailty empirically using a technique called factor analysis. They identified nine variables that loaded heavily on a factor named frailty: age more than 80 years, depression, use of sedative drugs, sedentary lifestyle, reduced muscle strength in shoulder or knee, visual loss, impaired gait, impaired balance and lower limb impairments. In this view, frailty might be seen as a kind of precursor state for disability.

Conclusion

My aim in this chapter was neither to review theories of aging nor to provide an exhaustive catalogue of age-related changes. For these, the interested reader is referred to any of the major textbooks of geriatric medicine and gerontology. Such descriptions would have had little relevance to a book devoted to how an aged individual might respond to the stress of physical injury. My intention was rather to emphasise that the medical problems of the old are of immense importance because old people represent a considerable proportion of the population and place disproportionate demands on health services, including trauma services. Justice demands that their problems are taken seriously, particularly at a time of rising costs of health care, so that the most effective and economic treatments can be given. Their interests and the interests of society are not well served by giving inappropriate interventions, even with the best of intentions.

Old trauma victims are not the same as younger ones, nor do old trauma victims have the same needs as one another. The old are not a homogeneous population. Quite unlike the prevalent stereotype of sameness, the old are much more characterised by their variation. As well as ill-defined intrinsic processes that may affect all organs and systems in the body, they will have accumulated the effects of a lifetime of environmental exposures and the consequences of their lifestyle. It has been argued that some of us are especially resistant to acquiring some of these conditions and that nonagenarians tend to be more vigorous than expected with lower than predicted mortality rates. The less resistant of us, it is argued, will already have died. This phenomenon of differential survival with retained functional abilities is poorly researched and very few studies in aging include people so old. This notion is supported by the superior outcome after hip fractures in the oldest old reported by Folman *et al.* (1994).

The differences between young and old will influence how the old respond to the stress of physical injury and the heterogeneity among the old may be associated with heterogeneous injury responses. The differences should also influence how their problems are best managed. For some, this will mean that no restorative intervention is likely to influence the ultimate outcome and no treatments other than palliative ones should be given. This view is supported by the study of Folman *et al.* (1994) who propose that nonoperative management might be the most appropriate way to treat hip fractures in the most disabled. To deprive individuals of a treatment that will substantially benefit them merely on the basis of age is a gross injustice. It behoves all of us involved in trauma care to recognise the specific needs of elderly patients, to research the unknown and to translate research findings into clinical practice. These issues form the basis for the remaining chapters of this book.

References

Abrams, M. (1985). The health of the very elderly. In *Recent Advances in Geriatric Medicine* 3, ed. B. Isaacs, pp. 217–26. Edinburgh: Churchill Livingstone.

Blumenthal, H. T. (1993). The aging-disease dichotomy is alive, but is it well? *J Am Geriat Soc*, **41**, 1272–3.

Campbell, A. J. (1976). Femoral neck fractures in elderly women: a prospective study. *Age Ageing*, **5**, 102–9.

Champion, H. R., Copes, W. S., Buyer, D., Flanagan, M. E., Bain, L. & Sacco, W. J. (1989). Major trauma in geriatric patients. *Am J Publ Health*, **79**, 1278–82.

Champion, H. R., Lopes, W. S. & Sacco, W. J. (1990). The major trauma outcome study: establishing national norms for trauma care. *J Trauma*, **30**, 1356–65.

Curb, J. D., Guralnik, J. M., LaCroix, A. Z., Korper, S. P., Deeg, D., Miles, T. & White, L. (1990). Effective aging: meeting the challenge of growing older. *J Am Geriatr Soc*, **38**, 827–8.

Denham, M. J. (1990). Adverse drug reactions. *Br Med Bull*, **46**, 53–62.

Eastwood, H. D. (1987). Delayed diagnosis of femoral neck fractures in the elderly. *Age Ageing*, **16**, 378–82.

Evans, J. G. (1988a). Falls and fractures. *Age Ageing*, **17**, 361–4.

Evans, J. G. (1988b). Aging and disease. In *Research and the Aging Population*, ed. D. Evered & J. Whelan. pp. 38–57. Ciba Foundation Symposium No. 134. Chichester: John Wiley.

Fife, D. (1987). Time from injury to death (survival time) among fatally injured pedestrians. *Injury*, **18**, 315–18.

Finelli, F. C., Jonsson, J., Champion, H. R., Morelli, S. & Fouty, W. J. (1989). A case control study for major trauma in geriatric patients. *J Trauma*, **29**, 541–8.

Folman, Y., Gepstein, R., Assaraf, A. & Liberty, S. (1994). Functional recovery after operative treatment of femoral neck fractures in an institutionalized elderly population. *Arch Phys Med Rehabil*, **75**, 454–6.

Goss, R. J. (1994). Why study ageing in cold-blooded animals? *Gerontology*, **40**, 65–9.

Guralnik, J. M., LaCroix, A. Z., Everett, D. F. & Kovar, M. G. (1989). Aging in the eighties: the prevalence of co-morbidity and association with disability. Advance Data from Vital and Health Statistics, No. 170. Hyattsville MD: National Center for Health Statistics.

Gustilo, R. B., Corpuz, V. & Sherman, R. E. (1985). Epidemiology, mortality and morbidity in multiple trauma patients. *Orthopaedics*, **8**, 1523–8.

Holmberg, S., Conradi, P., Kalen, R. & Thorngren, K. G. (1986). Mortality after cervical hip fracture: 3002 patients followed for 6 years. *Acta Orthop Scand*, **57**, 8–11.

Jensen, J. S. & Tøndevold, E. (1979). Mortality after hip fractures. *Acta Orthop Scand*, **50**, 161–7.

Knaus, W. A., Wagner, D. P. & Lynn, J. (1991a). Short-term mortality predictions for critically ill hospitalized adults: science and ethics. *Science*, **254**, 389–94.

Knaus, W. A., Wagner, D. P., Draper, E. A., Zimmerman, J. E., Bergner, M., Bastos, P. G., Sirio, C. A., Murphy, D. J., Lotring, T., Damiano, A. & Harrell, F. E. (1991b). The APACHE III prognostic system: risk prediction of hospital mortality for critically ill hospitalized adults. *Chest*, **100**, 1619–36.

Macfadyen, D. (1990). International demographic trends. In *Improving the Health of Older People. A World View*, ed R. L. Kane, J. G. Evans & D. Macfadyen, pp. 19–29. Oxford: Oxford University Press.

Magaziner, J., Simonsick, E. M., Kashner, T. M., Hebel, J. R. & Kenzora, J. E. (1989). Survival experience of aged hip fracture patients. *Am J Publ Health*, **79**, 274–8.

Marottoli, R. A., Berkman, L. F. & Cooney, L. M. (1992). Decline in physical function following hip fracture. *J Am Geriatr Soc*, **40**, 861–6.

McCoy, G. F., Johnstone, R. A. & Duthie, R. B. (1989). Injury to the elderly in road traffic accidents. *J Trauma*, **29**, 494–7.

Miller, C. W. (1978). Survival and ambulation following hip fracture. *J Bone Joint Surg (Am)*, **60**, 930–4.

Mooradian, A. D. (1990). Biomarkers of aging: do we know what to look for? *J Gerontol*, **45**, B183–B186.

Oreskovich, M. R., Howard, J. D., Copass, M. K. & Carrico, C. J. (1984). Geriatric trauma: injury patterns and outcome. *J Trauma*, **24**, 565–9.

Osler, T., Hales, K., Baack, B., Bear, K., Hsi, K., Pathak, D. & Demarest, G. (1988). Trauma in the elderly. *Am J Surg*, **156**, 537–43.

Rose, M. R. (1991). *Evolutionary Biology of Aging*. Oxford: Oxford University Press.

Ruiz-Torres, A., Agudo, A., Vicent, D. & Beier, W. (1990). Measuring human aging using a two compartment mathematical model and the vitality concept. *Arch Gerontol Geriatr*, **10**, 69–76.

Scalea, T. M., Simon, H. M., Duncan, A. O., Atweh, N. A., Sclafani, S. J. A., Phillips, T. F. & Shaftan, G. W. (1990). Geriatric blunt multiple trauma: improved survival with early invasive monitoring. *J Trauma*, **30**, 129–34.

Schneider, E. L. & Guralnik, J. M. (1990). The aging of America: impact on health care costs. *JAMA*, **263**, 2335–40.

Seeman, T. E., Guralnik, J. M., Kaplan, G. A., Knudsen, L. & Cohen, R. (1989). The health consequences of multiple morbidity in the elderly. The Alameda County Study. *J Aging Health*, **1**, 50–66.

Shock, N. W. (1983). Aging and physiological systems. *J Chron Dis*, **36**, 137–42.

Sklar, D. P., Demarest, G. B. & McFeeley, P. (1989). Increased pedestrian mortality among the elderly. *Am J Emerg Med*, **7**, 387–90.

Speechley, M. & Tinetti, M. (1991). Falls and injuries in frail and vigorous community elderly persons. *J Am Geriatr Soc*, **39**, 46–52.

Timiras, P. S. (1972). *Developmental Physiology and Aging*, pp. 411–29. New York: Macmillan.

Tubbs, N. (1976). A comparison of deaths from injury: 1947–56 compared with 1962–71. *Injury*, **7**, 233–41.

US Bureau of the Census: Population profile of the United States: 1989. Current Population Reports Series P-23, No 159. Washington, DC: US Government Printing Office.

Wilson, L. A., Lawson, I. R. & Bray, W. (1962). Multiple disorders in the elderly: a clinical and statistical study. *Lancet*, **2**, 841–3.
Woodhouse, K. W. & James, O. F. W. (1990). Hepatic drug metabolism and ageing. *Br Med Bull*, **46**, 22–35.

3

Epidemiology of trauma in the elderly

J. GRIMLEY EVANS

Mortality

The most readily available data on injury relate to mortality. In the USA, injury deaths are the fourth commonest cause of mortality overall. Among people aged 65 years and over in the USA the two most common causes of injury deaths are those due to falls, occurring at an annual rate of 28.5 per 100000, and motor vehicle accidents at 22 per 100000 (Sattin & Nevitt, 1992). Annual mortality rates from burns among people aged 65 years and over in the USA are around 5 per 100000. In England and Wales in 1993 there were 15700 deaths from injury and poisoning (31 per 100000) of which 39% were of people aged 65 years and over. These figures represent annual mortality rates of 31 per 100000 for all ages and 78 per 100000 for men and 73 per 100000 for women at ages over 65 years. A quarter of the 2900 people dying from motor vehicle accidents in England and Wales in 1993 were aged 65 years or over.

Few direct comparisons of the epidemiology of injury in different countries have been presented. Li & Baker (1992) report that age-adjusted death rates from all injuries in a population sample in China were 12.6% higher than in the USA. Death rates from motor vehicle injuries and homicide were higher in the USA, particularly among young adults. In China deaths from drowning were very high among children and old people. Deaths from suicide were also much higher in China where suicide rates among young women were as high as motor vehicle death rates among young men in the USA. Suicide rates among old people of China were higher in both sexes than among elderly men in the USA. It is not too difficult to deduce that both the physical and cultural environment are important determinants of injury rates at all ages and particularly among the more vulnerable young and old. The need to identify what those determinants are is implicit in the many calls for a reduction in injuries as a cause of ill-health and disability in the UK (Secretary of State for Health, 1992) and elsewhere (Centers for Disease Control, 1989; Li & Baker, 1992).

Hospital care

In addition to the personal sufferings induced by injuries in later life, there are also more tangible costs. Hospital discharge data in the USA indicated that although people aged 65 years and over comprised only 12% of the population, they accounted for a quarter of hospital expenditure on treatment of injuries in 1985 (MacKenzie *et al.*, 1990).

There are striking differences between the USA and the UK in the pattern of hospital use associated with trauma. Gorman *et al.* (1995) studied the epidemiology of major injuries in Mersey and North Wales. Death rates from injury were 23 per 100000 compared with 63 per 100000 in the USA. For each death from injury in the USA there are 23 patients admitted to hospital for a mean of 7.5 days whereas in Mersey for each injury death only 1.2 patients with major blunt injuries were admitted to hospital but with a mean stay of 31 days. These differences are likely to reflect differences in the pattern of trauma and in the distribution of its medical management between hospital and primary care settings. In the USA nearly three-quarters of the hospitalisations and one-half of the hospital costs were for minor injuries (ICD/AIS grades 1 and 2) (MacKenzie *et al.*, 1990).

Fatality

The defining feature of aging in the sense of senescence is loss of adaptability of an organism with time and is manifest as a broadly exponential increase in total mortality rates with age (Fairweather & Grimley Evans, 1990). The fatality associated with a given level of physical trauma also increases with age as a broadly exponential function of age and is 25% higher for women over the age range 15–45 years, but higher for males above and below that range (Evans, 1988). The association of fatality with age has led to suggestions that age should be used in the triage of injured patients for the allocation of treatment resources (Martin & Teberian, 1990). This would be to let agism masquerade as medical science. It is not age that determines the fatality of injury, it is the age-associated changes in physiology and these vary enormously between individuals. Scalea *et al.* (1990) have urged that age-associated loss of adaptability should be anticipated and partly compensated for by earlier, more intensive and invasive monitoring of older trauma patients. There is certainly evidence that the quality of care for elderly trauma patients has an important influence on mortality. Declining mortality rates from accidental falls in the elderly population of the USA indicate that trauma management improved outcomes over the period 1962–88 by 2.74 times in men and 4.22 times in women (Riggs, 1993). Johnson *et al.* (1994) studied admissions to a tertiary surgical intensive care unit over a 5-year period and showed that on average older patients showed higher Simplified Acute Physiology Scores

24   *J. Grimley Evans*

(SAPS) for given Injury Severity Scores (ISS) than younger patients, and this difference remained if age was omitted from the SAPS calculation. The higher proportion of older than of younger patients dying in intensive care was almost entirely attributable to differences in SAPS and not to age. Mortality rates after discharge from the intensive care unit were, as in the general population, higher among older than younger patients.

Incidence

There have been few studies of the age-specific incidence of injuries of all types in general populations. Sahlin *et al.* (1990) report a year's experience in 1985–86 at the Trondheim University Hospital in Norway where a single accident service provides all hospital-based care for injuries in a definable population. Age-specific incidence rates (Figure 3.1) are high in early adult life declining later to rise again into extreme old age. Rates were higher in males up to the age of 50 years, after which rates became higher in women.

Road traffic accidents furnished a high proportion of the injuries at young adult ages in the Trondheim study, but above the age of 65 years more than half of the injuries were caused by simple falls. As reviewed elsewhere in this volume falls are common among older people. In retrospective population surveys falls are found to have occurred in the preceding 12 months to more than a quarter of people aged 65 years

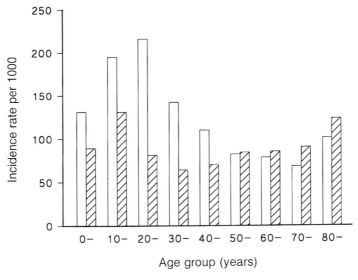

Figure 3.1. Sex- and age-specific incidence rates for injuries, Trondheim, Norway 1985–86. □, male; ▨, female. Redrawn from Sahlin *et al.* (1990).

and over and 40% of those aged 80 years and over (Prudham & Grimley Evans, 1981). The majority of falls experienced by older people do not cause significant injury. In one study only 6% of 539 prospectively identified falls among a sample of elderly volunteers in a San Francisco community resulted in fracture or dislocation but 55% caused minor soft tissue injuries (Nevitt *et al.*, 1991). In a study of a population aged 65 years and over in Miami Beach, Florida, estimated incidence rates of fall injury events were 96 per 1000 person-years in women and 84 per 1000 person-years in men. Slightly over 40% of the injuries were severe enough to lead to hospital admission and 2% were fatal (Sattin *et al.*, 1990). These figures concerned with overt injury underestimate the total burden of morbidity imposed on the older population by falls, which may lead to disabling anxiety and immobility or institutionalisation.

Head injury

There are many methodological differences between the published studies on head injury, particularly in the methods of ascertainment and in the definitions of what constitutes head trauma. Some studies have included all forms of head trauma, some have restricted consideration to brain injuries with or without skull fractures. Others have excluded gunshot wounds. These differences of definition have an effect on the age association of head injury as there are widespread differences between countries, particularly in the relative importance of road traffic accidents and gunshot wounds in generating head injuries at different ages.

Despite such culturally dependent differences in aetiological factors, the data present a broadly coherent picture. Incidence rates for all forms of head trauma as exemplified in the data from Aquitaine, France, in 1986 (Figure 3.2) show moderately high levels in childhood, a massive peak round the age of 20 years followed by a decline into late middle age and then a rise into old age (Tiret *et al.*, 1990). Rates are consistently higher in males than females. The sharp peak in early adult life is largely attributable to road traffic accidents and the pattern of head injury due to falls is U-shaped with very high rates in childhood, falling to much lower levels throughout most of adult life and rising again in old age. The rates in children probably reflect a high rate of referral of minor injuries to hospital compared with later age groups. In terms of death rates from head trauma, there is also a U-shaped relation to age but rates are extremely low in childhood.

Fractures

Total incidence rates of fractures show a bimodal relation with age with high rates in adolescence declining to a nadir in middle age followed by an increase into old age. This is demonstrated in Figure 3.3 with data redrawn from a study from Trondheim

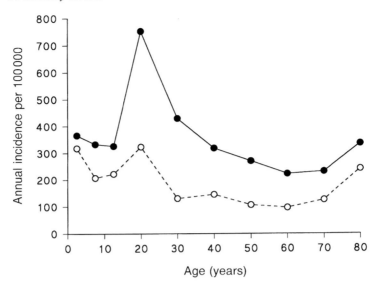

Figure 3.2. Sex- and age-specific rates for head injury, Aquitaine, France 1986. ●, male; ○, female. Redrawn from Tiret *et al.* (1990).

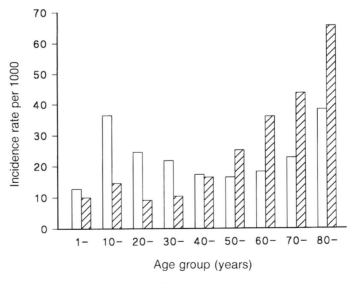

Figure 3.3. Sex- and age-specific incidence rates for fractures (all types) Trondheim, Norway 1985–6. □, male; ▨, female. Redrawn from Sahlin 1990.

(Sahlin, 1990) and a similar pattern is seen in England (Donaldson *et al.*, 1990). Except at ages above 80 years, the great majority of fractures are dealt with on an outpatient basis and hospital discharge data are of limited epidemiological value.

Osteoporosis is assumed to be one of the responsible factors for the rise in fracture rates in later life. Osteoporosis has both genetic and environmental factors and is produced by an age-associated loss of bone acting on a peak bone mass reached in early adult life. Fractures of the vertebrae, distal forearm and the proximal femur are regarded as particularly characteristic of osteoporosis but several other fractures show a pattern of increasing rates in later life, with higher rates in women that one would expect as a manifestation of osteoporosis. There is more to the pathogenesis of fractures than bone weakness however. Figure 3.4 shows representative age-specific incidence rates for the three 'osteoporotic' fractures and indicates that they cannot be simply regarded to result from the same single cause. In later life, rates for all three are higher in women than in men and this is due to both lower peak bone mass in women and accelerated loss of bone associated with oestrogen withdrawal at the menopause.

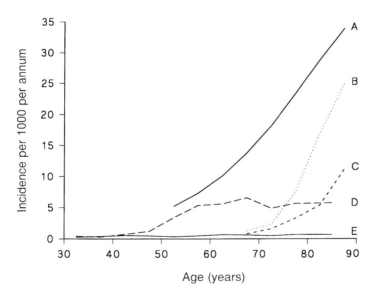

Figure 3.4. Sex- and age-specific incidence rates for specific fractures in adult life. (A) Vertebral fractures in women (Melton *et al.*, 1989); (B) proximal femoral fractures in women and (C) men (Grimley Evans *et al.*, 1979a). (D) Distal forearm fractures in women and (E) men (Alffram & Bauer, 1962).

Vertebral fractures

Studies of the prevalence and incidence of vertebral fractures require radiographic surveys rather than questionnaires. In one study 50% of women experiencing a vertebral fracture were unaware that it had occurred (Melton *et al.*, 1989). A small number of women, 3% of those with fractures in one series (Melton *et al.*, 1989), suffer vertebral fractures from definable severe trauma but most osteoporotic vertebral fractures seem to be 'spontaneous'. Vertebrae are subjected to considerable stresses; during bending, for example, they may be subjected to forces greater than total body weight. Age-associated changes in the structure and compliance of the intervertebral discs may impair their function in redistributing forces through adjacent vertebrae. Fractures are most common in the midthoracic region and around the thoracolumbar junction. Data from Rochester (Melton *et al.*, 1989) showed that some 18% of women aged over 50 years and 27% of women aged over 65 years had one or more vertebral fractures, and the prevalence rose towards 60% in extreme old age.

It seems clear that oestrogen deficiency, and androgen deficiency in men, is one of the important causes of osteoporotic vertebral fractures. In terms of identifying women at particular risk of vertebral fractures studies show that both the presence of a fracture and low bone mineral density are predictors of further fractures (Ross *et al.*, 1991a). Women with a history of ovulatory disturbances may be at above average risk of vertebral osteoporosis (Prior *et al.*, 1990), perhaps because of a degree of hypogonadism. Cigarette smoking also emerges as a significant risk factor for vertebral fractures in case-control studies. None the less, a case-control study of prevalent vertebral fractures among women attending British general practitioners was unable to identify a useful screening method based on personal risk factors. In this study, women with vertebral fractures were on average older and shorter, had experienced an earlier menopause and had more frequently a history of hyperthyroidism (Cooper *et al.*, 1991). A Dutch study also found that screening on the basis of a personal risk score did not produce useful levels of sensitivity or specificity for vertebral and wrist fractures during a 9-year follow-up (van Hemert *et al.*, 1990).

Distal forearm fractures

Distal forearm fractures occur with low incidence in children but show a sharp peak in adolescents of both sexes before returning to lower levels in early adult life (Alffram & Bauer, 1962). The adolescent peak is generally attributed to sporting and other accidents but a phase of relative osteoporosis associated with the adolescent growth spurt may be relevant. A study of Japanese children has shown that the age of peak incidence of wrist fractures corresponds to the age of lowest forearm bone density: 11 years in girls and 13 years in boys (Hagino *et al.*, 1990).

In adult life, the striking feature of the age-specific rates of distal forearm fracture is the large stepwise increase in risk in middle life in women. There is also a striking degree of consistency in the pattern of oscillation of rates at ages above 60 years (Alffram & Bauer, 1962; Miller & Grimley Evans, 1985; Riggs & Melton, 1986). Part of this pattern may be due to an interaction between bone weakness from osteoporosis and the age-specific incidence of falls which shows a localised increase and then decrease among women aged 45–60 years (Winner *et al.*, 1989). The reasons for this transient increase in risk of falling among middle-aged women are unknown but may include a hitherto unrecognised manifestation of the menopause, medication such as hypnotics or tranquillisers or physical factors such as reduced muscle strength or a change in body image consequent on a redistribution of body fat.

Variations in the absolute levels of incidence for distal forearm fracture have been noted; rates in Newcastle, UK, in the 1980s (Miller & Grimley Evans, 1985) were higher than in Malmö, Sweden, 30 years before (Alffram & Bauer, 1962) and rates in Nigeria seem much lower still (Adebajo *et al.*, 1991). To what extent this reflects differences in the prevalence of osteoporosis or differences in patterns of trauma is unknown. In adult life in temperate zones, one determinant of the injury is freezing weather and each year in the UK the onset of icy conditions underfoot causes a mini-epidemic of distal forearm fracture (Miller & Grimley Evans, 1985). This epidemic fades despite the continuation or early return of icy conditions but whether this is because the populace becomes cautious enough to stop falling over or because a susceptible osteoporotic subpopulation of fallers is 'used up' is not known.

Proximal femoral fracture

Proximal femoral fracture (PFF) affects some 45000 UK residents each year and approximately 2% of men and 3% of women will experience a PFF before the age of 75 years (Law *et al.*, 1991). It is a clinically significant fracture. In epidemiologically valid series, 25–30% of older patients die in the 6 months following injury (Greatorex, 1988) and only a half of survivors return to their original levels of functioning. Ten per cent are still in hospital 6 months after the injury and more than a half of survivors are suffering complications, including loss of mobility, pain and leg swelling, at that stage (Grimley Evans *et al.*, 1979a). In the USA at least half the survivors of PFF enter nursing home care (Riggs & Melton, 1986).

At ages up to about 55 years PFF are usually associated with severe degrees of trauma, particularly as incurred in road traffic accidents, and are more frequent in men than in women. From around the age of 55 years rates start to rise in women and from the age of 65 years increase exponentially, doubling with every 7 years of age approximately. An exponential increase in incidence rates of approximately similar slope begins in men around 10 years of age later.

Although virtually all cases of PFF come to medical attention there are some methodological difficulties in obtaining valid incidence and fatality rates. Mortality data are likely to be useless; in one British study less than one-fifth of patients dying in hospital following admission with PFF had the fracture certified as the underlying cause of death (Donaldson *et al.*, 1989). Hospital series of cases can be misleading because of selection factors determining which cases go to which hospital. Even within a single city two hospitals in the same city may receive a very different selection of patients with PFF (Grimley Evans *et al.*, 1980). Patients injured in public places such as shops and bus stations may not be normally resident in a hospital's catchment area and will be fitter than old people who do not leave their homes or are resident in institutions. Some residents in mental hospitals, where incidence rates of PFF have in the past been particularly high (Leitch *et al.*, 1964), may be treated conservatively without transfer to an orthopaedic unit. Routine data may also be inaccurate; Rees (1982) showed that the accuracy of coding of PFF varied greatly in different hospitals. Routine data may also not distinguish between a new case and a patient admitted for revision of an operatively treated PFF from some time before. A transfer of an old person from an orthopaedic unit to a geriatric rehabilitation unit may be recorded as two admissions for PFF rather than one. A valid study requires the identification of all and only the fractures affecting people resident in a geographically defined population within a specified time period.

Risk factors for proximal femoral fracture

Identification of risk factors for PFF is an important issue for public health approaches to control of the injury. At a clinical level, prediction of risk may have benefits for the individual. Cummings *et al.* (1995) identified a number of risk factors in a prospective observational study of women aged 65 years and over. For women with no more than two risk factors incidence rates of PFF were 1.1 per 1000 person-years; for women with five or more risk factors incidence rates were 27 per 1000 person-years.

Problems in identifying risk factors

The easiest and cheapest way of identifying risk factors for PFF is by case-control studies but there are at least two important problems. First, PFF has a multifactorial pathogenesis and various aetiological factors relate to more than one of the pathogenic processes. In Western societies most fractures in later life result from simple falls on the same level (as distinct from falls down stairs or off ladders). Whether a given fall results in a fracture depends on bone strength and what protective factors may be acting. The fact that falls (Prudham & Grimley Evans, 1981) and PFF increase steeply in incidence through old age but distal forearm fractures do not suggest that as people grow older they are more likely to fall but less likely to use their arms to break their fall (and their wrists) and protect their hips (Grimley Evans, 1982). As to be predicted from this model, elderly people injuring themselves in a fall have more preceding cognitive and neuromuscular impairment than those who fall without injury (Nevitt *et al.*, 1991). In addition to neuromuscular responses to falling there may be other more passive factors such as the cushioning effects of subcutaneous fat, clothing or floor covering that determine whether a particular fall results in fracture. The direction of falling may also contribute to the differences in injuries sustained by young and old. Younger people may more often fall forwards on to outstretched hands when hurrying and tripping while older people may more often lose balance and fall sideways on to a hip (Nevitt & Cummings, 1993).

The second problem is heterogeneity of the people who suffer PFF who can be broadly polarised between two groups. At one extreme is the frail old person with physical and mental impairment who breaks her hip in a fall in her own home or while resident in an institution and does badly after treatment. At the other extreme is the physically and mentally fit older person who breaks her hip in a fall down a department store escalator or hurrying to catch a bus. She usually does well after the fracture. In one series of studies the difference between the two could be discerned by the place of fracture and the mental test score on admission to hospital, which was on average higher in those suffering their PFF out of doors (Grimley Evans *et al.*, 1979b). As discussed later there was also a difference between the two groups in seasonal incidence. Case-control studies without an adequate epidemiological base may produce varying results depending on what mix of these two types of cases are enrolled. This is apparent in the varying relation identified in studies between PFF and health or contact with health services. In some studies PFF patients emerge as fitter than the general population, in others as less fit.

Both these problems probably contribute to the conflicting results reported for the relation between thiazides and risk of PFF. The use of thiazide diuretics is associated with preservation of bone density but results of case-control studies of their relation to PFF have been variable (Ray *et al.*, 1989b; LaCroix *et al.*, 1990; Heidrich *et al.*, 1991). The use of diuretics is associated with propensity for falls presumably because of their being prescribed for cardiovascular diseases that cause falls and immobility (Prudham & Grimley Evans, 1981). Depending on the proportions of the 'fit' and the 'unfit' subpopulations of old people recruited into a case-control study, thiazides may emerge as causative of or protective against PFF (or neither).

Osteoporosis

Osteoporosis is the most prevalent form of bone weakness and therefore likely to be involved in the pathogenesis of PFF. Most but not all studies have found lower bone density in cases of PFF than in controls but the differences are on average small and what difference there is between cases and controls diminishes with age (Law *et al.*, 1991). Case-control studies underestimate the significance of osteoporosis as a risk factor for PFF in later life. Bone density falls with age to a degree where nearly all women past the age of 80 years have bones below the fracture threshold defined by the likelihood of the bone breaking under the kinetic energy developed by a simple fall, which is the cause of more than 90% of such fractures. Although at younger ages cases and controls will differ in bone density, at later ages both cases and controls will have bone densities within the zone of fracture risk. The variance between cases and controls at this higher age will therefore be explained by the factors other than bone density which determine fracture risk. None the less, the overall incidence of fractures may be determined by the proportion of the population whose bone strength falls below fracture threshold, in other words the prevalence of osteoporosis. This failure of the case-control method to quantify accurately a major determinant of fracture incidence comes about through the technical problem of 'over-matching' whereby in matching cases and controls for age and sex one has also matched for the variable of interest, namely osteoporosis.

Locality and race

There are local, regional and racial differences in the incidence of PFF. Rates are generally higher in urban than in rural environments (Madhok *et al.*, 1993). This may reflect lower levels of exercise in urban areas, or possibly higher prevalence rates of pre-existing morbidity due to ill or disabled older people migrating into towns. In terms of regions and race, rates are highest in the white populations of Scandinavia, New Zealand and the USA and somewhat lower in the UK and Finland (Maggi *et al.*, 1991). Rates are lower among black people than in white people in the USA (Kellie & Brody, 1990) and in South Africa (Solomon, 1979) and among Maori compared with European New Zealanders (Stott & Stevenson, 1980). Rates have also been lower in Asiatic populations in Singapore (Wong, 1966) and Hong Kong (Chalmers & Ho, 1970). In general, where rates are high, they are higher in women than in men but this may not be the case in populations of low incidence. In Hong Kong rates were higher in men than women in the 1960s (Chalmers & Ho, 1970) but since then rates have increased in both sexes with the emergence of higher rates in women (Lau, 1988).

One contributor to racial difference in PFF incidence may be body height. Several studies have shown that the incidence is higher in taller than in shorter people (Meyer *et al.*, 1993). This may reflect increased energy of impact; the kinetic energy transmitted to the femur in a fall will be equal to the potential energy of the person before the fall. This will be the product of the person's weight and the height of his or her centre of gravity above the ground. Assuming that the centre of gravity is at the midpoint of the body and that body weight increases in proportion to the square of height, as assumed in the computation of the Body Mass (Quetelet's) Index, an increase in mean height of women by 2.5 cm would lead, other things being equal, to an increase in the energy generated in a fall of 4–5%. This is less than the regression of fracture risk on height found in studies of American populations (Hemenway *et al.*, 1994, 1995) but it is possible that in America the effect of height is confounded by an association of height with mechanisms of risk linked to ethnic origin. The kinetic energy effect of increasing height may also be amplified by an increase in the length and fragility of the femoral neck associated with height (Reid *et al.*, 1994).

The incidence among Japanese living in Hawaii is similar to that of Japanese living in Japan but lower than that of USA white people (Ross *et al.*, 1991b). The differences might therefore be genetic in origin or due to lifestyle factors that are culturally preserved among migrant Japanese. Genetic differences are thought to contribute to the difference in incidence between black and white peoples in the USA. Black people are found to have higher bone densities (Trotter *et al.*, 1960) and lower bone turnover rates (Weinstein & Bell, 1988), and a racial difference in the anatomical angle at the femoral neck has also been suggested as a relevant factor (Walensky & O'Brien, 1968). There may also be differences in vitamin D metabolism between black and white peoples (Bell *et al.*, 1985).

Data on deaths from falls and fractures used to show higher rates in the north than in the south of the UK (Eddy, 1972). This gradient is seen for a wide variety of causes of mortality and may have been due to a fatality rather than an incidence difference. A direct comparison of PFF incidence rates in Newcastle upon Tyne and Oxford in the early 1980s showed identical incidence rates (Grimley Evans, 1985). Two studies of Medicare and Insurance enrolees in the USA show states (Stroup *et al.*, 1990) and counties (Jacobsen *et al.*, 1990) with highest rates tending to cluster towards the southeast of the country.

Increasing incidence of femoral fracture

The incidence of proximal femoral fracture has increased in the UK over the last 30 years (Boyce & Vessey, 1985). Hospital discharge data from the Hospital Inpatient Enquiry (HIPE) suggest that rates in both sexes may have levelled off since 1979 (Spector *et al.*, 1990). More detailed analysis of HIPE data suggests that in addition to a secular increase in rates in the 1970s, there may have been a cohort effect with successive generations of people born from the 1880s into the 20th century reaching later life with increasing risk of fracture (Grimley Evans *et al.*, 1997).

Incidence has been increasing in other countries, notably Hong Kong (Lau, 1988), Sweden (Sernbo & Johnell, 1989), Finland (Parkkari *et al.*, 1994) and also Spain, Norway, Denmark, USA and Canada (Maggi *et al.*, 1991). The reports differ somewhat in how the incidence changes have affected the two sexes. Data from successive incidence studies in Newcastle upon Tyne from 1971 to 1983 (Grimley Evans, 1985) suggested that although rates in men had apparently risen in the preceding decade (as shown by a comparison with rates from Oxford in 1963–64) rates during the 1970s were stable in men but were still increasing in women at a rate similar to that deduced by Boyce & Vessey (1985) in Oxford. As already noted, rates in Oxford and Newcastle in 1983 were identical. This pattern would be compatible with a long-term effect of cigarette smoking which is associated with lower bone density in postmenopausal women (Krall & Dawson-Hughes, 1991) and in 70-year-old men (Mellstrom *et al.*, 1982). Historically, the prevalence rate of cigarette smoking increased among men during the first part of the 20th century but then stabilised around 30–40 years ago when the habit was still increasing among women.

While it seems reasonable to suggest that the increase in incidence of femoral fractures reflects a rising prevalence of osteoporosis there is little direct evidence for this. Age-associated loss of bone seems to be universal in the human species (Garn *et al.*, 1967) and osteoporosis has been documented in a woman from the Bronze Age (Frigo & Lang, 1995). An archaeological study of skeletons from a London crypt has shown that average bone mineral density has declined in England over the past 200 years but it is not known if this is a recent change (Lees *et al.*, 1993). Sernbo & Johnell (1989) compared the Femoral Neck Index (FNI) of radiographs from cases of proximal femoral fracture in the 1950s and 1980s from Malmö, Sweden. The data suggested higher FNI (i.e. less osteoporosis) in the 1950s sample. This might indicate a shift towards a greater prevalence of osteoporosis in the general population, but equally it might reflect changes in the nature or incidence of trauma or in protective factors in falling. While there are no data bearing directly on the possibility of secular changes in the incidence of falls, Wickham *et al.* (1989) have suggested that factors such as housing may have a general effect on the population risk of falling. Secular changes in levels of obesity, and even in use of medications, could also be relevant to the incidence and consequences of falls. Several authors have suggested that reduction in levels of habitual physical exercise may be the main cause of the increase in femoral fracture incidence in the past 30 years. All these factors might affect incidence of PFF by an effect on osteoporosis or on falls and protective responses. Epidemiological experience suggests that it is unlikely that any single factor will prove to be the entire explanation for the secular trend.

Seasonal variation in incidence

The incidence of PFF is higher in the winter months than in the summer, and as this is true for injuries that occur indoors it cannot be attributed simply to the effect of falling on snow and ice as in the case of distal forearm fracture. In a hospital series of cases in

Nottingham (Bastow *et al.*, 1983) the seasonal effect was attributable to a link between numbers of cases and daily temperature and was greatest in thin people. The authors postulated that some thin old people suffer minor degrees of hypothermia in cold weather that impairs neuromuscular function and causes them to fall. The thin subjects certainly had lower body temperatures than those of fatter patients on arrival at hospital but this difference may have originated after rather than before the fracture. Other data suggest that temperature cannot be the whole explanation for seasonal effects. In a USA study of Medicare patients with PFF (Jacobsen *et al.*, 1991) the seasonal pattern of high rates in winter and low in summer was constant in timing and magnitude across age groups from 65 years upwards and over five geographical areas from north of latitude 45° to south of 30 °N. This suggests that temperature may not be the relevant factor, particularly given North American standards of house heating even among a Medicare population.

In Newcastle upon Tyne the timing of the seasonal peak differed between patients who suffered PFF from falling indoors and those who fell out of doors. While both types showed a summer nadir, the out-of-the-home fractures were most common in December and January and the in-home fractures peaked in March and April (Grimley Evans, 1993). The fractures in the active groups are thought to represent the dangers of Christmas shopping and January sales; a similar effect has been noted in association with preparation for Jewish religious festivals in Jerusalem (Pogrund *et al.*, 1977) although there is some doubt about the accuracy of the calculated population at risk in that study. The spring peak in the indoor fractures does not correspond with the coldest months in Newcastle but does correspond with the end of the seasonal period of lowest blood vitamin D levels in old people (Lawson *et al.*, 1979). One possible explanation therefore is a subclinical neuromyopathy from vitamin D deficiency in a predominantly housebound group of a northern population. The data also showed an unexpected and unexplained peak in September.

Oestrogens

Although bone loss occurs throughout life from the age of around 25 years, there is a period of accelerated loss in women for the 5–10 years after the menopause. This accelerated loss is delayed by the administration of exogenous oestrogen, but it is not yet clear whether a long-term gain in bone density is obtained if the oestrogens are subsequently discontinued (Law *et al.*, 1991). Oestrogens may also maintain muscle strength (Phillips *et al.*, 1993) and may therefore have an effect in preventing falls and increasing the effectiveness of protective responses in falling. Both case-control studies and prospective studies of the natural menopause suggest that exogenous oestrogen therapy reduces the incidence of PFF, although possibly only while the therapy is being taken. The serious methodological problem is that the studies reported on the natural menopause have been observational and based on women who selected themselves for perimenopausal oestrogen therapy. Barrett-Connor (1991) has drawn attention to the possible importance of this selection bias by demonstrating that women who report perimenopausal oestrogen therapy had more physician contacts and undertook significantly more preventive health care procedures, including daily exercise, than women who did not take hormone replacement therapy (HRT).

Other aspects of reproductive functioning may also have an effect on risk of PFF. Some case-control studies suggest that risk diminishes with the number of children born (Wyshak, 1981) and that breast feeding of children is associated with lower risk (Kreiger *et al.*, 1982).

Alcohol intake

Alcoholics have low bone density (Lalor *et al.*, 1986) and a high incidence of PFF. Moderate alcohol intake is not strongly associated with an increased risk of PFF. One study of middle-aged nurses found a 24% increase in risk of PFF among the women drinking more than two units of alcohol daily but the increased risk was restricted to the group who were also underweight (Hemenway *et al.*, 1988). While an increased propensity to falling might contribute to the incidence of PFF in alcoholics, no association has been found between falls and the ordinary levels of alcohol intake observed in population studies of elderly people in Britain (Prudham & Grimley Evans, 1981) or in North America (Tinetti *et al.*, 1988).

Drugs

Some forms of medication are associated with the risk of falling and may therefore be expected to emerge as risk factors for PFF. Hypnotics and sedatives are consistently associated with risk, and long-acting sedative drugs (Ray *et al.*, 1989) and cyclic antidepressants (Ray *et al.*, 1991) seem to be particularly important.

Some other drugs may act through an effect on osteoporosis. In some studies caffeine intake has been found to be positively linked with the risk of PFF (Kiel *et al.*, 1990; Cummings *et al.*, 1995) but in Swedish data it was found that when adjustment was made for cigarette smoking and other factors the effect of coffee drinking on bone loss and fractures was very small (Johansson *et al.*, 1992). On the positive side, as already noted, some studies have demonstrated that thiazide diuretics have a favourable effect on bone density and on the incidence of fractures (Ray *et al.*, 1989a; LaCroix *et al.*, 1990), although there are some opposing findings (Heidrich *et al.*, 1991). The effect is of sufficient magnitude, a possible reduction of a third in the risk of PFF, that it is a reason, where clinically appropriate, for choosing thiazides as first line treatment for hypertension in patients in middle age and beyond.

Fluoride

The relation between fluoride and fractures has been widely debated over the years. Although some epidemiological studies have suggested that the frequency of osteoporosis-related fractures is higher in areas with low fluoride content in the drinking water, others have produced opposite findings. Most studies have examined fluoride intake in drinking water only but there are many other dietary sources. A review from a Workshop of the US National Institutes of Health (Gordon & Corbin, 1992) concluded that it was not possible to draw conclusions relating fluoride levels in drinking water to fracture rates or osteoporosis.

Physical activity

Problems in mobility are associated with increased risk of falls (Prudham & Grimley Evans, 1981) and therefore not surprisingly with risk of PFF (Cummings *et al.*, 1995). Over and above this, a range of studies (Law *et al.*, 1991) have shown an inverse relation between habitual exercise levels and risk of hip fractures. In broad terms, compared with the risk in women with low levels of activity, moderate activity is associated with a 40–50% lower risk and high levels of activity with a 70% lower risk. Several intervention studies have shown short-term benefits from exercise regimes. Animal work has also shown that even small loading stresses applied to bones in immobilised limbs can bring about measurable reductions in disuse bone loss (Lanyon, 1990). The benefits of exercise probably arise partly through an effect on the maintenance of bone mass but also by reducing the risk of falls and improving protective responses to falling. Although many of the studies on exercise and propensity to falls have been too small or methodologically flawed, a meta-analysis of seven coordinated trials suggests a beneficial effect (Province *et al.*, 1995).

Dietary calcium

There has been a prolonged controversy over the relevance of dietary calcium levels to the genesis of osteoporosis and the incidence of fractures. A much-quoted Yugoslavian study compared cross-sectional findings in the adults of two geographical areas with different mean levels of dietary calcium intake (Matkovic *et al.*, 1979). In both areas mean metacarpal indices declined similarly with age but were higher at all ages in the region with the higher calcium intake. Forearm and hip fracture incidence rates were lower in the region with higher calcium intakes. There were however other differences in diet and lifestyle between the two populations. Energy intake was higher in the high calcium group and this may reflect higher levels of physical activity for example. What the data do suggest, however, is that if dietary calcium intake were important in the genesis of osteoporosis its action at the levels studied in the two Yugoslavian populations is through an increase in bone mass laid down in childhood and adolescence not through retarding subsequent age-associated loss.

Despite some support for an association between low dietary calcium intake and risk of PFF (Holbrook *et al.*, 1988) the evidence is not compelling for the USA and the UK. The situation may be different in populations with low average intakes. Among elderly Chinese women in Hong Kong average daily intakes are below 400 mg and cases of PFF were found to have lower intakes than controls (Lau *et al.*, 1988). Calcium supplements given to elderly Hong Kong women with very low intakes reduced bone mineral loss measured at the hip (Lau *et al.*, 1988).

Little is known about individual variation in the ability to adapt to a low calcium diet and there may also be variation in the absorption of calcium (Heaney, 1991). Although average calcium intake in Western populations seems adequate some people may therefore be at suboptimal levels. Overall, it seems prudent to recommend dietary calcium intakes of the order of 800–1000 mg per diem for the population as a whole, but the scope for affecting fracture incidence in economically advanced nations through the manipulation of dietary calcium or the prescription of calcium supplements in adult life seems limited.

Vitamin D

Severe deficiency of vitamin D activity produces the histological picture of osteomalacia which has been found in a proportion of old people with PFF in the UK, although it now seems rarer than in the past (Compston *et al.*, 1991). In the UK old people with PFF show lower serum vitamin D levels than are found in controls (Baker *et al.*, 1979). While this might indicate the presence of osteomalacia in a proportion, it might merely reflect the lower exposure to ultraviolet light of that proportion of patients with PFF who are less mobile out of doors than the general population. It seems that sunlight exposure makes a greater contribution to serum vitamin D levels in the aged of the UK than does dietary intake (Lawson *et al.*, 1979) and being immobile and housebound is associated with a greater than average risk of falls (Prudham & Grimley Evans, 1981). There is however the possibility that milder forms of vitamin D deficiency may produce osteoporosis rather than osteomalacia by inducing a compensatory rise in parathyroid hormone. It has been noted that levels of vitamin D intake common in a general population sample of middle-aged women in

North America are not sufficient to prevent a rise in serum parathyroid hormone levels during the winter months (Krall *et al.*, 1989). The implication could be that increased bone absorption during the winter could over the years contribute to age-associated bone loss. In support of this hypothesis, a negative correlation has been shown between serum hydroxyvitamin D levels and bone mineral density in a population sample of British women (Khaw *et al.*, 1992). Seasonal supplements of vitamin D can prevent the wintertime rise in parathyroid hormone levels and reduce bone loss (Dawson-Hughes *et al.*, 1991).

Some interventive studies in selected population samples have shown a reduction in fracture rates following administration of vitamin D, with or without calcium supplements (Heikinheimo *et al.*, 1992; Chapuy *et al.*, 1994). The onset of apparent benefit in these studies was rapid, and it is possible that part of the benefit might have arisen through a reduction in risk of falls by cure of the neuromyopathy of more severe degrees of vitamin D deficiency in some of the subjects. Larger trials in general populations are needed.

Other fractures

Other specific fractures in later life have received less epidemiological attention. Fractures of the pelvis increase steeply in incidence in later life with higher rates in women (Ragnarsson & Jacobsson, 1992). This pattern suggests an important aetiological contribution from osteoporosis. Fractures of the proximal humerus start to increase steeply in women around the age of 50 years but do not rise in men until the eighth decade of life (Donaldson *et al.*, 1990). In a population sample of elderly women, Kelsey *et al.* (1992) found that women who incurred proximal fractures of the humerus tended to be less healthy and active than those who broke their wrists. This could be a further manifestation of the postulated failure of some older people to react by extending their arms in response to falling.

Bengnér *et al.* (1990) compared the incidence of fractures of the shaft of the femur and tibia in Malmö in the 1950s and 1980s. Fractures of the femoral shaft showed a U-shaped relation to age in both sexes with highest rates in male children and adolescents. From the 1950s to the 180s incidence rates increased in older women but fell in men. Supracondylar femoral fracture rates were low but with a perceptibly U-shaped relation to age and with an increase with time in both men and women aged over 60 years. As in English data (Donaldson *et al.*, 1990) tibial shaft fractures decrease with age throughout adult life in men; in women they fall from high rates in childhood but remained fairly constant in incidence for the rest of adult life with perhaps a slight rise above age 75 years. There was no secular trend.

Burns

Feller *et al.* (1982) calculated comparative risks of burns by comparing the proportions of specific age groups in patients with the proportions in the general population in the USA. The data (Figure 3.5) show high risks in early childhood for both sexes and in early adult life in men. From the age of 70 years there is an increase in risk for both men and women. In this last age group cooking injuries accounted for around 17% of cases and incinerating rubbish, hot bathing water and falling asleep while smoking accounted for 10–11% each. Ignition of clothing seems a greater risk for older people than younger (Rossignol *et al.*, 1985). Alcohol consumption may be a less frequent contributor to burn accidents in later life than at younger ages, at least in fatal household fires (Elder *et al.*, 1996).

The fatality rate from burns increases steeply with later age. The US National Burn Information Exchange has data linking age and percentage of body surface affected with survival following burns (Figure 3.6) (Feller *et al.*, 1980). These data are from participating hospitals with specialised burn treatment facilities and presumably represent the best of care that is available. The generality of results may be even less impressive. As in other fields, there is evidence that older patients may receive less effective treatment than younger patients on the unjustified presumption that they will inevitably be unable to respond to energetic therapy (Linn, 1980).

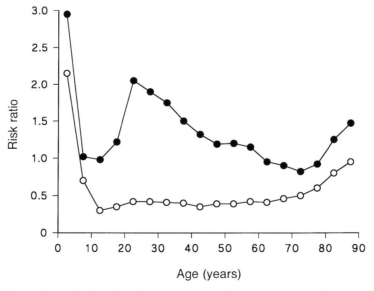

Figure 3.5. Relative risk of burns by sex and age. ●, male; ○, female. Redrawn from Feller *et al.* (1982).

Road traffic accidents

Road traffic accidents are an important cause of injury at all ages in economically developed nations. In the UK the probability of a car driver being involved in an injury accident has been calculated as 0.335 for a man and 0.242 for a woman during an average driving career (Broughton, 1987). Three male drivers in a thousand and one female driver in a thousand will end their driving careers by being killed in a traffic accident.

Driver casualties per head of population initially decrease with age but start to rise after the middle years. The rise in rates appears earlier for the more serious accidents and is more apparent if the distance travelled is taken into account (Broughton, 1987). In later life rates are higher for female than for male drivers for all grades of accident. A complicating factor in interpreting these trends is a non-linear relation between mileage and accidents (Janke, 1991) in that high-mileage drivers gain most miles on motorways, where the accident rate per distance travelled is lower than on smaller roads.

The types of accident vary with age. In early adult life accidents tend to be associated with speeding and alcohol ingestion. In later life accidents tend to occur at slower speeds and involve collisions at intersections (McFarland *et al.*, 1964; Sattin & Nevitt, 1992). The contribution to accidents of alcohol ingestion by car drivers and passengers seems to be much smaller than at younger ages (Holubowycz & McLean, 1995).

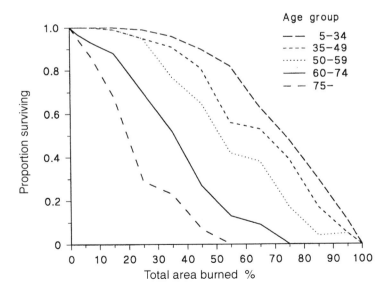

Figure 3.6. Fatality of burns by age and body surface area affected. After Feller *et al.* (1980).

There is evidence of an association in later life between the risk of driving accidents and visual problems. These include poor acuity, particularly at low levels of illumination (Sturr & Taub, 1990), and objective or functional restriction of visual fields. In a study of Californian drivers, Keltner & Johnson (1987) found visual field loss in 3.0–3.5% of those aged under 60 years, but 7% of those aged 60–65 years and 13% of those over 65 years. Nearly 60% of those with visual field loss had been unaware of the loss of peripheral vision. Drivers with visual field loss in both eyes had twice as high accident and conviction rates as an age- and sex-matched control group with normal visual fields.

To some extent older drivers recognise their problems and compensate for them. They may restrict driving to daylight and times of low traffic. They tend to drive more slowly than young adults and to drink less alcohol. Holland & Rabbitt (1994) found that individuals who had been made aware of visual or hearing losses reported making changes in their driving behaviour to compensate. Rabbitt (1991) also found that accident rates proved to be lower among those who had altered their driving behaviour because of noticing a change in their sensory abilities. There is also evidence that older people can improve their visual performance by specific practice (Ball & Sekuler, 1986).

There are some negative factors however; older drivers may be more likely to be taking medications, and a relation has been shown between road traffic accidents and the prescription of minor tranquillisers (Skegg *et al.*, 1979). Older drivers (and pedestrians) may not have accurate insight into their particular problems. Sattin & Nevitt (1992) note that older drivers ranked failure to give way at intersections as the ninth problem out of ten although it is the major cause of accidents involving older drivers. Compatible findings have been reported in the UK (AA Foundation, 1988).

Cognitive impairment of drivers can be assumed to be a risk factor for road traffic accidents, although its significance has not been well quantified (Parasuraman, 1991). It is clear that many older people with dementia continue to drive and to be involved in accidents (O'Neill *et al.*, 1992), and there is a need for standardised tests of driving ability for such patients (Fitten *et al.*, 1995).

There are ways in which traffic regulations and the design of roadways make things unnecessarily difficult for older drivers and pedestrians. Traffic in urban areas is allowed to move faster than is appropriate, and often faster than is lawful; bus stops should be placed beyond intersections rather than before them and pedestrian crossings should allow enough time for older and slower people to cross the road in safety.

Several commentators have suggested that the conventional form of seat belt provided in cars has been designed for younger motorists and in collisions can fracture the more rigid rib cage of older people. The Volvo Car Crash Register data show that the risk of sustaining fracture, particularly rib cage fracture, increases steeply with age for drivers and front seat passengers involved in frontal collisions (Brorsson, 1989). The risk of fracture is 3.2 times higher in people aged 65–74 years than in people aged

18–24 years, and for rib cage fracture the risk is 10.9 times higher in the older age group.

Comment

The epidemiology of trauma in later life is dominated by age-associated decline in adaptability leading both to an increase in the incidence of trauma and to poorer outcomes from treatment. There is a need for a more rational approach to selection of treatment for older patients but if the suffering and costs of trauma in later life are to be reduced efforts will need to be directed at prevention. Traditional approaches to prevention of falls by removing recognisable hazards from an old person's environment are unlikely to produce much benefit at a population level (Campbell *et al.*, 1990). Multidisciplinary assessment of old people who fall while resident in institutions may confer some benefits but preventing further falls does not seem to be among them (Rubenstein, *et al.*, 1990). We do not know if the same would be true in the general population. Although there are some promising findings for high risk groups (Tinetti *et al.*, 1994) falls are so common that it would not be feasible to investigate all old people who fall. A more selective approach needs to be evaluated, focusing perhaps on those who fall for no identifiable reason (Campbell *et al.*, 1989) or on those who fall twice or more within a year (Grimley Evans, 1990). There are undoubtedly aspects of the public environment, particularly in the design of stairways and steps, which merit attention in preventing unnecessary falls (Archea, 1985).

Finally there seems to be scope for a more systematic approach to preventing and reducing the severity of road traffic accidents in later life. Here, as in the deployment of treatment for older people, there is need for a wider recognition and analysis of the heterogeneity of functioning in later life. We should stop talking about 'the elderly' and think about old people.

References

AA Foundation for Road Safety Research. (1988). *Motoring and the Older Driver*. Basingstoke, Hants: Automobile Association.

Adebajo, A. O., Cooper, C. & Grimley Evans, J. (1991). Fractures of the hip and distal forearm in West Africa and the United Kingdom. *Age Ageing*, **20**, 435–8.

Alffram, P.-A. & Bauer, G. C. H. (1962). Epidemiology of fractures of the forearm. *J Bone Joint Surg*, **44A**, 105–14.

Archea, J. C. (1985). Environmental factors associated with stair accidents by the elderly. *Clin Geriatr Med*, **1**, 555–68.

Baker, M. R., McDonnell, H., Peacock, M. & Nordin, B. E. C. (1979). Plasma 25–hydroxy vitamin D concentrations in patients with fractures of the femoral neck. *Br Med J*, **1**, 589.

Ball, K. & Sekuler, R. (1986). Improving visual perception in older observers. *J Gerontol*, **41**, 176–82.

Barrett-Connor, E. (1991). Postmenopausal estrogen and prevention bias. *Ann Intern Med*, **115**, 455–6.

Bastow, M. D., Rawlings, J. & Allison, S. P. (1983). Undernutrition, hypothermia, and injury in elderly women with fractured femur: an injury response to altered metabolism? *Lancet*, **1**, 143–6.

Bell, N. H., Greene, A., Epstein, S., Oexman, M. J., Shaw, S. & Shary, J. (1985). Evidence for alteration of the vitamin D-endocrine system in blacks. *J Clin Invest*, **76**, 470–3.

Bengnér, U., Ekbom, T., Johnell, O. & Nilsson, B. E. (1990). Incidence of femoral and tibial shaft fractures. Epidemiology 1950–1983 in Malmö, Sweden. *Acta Orthop Scand*, **61**, 251–4.

Boyce, W. J. & Vessey, M. P. (1985). Rising incidence of fracture of the proximal femur. *Lancet*, **1**, 150–1.

Brorsson, B. (1989). Age and injury severity. *Scand J Soc Med*, **17**, 287–90.

Broughton, J. (1987). Casualty rates by age and sex. In *Road Accidents of Great Britain* 1987: *the Casualty Report*, pp. 60–4. London: HMSO.

Campbell, A. J., Borrie, M. J. & Spears, G. F. (1989). Risk factors for falls in a community-based prospective study of people 70 years and older. *J Gerontol*, **44**, M112–M117.

Campbell, A. J., Borrie, M. J., Spears, G. F., Jackson, S. L., Brown, J. S. & Fitzgerald, J. L. (1990). Circumstances and consequences of falls experienced by a community population 70 years and over during a prospective study. *Age Ageing*, **19**, 136–41.

Centers for Disease Control. (1989). Cost of injury – United States: a report to Congress, *JAMA*, **262**, 2803–4.

Chalmers, J. & Ho, K. C. (1970). Geographical variations in senile osteoporosis. The association with physical activity. *J Bone Joint Surg*, **52B**, 667–75.

Chapuy, M. C., Arlot, M. E., Delmas, P. D. & Meunier, P. J. (1994). Effect of calcium and cholecalciferol treatment for three years on hip fractures in elderly women. *Br Med J*, **308**, 1081–2.

Compston, J. E., Vedi, S. & Croucher, P. I. (1991). Low prevalence of osteomalacia in elderly patients with hip fracture. *Age Ageing*, **20**, 132–4.

Cooper, C., Shah, S., Hand, D. J., Adams, J., Compston, J., David, M. & Woolf, A. (1991). Screening for vertebral osteoporosis using individual risk factors. *Osteop Int*, **2**, 48–53.

Cummings, S.R., Nevitt, M. C., Broloher, W. S. *et al.* (1995). Risk factors for hip fractures in white women. *New Engl J Med*, **332**, 767–73.

Dawson-Hughes, B., Dallal, G. E., Krall, E. A., Harris, S., Sokoll, L. J. & Falconer, G. (1991). Effect of vitamin D supplementation on wintertime and overall bone loss in healthy postmenopausal women. *Ann Intern Med*, **115**, 505–12.

Donaldson, L. J., Cook, A. & Thomson, R. G. (1990). Incidence of fractures in a geographically defined population. *J Epidemiol Comm Hlth*, **44**, 241–5.

Donaldson, L. J., Parsons, L. & Cook, A. J. (1989). Death certification in fractured neck of femur. *Publ Hlth* (*Lond*), **103**, 237–43.

Eddy, T. P. (1972). Deaths from falls and fractures. *Br J Prev Soc Med*, **26**, 173–9.

Elder, A. T., Squires, T. & Busuttil, A. (1996). Fire fatalities in elderly people. *Age Ageing*, **25**, 214–16.

Evans, L. (1988). Risk of fatality from physical trauma versus sex and age. *J Trauma*, **28**, 368–77.

Fairweather, D. S. & Grimley Evans J. (1990). Ageing. In *The Metabolic and Molecular Basis of Acquired Disease*, ed. R. D. Cohen, B. Lewis & K. G. M. M. Alberti, pp. 213–36. London: Bailliere Tindall.

Feller, I., James, M. H. & Jones, C. A. (1982). Burn epidemiology: focus on youngsters and the aged. *J Burn Care Rehab*, **3**, 285–329.

Feller, I., Tholen, D. & Cornell, R. G. (1980). Improvements in burn care, 1965 to 1979. *JAMA*, **244**, 2074–8.

Fitten, L. J., Perryman, K. M., Wilkinson, C. J., Little, R. J., Burns, M. M., Pachana, N., Mervis, J. R., Malmgren, R., Siembieda, D. W. & Ganzell, S. (1995). Alzheimer and vascular dementias and driving. A prospective road and laboratory study. *JAMA*, **273**, 1360–5.

Frigo, P. & Lang, C. (1995). Osteoporosis in a woman of the early Bronze Age. *New Engl J Med*, **333**, 1468.

Garn, S. M., Rohmann, C. G. & Wagner, B. (1967). Bone loss as a general phenomenon in man. *Fed Proc*, **26**, 1729–36.

Gordon, S. L. & Corbin, S. B. (1992). Summary of Workshop on Drinking Water Fluoride Influence on Hip Fracture and Bone Health (National Institutes of Health, 10 April 1991). *Osteop Int*, **2**, 109–17.

Gorman, D. F., Teanby, D. N., Sinha, M. P., Wotherspoon, J., Boot, D. A. & Molokhia, A. (1995). The epidemiology of major injuries in Mersey Region and North Wales. *Injury*, **26**, 51–4.

Greatorex, I. F. (1988). Proximal femoral fractures: an assessment of the outcome of health care in elderly people. *Commun Med*, **10**, 203–10.

Grimley Evans, J. (1982). Epidemiology of proximal femoral fracture. In *Recent Advances in Geriatric Medicine* 2, ed. B. Isaacs, pp. 201–14. Edinburgh: Churchill Livingstone.

Grimley Evans, J. (1985). Incidence of proximal femoral fracture. *Lancet*, **1**, 925–6.

Grimley Evans, J. (1990). Fallers, non-fallers and poison. *Age Ageing*, **19**, 268–9.

Grimley Evans, J. (1993). The epidemiology of osteoporosis. *Rev Clin Gerontol*, **3**, 13–30.

Grimley Evans, J., Prudham, D. & Wandless, I. (1979a). A prospective study of proximal femoral fracture: incidence and outcome. *Publ Hlth (Lond)*, **93**, 235–41.

Grimley Evans, J., Prudham, D. & Wandless, I. (1979b). A prospective study of fractured proximal femur: factors predisposing to survival. *Age Ageing*, **8**, 246–50.

Grimley Evans, J., Prudham, D. & Wandless, I. (1980). A prospective study of fractured proximal femur: hospital differences. *Publ Hlth (Lond)*, **94**, 149–54.

Grimley Evans, J., Seagroatt, V. & Goldacre, M. J. (1997). Secular trends in proximal femoral fracture, Oxford Record Linkage Study area and England 1968–85. *J Epidemiol Comm Health*, **151**, 424–9.

Hagino, H., Yamamoto, K., Teshima, R., Kishimoto, H. & Nakamura, T. (1990). Fracture incidence and bone mineral density of the distal radius in Japanese schoolchildren. *Arch Orthop Traum Surg*, **109**, 262–4.

Heaney, R. P. (1991). Calcium supplements: practical considerations. *Osteop Int*, **1**, 65–71.

Heidrich, F. E., Stergachis, A. & Gross, K. M. (1991). Diuretic drug use and the risk for hip fracture. *Ann Intern Med*, **115**, 1–6.

Heikinheimo, R. J., Inkovaara, J. A., Harju, E. J., Haavisto, M. V., Kaarela, R. H., Kataja, J. M., Kokko, A. M.-L., Kolho, L. A. & Rajala, S. A. (1992). Annual injection of vitamin D and fracture of aged bones. *Calcif Tissue Int*, **51**, 105–10.

Hemenway, D., Azrael, D. R., Rimm, E. B., Feskanich, D. & Willen, D. C. (1994). Risk factors for hip fracture in US men aged 40 through 75 years. *Am J Publ Hlth*, **84**, 1843–5.

Hemenway, D., Colditz, G. A., Willett, W. C., Stampfer, M. J. & Speizer, F. E. (1988). Fractures and lifestyle: effect of cigarette smoking, alcohol intake, and relative weight on the risk of hip and forearm fracture in middle-aged women. *Am J Pub Hlth*, **78**, 1554–8.

Hemenway, D., Feskanich, D. & Colditz, G. A. (1995). Body height and hip fracture: a cohort study of 90000 women. *Int J Epidemiol*, **24**, 783–6.

Holbrook, T. L., Barrett-Connor, E. & Wingard, D. L. (1988). Dietary calcium and hip fracture: 14–year prospective population study. *Lancet*, **ii**, 1046–9.

Holland, C. A. & Rabbitt, P. M. A. (1994). The problems of being an older driver: comparing the perceptions of an expert group and older drivers. *Applied Ergonomics*, **25**, 17–27.

Holubowycz, O. T. & McLean, A.J. (1995). Demographic characteristics, drinking pattern and drink-driving behaviour of injured male drivers and motorcycle riders. *J Stud Alcohol*, **56**, 513–21.

Jacobsen, S. J., Goldberg, J., Miles, T. P., Brody, J. A., Stiers, W. & Rimm, A. A. (1990). Regional variation in the incidence of hip fracture. *JAMA*, **264**, 500–2.

Jacobsen, S. J., Goldberg, J., Miles, T. P., Brody, J. A., Stiers, W. & Rimm, A. A. (1991). Seasonal variation in the incidence of hip fracture among white persons aged 65 years and older in the United States, 1984–1987. *Am J Epidemiol*, **133**, 996–1004.

Janke, M. K. (1991). Accidents, mileage and the exaggeration of risk. *Accid Anal Prev*, **23**, 183–8.

Johansson, C., Mellström, D., Lerner, U. & Österberg, T. (1992). Coffee drinking: a minor risk factor for bone loss and fractures. *Age Ageing*, **21**, 20–6.

Johnson, C. L., Margulies, D. R., Kearney, T. J., Hiatt, J. R. & Shabot, M. M. (1994). Trauma in the elderly: an analysis of outcomes based on age. *Am Surg*, **60**, 899–902.

Kellie, S. E. & Brody, J. A. (1990). Sex-specific and race-specific hip fracture rates. *Am J Publ Hlth*, **80**, 326–8.

Kelsey, J. L., Browner, W. S., Seeley, D. G., Nevitt, M. C. & Cummings, S. R. (1992). Risk factors for fractures of the distal forearm and proximal humerus. *Am J Epidemiol*, **135**, 477–89.

Keltner, J. L. & Johnson, C. A. (1987). Visual function, driving safety and the elderly. *Ophthalmology*, **94**, 1180–8.

Khaw, K.-T., Sneyd, M.-J. & Compston, J. (1992). Bone density parathyroid hormone and 25–hydroxyvitamin D concentrations in middle aged women. *Br Med J*, **305**, 273–7.

Kiel, D. P., Felson, D. T., Hannan, M. T., Anderson, J. L. & Wilson, P. W. F. (1990). Caffeine and the risk of hip fracture: the Framingham study. *Am J Epidemiol*, **132**, 675–84.

Krall, E. A. & Dawson-Hughes, B. (1991). Smoking and bone loss among post-menopausal women. *J Bone Mineral Res*, **6**, 331–7.

Krall, E. A., Sahyoun, N., Tannenbaum, S., Dallal, G. E. & Dawson-Hughes, B. (1989). Effect of vitamin D intake on seasonal variation in parathyroid hormone secretion in post-menopausal women. *New Engl J Med*, **321**, 1777–83.

Kreiger, N., Kelsey, J. L., Holford, T. R. & O'Connor, T. (1982). An epidemiologic study of hip fracture in postmenopausal women. *Am J Epidemiol*, **116**, 141–8.

LaCroix, A. Z., Wienpahl, J., White, L. R., Wallace, R. B., Scherr, P. A., George, L. K., Cornoni-Huntley, J. & Ostfeld, A. M. (1990). Thiazide diuretic agents and the incidence of hip fracture. *New Engl J Med*, **322**, 286–90.

Lalor, B. C., France, M. W., Powell, D., Adams, P. H. & Counihan, T. B. (1986). Bone and mineral metabolism and chronic alcohol abuse. *Q J Med*, **59**, 497–511.

Lanyon, L. E. (1990). Bone loading: the functional determinant of bone architecture and a physiological contributor to the prevention of osteoporosis. In *Osteoporosis 1990*, ed. R. Smith, pp. 63–78. London: Royal College of Physicians of London.

Lau, E., Donnan, S., Barker, D. J. P. & Cooper, C. (1988). Physical activity and calcium intake in fracture of the proximal femur in Hong Kong. *Br Med J*, **297**, 441–3.

Lau, E. M. C. (1988). Osteoporosis in elderly Chinese. *Br Med J*, **296**, 1263.

Law, M. R., Wald, N. J. & Meade, T. W. (1991). Strategies for prevention of osteoporosis and hip fracture. *Br Med J*, **303**, 453–9.

Lawson, D. E. M., Paul, A. A., Black, A. E., Cole, T. J., Mandal, A. R. & Davie, M. (1979). Relative contributions of diet and sunlight to vitamin D state in the elderly. *Br Med J*, **2**, 303–5.

Lees, B., Molleson, T., Arnett, T. R. & Stevenson, J. C. (1993). Differences in proximal femur bone density over two centuries. *Lancet*, **341**, 673–75.

Leitch, I. H., Knowelden, J. & Seddon, H. J. (1964). Incidence of fractures, particularly of the neck of the femur, in patients in mental hospitals. *Br J Prev Soc Med*, **18**, 142–5.

Li, G. & Baker, S. P. (1992). A comparison of injury death rates in China and the United States, 1986. *Am J Publ Hlth*, **82**, 605–9.

Linn, B. S. (1980). Age differences in the severity and outcome of burns. *J Am Geriatr Soc*, **28**, 118–22.

MacKenzie, E. J., Morris, J. A., Smith, G. S. & Fahey, M. (1990). Acute hospital costs of trauma in the United States: implications for regionalized systems of care. *J Trauma*, **30**, 1096–101.

Madhok, R., Melton, L. J., Atkinson, E. J., O'Fallon, W. M. & Lewallen, D. G. (1993). Urban vs rural increase in hip fracture incidence. Age and sex of 901 cases 1980–89 in Olmsted County USA. *Acta Orthop Scand*, **64**, 543–8.

Maggi, S., Kelsey, J. L., Litvak, J. & Heyse, S. P. (1991). Incidence of hip fractures in the elderly: a cross-national analysis. *Osteop Int*, **1**, 232–41.

Martin, R. E. & Teberian, G. (1990). Multiple trauma and the elderly patient. *Emerg Med Clin North Am*, **8**, 411–20.

Matkovic, V., Kostial, K., Simonovic, I., Buzina, R., Broderec, A. & Nordin, B. E. C. (1979). Bone status and fracture rates in two regions of Yugoslavia. *Am J Clin Nutr*, **32**, 540–9.

McFarland, R. A., Tune, G. S. & Welford, A. T. (1964). On the driving of automobiles by older people. *J Gerontol*, **19**, 190–7.

Mellstrom, D., Rundgren, D., Jagenburg, R., Steen, B. & Svanborg, A. (1982). Tobacco smoking, ageing and health among the elderly: a longitudinal population study of 70-year old men and an age cohort comparison. *Age Ageing*, **11**, 45–58.

Melton, L. J., Kan, S. J., Frye, M. A., Wahner, H. W., O'Fallon, W. M. & Riggs, B. L. (1989). Epidemiology of vertebral fractures in women. *Am J Epidemiol*, **129**, 1000–11.

Meyer, H. E., Tverdal, A. & Falch, J. A. (1993). Risk factors for hip fracture in middle-aged Norwegian women and men. *Am J Epidemiol*, **137**, 1203–11.

Miller, S. W. M. & Grimley Evans, J. (1985). Fractures of the distal forearm in Newcastle: an epidemiological survey. *Age Ageing*, **14**, 155–8.

Nevitt, M. C. & Cummings, S. R. (1993). Study of Osteoporotic Fractures Research Group. Type of fall and risk of hip and wrist fractures: the study of osteoporotic fractures. *J Am Geriatr Soc*, **41**, 1226–34.

Nevitt, M. C., Cummings, S. R. & Hudes, E. S. (1991). Risk factors for injurious falls: a prospective study. *J Gerontol*, **46**, M164–M170.

O'Neill, D., Neubauer, K., Boyle, M., Gerrard, J., Surmon, D. & Wilcock, G. K. (1992). Dementia and driving. *J R Soc Med*, **85**, 199–202.

Parkkari, J., Kannus, P., Niemi, S., Pasanen, M., Järvinen, M., Lüthje, P. & Vuori, L. (1994). Increasing age-adjusted incidence of hip fractures in Finland: the number and incidence of fractures in 1970–1991 and prediction for the future. *Calcif Tissue Int*, **55**, 342–5.

Parasuraman, R. (1991). Attention and driving skills in aging and Alzheimer's disease. *Hum Factors*, **33**, 539–57.

Phillips, S. K., Rook, K. M., Siddle, N. C., Bruce, S. A. & Woledge, R. C. (1993). Muscle weakness in women occurs at an earlier age than in men, but strength is preserved by hormone replacement therapy. *Clin Sci*, **84**, 95–8.

Pogrund, H., Makin, M., Manczel, J. & Steinberg, R. (1977). The epidemiology of femoral neck fracture in Jerusalem: a prospective study. *Clin Orthop*, **124**, 141–6.

Prior, J. C., Vigna, Y. M., Schechter, M. T. & Burgess, A. E. (1990). Spinal bone loss and ovulatory disturbances. *New Engl J Med*, **323**, 1221–7.

Province, M. A., Hadley, E. C., Hornbrook, M. C., Lipsitz, L. A., Miller, J. P., Mulrow, C. D., Ory, M. G., Sattin, R. W., Tinetti, M. E. & Wolf, S. L. for the FICSIT Group (1995). The effects of exercise on falls in elderly patients. A preplanned meta-analysis of the FICSIT trials. *JAMA*, **273**, 1341–7.

Prudham, D. & Grimley Evans, J. (1981). Factors associated with falls in the elderly: a community study. *Age Ageing*, **10**, 264–70.

Rabbitt, P. (1991). Factors promoting accidents involving elderly pedestrians and drivers. In *Behavioural Research in Road Safety*, ed. G. B. Grayson & J. F. Lester, pp. 167–83. Proceedings of a Seminar held at Nottingham University, Crowthorne, Berkshire: Transport and Road Research Laboratory.

Ragnarsson, B. & Jacobsson, B. (1992). Epidemiology of pelvic fractures in a Swedish county. *Acta Orthop Scand*, **63**, 297–300.

Ray, W. A., Griffin, M. R. & Downey, W. (1989a). Benzodiazepines of long and short elimination half-life and the risk of hip fracture. *JAMA*, **262**, 3303–7.

Ray, W. A., Griffin, M. R., Downey, W. & Melton, L. J. (1989b). Long-term use of thiazide diuretics and risk of hip fracture. *Lancet*, **1**, 687–90.

Ray, W. A., Griffin, M. R. & Malcolm, E. (1991). Cyclic antidepressants and the risk of hip fracture. *Arch Intern Med*, **151**, 754–6.

Rees, J. L. (1982). Accuracy of Hospital Activity Analysis data in estimating the incidence of proximal femoral fracture. *Br Med J*, **284**, 1856–7.

Reid, I. R., Chin, K., Evans, M. C. & Jones, J. G. (1994). Relation between increase in length of hip axis in older women between 1950s and 1990s and increase in age specific rates of hip fracture. *Br Med J*, **309**, 508–9.

Riggs, B. L. & Melton, L. J. (1986). Involutional osteoporosis. *New Eng J Med*, **314**, 1676–86.

Riggs, J. E. (1993). Mortality from accidental falls among the elderly in the United States, 1962–1988: demonstrating the impact of improved trauma management. *J Trauma*, **35**, 212–19.

Ross, P. D., Davis, J. W., Epstein, R. S. & Wasnich, R. D. (1991a). Pre-existing fractures and bone mass predict vertebral fracture incidence in women. *Ann Intern Med*, **114**, 919–23.

Ross, P. D., Norimatsu, H., Davis, J. W., Yano, K., Wasnich, R. D., Fujiwara, S., Hosoda, Y. & Melton, L. J. (1991b). A comparison of hip fracture incidence among native Japanese, Japanese Americans, and American Caucasians. *Am J Epidemiol*, **133**, 801–9.

Rossignol, A. M., Locke, J. A., Boyle, C. M. & Burke, J. F. (1985). Consumer products and hospitalised burn injuries among elderly Massachusetts residents. *J Am Geriatr Soc*, **33**, 768–71.

Rubenstein, L. Z., Robbins, A. S., Josephson, K. R., Schulman, B. L. & Osterweil, D. (1990). The value of assessing falls in an edlerly population. A randomized clinical trial. *Ann Int Med*, **113**, 308–16.

Sahlin, Y. (1990). Occurrence of fractures in a defined population: a 1-year study. *Injury*, **21**, 158–60.

Sahlin, Y., Stene, T. M., Lereim, I. & Balstad, P. (1990). Occurrence of injuries in a defined population. *Injury*, **21**, 155–7.

Sattin, R. W., Huber, D. A. L., DeVito, C. A., Rodriguez, J. G., Ros, A., Bacchelli, S., Stevens, J. A. & Waxweiler, R. J. (1990). The incidence of fall injury events among the elderly in a defined population. *Am J Epidemiol*, **131**, 1028–37.

Sattin, R. W. & Nevitt, M. C. (1992). Injuries in later life: epidemiology and environmental aspects. In *Oxford Textbook of Geriatric Medicine*, ed. J. Grimley Evans & T. F. Williams, pp. 81–7. Oxford: Oxford University Press.

Scalea, T. M., Simon, H. M., Duncan, A. O., Atweh, N. A., Sclafani, S. J. A., Phillips, T. F. & Shaftan, G. W. (1990). Geriatric blunt multiple trauma: improved survival with early invasive monitoring. *J Trauma*, **30**, 129–34.

Secretary of State for Health. (1992). *The Health of the Nation. A Strategy for Health in England*. Cm1986. London: HMSO.

Sernbo, I. & Johnell, O. (1989). Changes in bone mass and fracture type in patients with hip fractures. A comparison between the 1950s and the 1980s in Malmö, Sweden. *Clin Orthop*, **238**, 139–47.

Skegg, D. C. G., Richards, S. M. & Doll, R. (1979). Minor tranquillizers and road accidents. *Br Med J*, **1**, 917–19.

Solomon, L. (1979). Bone density in ageing Caucasian and African populations. *Lancet*, **2**, 1326–30.

Spector, T. D., Cooper, C. & Fenton Lewis, A. (1990). Trends in admission for hip fracture in England and Wales, 1968–85. *Br Med J*, **300**, 173–4.

Stott, S. & Stevenson, W. (1980). The incidence of femoral neck fracture in New Zealand. *New Zealand Med J*, **91**, 5–9.

Stroup, N. E., Freni-Titulaer, F. W. J., Schwartz, J. J. (1990). Unexpected geographic variation in rates of hospitalization for patients who have fracture of the hip. *J Bone Joint Surg*, **72A**, 1294–8.

Sturr, J. F. & Taub, H. A. (1990). Performance of young and older drivers on a static acuity test under photopic and mesopic luminance conditions. *Hum Factors*, **32**, 1–8.

Tinetti, M. E., Speechley, M. & Ginter, S. F. (1988). Risk factors for falls among elderly persons living in the community. *New Engl J Med*, **319**, 1701–7.

Tinetti, M. E., Baker, D. I., McAvay, G., Claus, E. B., Garrett, P., Gottschalk, M., Koch, M.L., Trainor, K. & Horwitz, R. I. (1994). A multifactorial intervention to reduce the risk of falling among elderly people living in the community. *New Engl J Med*, **331**, 821–7.

Tiret, L., Hausherr, E., Thicoipe, M., Garros, B., Maurette, P., Castel, J.-P. & Hatton, F. (1990). The epidemiology of head trauma in Aquitaine (France), 1986: a community-based study of hospital admissions and deaths. *Int J Epidemiol*, **19**, 133–40.

Trotter, M., Broman, G. E. & Peterson, R. R. (1960). Densities of white and negro skeletons. *J Bone Joint Surg*, **40A**, 50–8.

Van Hemert, A. M., Vandenbroucke, J. P., Birkenhäger, J. C. & Valkenburg, H. A. (1990). Prediction of osteoporotic fractures in the general population by a fracture risk score. *Am J Epidemiol*, **132**, 123–35.

Walensky, N. A. & O'Brien, M. P. (1968). Anatomical factors relative to the racial selectivity of femoral neck fracture. *Am J Phys Anthr*, **8**, 93–6.

Weinstein, R. S. & Bell, N. H. (1988). Diminished rates of bone formation in normal black adults. *New Engl J Med*, **319**, 1698–701.

Wickham, C., Cooper, C., Margetts, B. M. & Barker, D. J. P. (1989). Muscle strength, activity, housing and the risk of falls in elderly people. *Age Ageing*, **18**, 47–51.

Winner, S. J., Morgan, C. A. & Grimley Evans, J. (1989). Perimenopausal risk of falling and incidence of distal forearm fracture. *Br Med J*, **298**, 1486–8.

Wong, P. C. N. (1966). Fracture epidemiology in a mixed South-east Asian community (Singapore). *Clin Orthop*, **45**, 55–61.

Wyshak, G. (1981). Hip fracture in elderly women and reproductive history. *J Gerontol*, **36**, 424–7.

4

Pathology of deaths from femur fractures

J. McCLURE

Introduction

It is well recognised that fractures of the proximal femur are a considerable health care problem. In the UK it has been calculated that 40000 new cases will occur annually and, of these, 70% will be treated by operation requiring either pinning and plating or the implantation of a prosthesis (Lewis, 1981). There is a common view that unless active operative treatment is undertaken the morbidity and mortality rates for this condition are high. Even with active surgical intervention, however, a substantial number of patients will die in the first year (between 8 and 27% depending on the series) and anything up to 50% of the first year survivors will be unable to walk without assistance (Katz et al., 1967). Women who have sustained a fracture of the proximal femur show an excess mortality (8% after 2 years) when compared with similar groups of women who have sustained a fracture of the forearm and in the population generally (Weiss et al., 1983). It is now apparent from epidemiological studies that there is a high early mortality rate after fracture of the proximal femur. Typical values are 17% after 3 months and 21.5% after 6 months. Rather disturbingly, it has been suggested that these values have changed little over a 15 year period during which active operative treatment has become more common (Jensen & Tøndevold, 1979).

There have been few systematic necropsy studies of the early and later events that are associated with the mortality due to fractures of the proximal femur. Pathologists are mostly concerned with establishing the cause of death and there is little interest in detailed examination of the fracture site and of the skeleton generally. Over a 9 month period consecutive, unselected cases of fracture of the proximal femur coming to post-mortem examination were studied in particular detail. In addition to a complete examination of soft visceral structures the fracture site was exposed by a lateral incision, the shaft of the femur divided at its midpoint, the joint capsule interrupted, the ligamentum teres divided (if appropriate) and the proximal portion of the bone removed in toto. The acetabulum was also excised and the synovium sampled for histological examination. If indicated, samples were recovered for microbiological examination. All bone specimens were cleaned of soft tissue and fixed in 10% buffered formalin and contact radiographs were made in a Faxitron cabinet X-ray machine. The lower vertebral column was examined by making parallel saw cuts (1 cm apart) in an anteroposterior direction, the resulting strip removed and a contact radiograph prepared. A transiliac core of bone was removed from the left anterior superior iliac spine at a standardised point with a Bordier trephine instrument. The core was embedded in a plastic resin and thin (5 μm) undecalcified sections were cut on a Polycut sledge microtome. Sections were stained by the von Kossa technique with various counterstains. Cortical thickness, trabecular bone volume, osteoid volume and the extent of calcification fronts (McClure, 1982) and resorbing surfaces were measured using eyepiece graticules. In addition, the marrow space was assessed to determine the presence or absence of intercurrent disease. The samples from the vertebral column were divided into smaller portions, decalcified in a solution of EDTA (with X-ray control), processed for conventional wax histology and examined after staining with haematoxylin and eosin (HE).

Materials and methods

The specimens recovered from the proximal femur presented particular technical challenges. After prolonged fixation (weeks) to obtain optimal preservation the blade/plate implants were removed from the specimens. A median slab (1 cm wide) cut in the coronal plane was prepared with a bandsaw and contact radiographs prepared. Prosthetic implants (a small number) had been embedded in bone cement and this was dissolved in chloroform (a process taking 6–9 months) and again median slabs were prepared and radiographed after removal of the metallic implant. All slabs were decalcified in EDTA again with X-ray control and embedded in paraffin wax to which dental wax had been added. Thin sections (5–6 μm) were cut on a sledge microtome and stained with various histological/histochemical techniques. The resultant glass slides were of considerable size and best examined by a hand lens although the adaptation of a microscope stage allowed examination with higher power objectives. Particular attention was paid to the presence or absence of bone trabecular structures and to the responses to parts of the implant such as screw nails and the head of the blade. The tissue responses close to the site of prosthetic implants were also noted.

   In the series there were 34 females and 16 males confirming the preponderance of females in the age group under study. The mean age of the group was 83 years (ranging from 58 to 96 years). The mean age of the females was 86 years (range 69–96 years) and that of the males was 76 years (range 58–90 years). Forty-two cases were treated

operatively and the eight cases which were treated conservatively were considered
unfit for operation. These latter patients all died within 12 hours of admission to
hospital and the majority died within the first 5 hours. Three cases had an established
recent myocardial infarct recognisable both macroscopically and microscopically. The
other five cases had histologically proved bronchopneumonia. While it was difficult to
ascertain the precise circumstances in which these patients sustained their fractures
there was evidence that the organic disorders mentioned above antedated the fractures. The macroscopic examination of the fracture site in these cases showed five
intertrochanteric and three subcapital fractures. Microscopic examination of the site
showed that all fractures were very recent as characterised by the presence of fresh
haematoma without a cellular response and with no evidence of any repair process.

In those patients treated by operative intervention there were 34 intertrochanteric
and transcervical fractures compared with 16 subcapital lesions. In the first group
there were 20 females and 14 males and in the second 14 females and two males. Again
the preponderance of females is noted. There is no satisfactory explanation for the very
marked predominance of females (7:1) in those patients with subcapital fractures. In
accordance with conventional approaches to treatment the femoral head in subcapital
fractures had been excised and replaced by a prosthesis. All excised femoral heads had
been examined pathologically. All showed recent haematoma with no evidence of a
cellular response. The marrow spaces were uniformly free of metastatic tumour. The
articular cartilages were intact and there was no evidence of osteoarthrosis. The latter
findings reinforced the view that patients with fractures of the proximal femur tend not
to have osteoarthrosis of the hip joint.

General post-mortem findings

In the series the overall survival time from the operation was 18 weeks with a range
from 0 to 156 weeks. The fact that all 50 cases had died within the year led to the fact of
the deaths being reported to HM Coroner and because of local practice this was
followed by a post-mortem examination. The series is therefore highly selected but it
does illustrate the observation, made earlier, that there is a significant death rate after
operative repair of fractured neck of femur. In 28 cases death could be confidently
linked from clinical and pathological considerations to the fracture. In these cases
there was either bronchopneumonia (75%) or pulmonary embolism. The bronchopneumonia was evident macroscopically and confirmed histologically. In 5% of cases
the disorder had become confluent in both lower lobes. In those cases with pulmonary
embolism the ante-mortem nature of the emboli was confirmed by histological examination. In half of the cases the emboli affected peripheral branches of pulmonary
arteries and were associated with zones of pulmonary infarction indicating that in

these cases the embolisation had occurred sufficiently long before death for ischaemic necrosis to become manifest. In all instances of pulmonary embolism venous thrombi were discovered after careful search in the peripheral venous system. In 60% of cases the thrombi were present in deep veins of the ipsilateral calf and in 40% they were present in the deep pelvic veins. All examples of ante-mortem venous thrombi were confirmed histologically by presence of organisation.

In the remaining cases death was due to a cardiovascular disorder, most commonly heart failure due to ischaemic heart disease. In these 22 cases there were ten instances of recent myocardial infarction with appropriate recent coronary artery thrombosis in six and diffuse coronary artery atheroma in four. In the remaining 12 cases there was extensive coronary artery atheroma, diffuse ischaemic myocardial fibrosis and evidence of acute pulmonary oedema.

In those cases (56%) with either bronchopneumonia or pulmonary embolism there was an evident link both in anatomical and clinical terms with the fracture of the proximal femur. In the other cases in which death was essentially due to ischaemic heart disease it was impossible to link the death with the fracture on purely morbid anatomical grounds although there may well have been an association. In all cases extensive sampling of the lungs for histological examination was performed. The sections were searched carefully for the presence of fat and/or marrow embolism. Significant degrees of these were not observed. Only occasionally were there a small number of cleared lipidic spaces.

It is evident from these observations that the major cause of death within a short time of operative repair of fractured neck of femur is a pulmonary disorder. These observations are not unexpected and the findings reinforce intuitive expectation. The high incidence of pulmonary embolism raises the question of a more aggressive diagnostic effort after surgery in the patients at risk. The high incidence of ischaemic heart disease probably reflects its prevalence in the group from which these patients were derived. The incidence of bronchopneumonia is also not unexpected and in many instances the clinical evidence was rather imprecise despite the fact that the condition was well established in the cases in which it was the attributable cause of death.

In the series there were two examples of intraoperative death. In both cases the patients were women with subcapital fracture in whom the femoral head had been resected with the implantation of a prosthesis. Bone cement had been used to secure and anchor the prosthesis and both patients had died in cardiopulmonary collapse. At post-mortem examination both had evidence of established ischaemic heart disease (coronary artery atheroma and diffuse myocardial fibrosis) and acute left ventricular failure (ventricular and atrial dilatation and acute pulmonary oedema). There was no evidence of established acute myocardial necrosis and no evidence of acute coronary artery occlusion. There have been reported cases of cardiopulmonary arrest associated with the use of bone cement but these are uncommon events and one doubts if the effect would be seen in two cases of a relatively small series of 50 cases. It is not possible to be definitive in this context.

Changes at the site of fracture repair

A striking feature of the study was the presence of local complications at the site of operative treatment. It is usually the situation that pathological examination of the fracture site and the operative repair is at best cursory. Local complications of significant degree were found in 41% of cases and the majority of these were found after internal fixation by blade and plate. In this process, which is used for transcervical and intertrochanteric fractures, the head and neck of the femur are penetrated from the lateral side by the blade of the implement which is fixed on the lateral aspect of the upper femur anchoring onto the cortical surface with screw nails. These screws penetrate the outer cortex and the medullary space of the proximal femur with variable penetration (depending on the width of the medullary cavity) of the opposite medial cortex. In many instances the tips of the screws had penetrated the full thickness of the medial cortex and investing periosteum with small areas of haematoma and new bone formation. The blade portion of the implant has a pointed free end and is triangular in cross section.

The positioning of the implant is of particular importance in relation to the extent of penetration of the neck and head of the femur (Figure 4.1). In 21% of cases the phenomenon of 'cutting-out' was observed. In this the pointed end of the blade penetrated the subchondral bone and articular cartilage of the head of the femur. The process was observed in intertrochanteric fractures with at least some degree of fragmentation of the cortical bone of the neck of the femur. Cutting-out was observed only in women patients who had low trabecular bone volumes in iliac crest samples. Penetration of the subchondral bone and articular cartilage resulted in fragments of bone and cartilage ('shards') being released into the joint cavity. In all cases the tip of the blade impinged on the articular surface of the acetabulum again causing excoriation and fragmentation (Figure 4.2). The synovial membrane contained embedded cartilage and bone fragments with a related infiltrate of mononuclear cells (macrophages and lymphocytes) and moderate amounts of foreign body-type giant cells (macrophage polykaryons). There was significant hypertrophy and hyperplasia of synovial lining cells. All these are the features of detritus or traumatic synovitis. Cutting-out has a severe disruptive mechanical effect on the hip joint exacerbated by weight-bearing and movement. Histological examination showed little bone tissue in the femoral head and neck of these cases and with general low trabecular bone volumes further collapse of bone tissue in the region contributes to the process. In addition the size of the implant in relation to the size of the proximal femur and the operative technique involved in the initial placing of the implant are important.

Microscopic examination of the site of implantation showed very little tissue reaction to the implant in those cases which died relatively soon after operation. Small areas of haematoma with minimal cellular accumulations were noted. With time the screw nails and the intramedullary component (blade) became invested initially with a membrane of collagenous (type 1) connective tissue. After 2–3 months this membrane had been replaced by woven bone undergoing lamellar transformation. Thus an investment of bone tissue around the intramedullary component formed a capsule linked to adjacent trabecular bone structures which resulted in the formation of a strutted structure which, given time, will effectively anchor the implant (Figure 4.3). Similar osseous changes were noted around the screw nails and the crimped pattern of

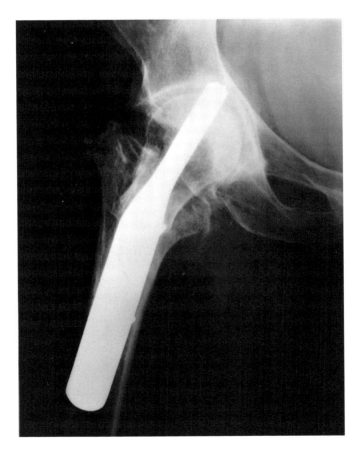

Figure 4.1. This X-radiograph shows 'cutting-out' of the blade of a blade/plate implant through the head of the femur and into the acetabulum.

the screw thread was faithfully replicated. In general there were few inflammatory cells in relation to the implant.

Except for the case of infection the site of prosthetic implantation did not show loosening. The bone cement had been in intimate contact with trabecular and cortical bone. Osteocyte lacunae in the structures close to the implant were generally empty. This is indicative of osteocyte necrosis. Osteocyte loss in bone is a feature of the aging process but in the context of prosthetic implantation it is considered that the process is accelerated by the exothermic reaction involved in the setting of the bone cement. It is not considered that these changes significantly impaired the mechanical integrity of the bone tissue. Again there was no significant cellular infiltration at the site of the prosthesis. In all cases the acetabular component was examined and similar features were observed in adjacent bone tissue.

In 21% of cases (other than those associated with cutting-out) there was evidence of infection and necrosis. Microbiological studies demonstrated anaerobic organisms with antibiotic sensitivity patterns strongly suggesting ante-mortem infection by patho-genetic organisms and not post-mortem bacterial overgrowth. There was frank pus formation within the joint cavity and extending through the capsule into para-articular

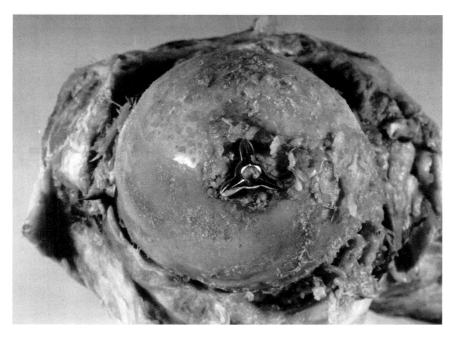

Figure 4.2. Blade tip has penetrated the articular cartilage. Note the marked irregularity and fragmentation of the articular surface.

structures. This was associated with tissue necrosis and fragmentation of bone. The synovium showed heavy infiltrates of neutrophil polymorphs together with smaller numbers of macrophages and lymphocytes. Extensive destruction of articular cartilage was present and microscopically there was loss of proteoglycan staining reactions and fragmentation of the cartilage matrix. In the case of the prosthetic replacement complicated by infection the femoral and acetabular components had become detached from bone and were lying free in what was effectively a large abscess cavity.

A number of other local complications were observed but much less frequently than cutting-out or infection. In two cases of internal fixation by blade and plate the blade

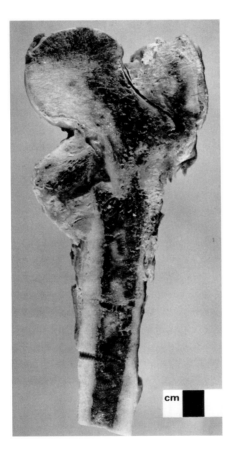

Figure 4.3. Median slab taken from the proximal femur with a healing intertrochanteric fracture. The plate of the blade/plate implant was in apposition to the lateral (left) aspect of the specimen. The screw nail tracks are present and the lower has penetrated the medial cortex.

was bent markedly reducing the inferior angle between the blade and the plate. Enquiry about the condition of the implement before implantation revealed no abnormality. The bent implant significantly altered the relation between the head, neck and shaft of the femur and would undoubtedly have caused abnormality of gait. At post-mortem examination it was impossible to straighten the blade manually. Both patients in whom this complication was noted were obese and it is concluded that attempted weight-bearing had caused the implant to bend.

In one case of blade and plate fixation new bone formation (heterotopic ossification) was found in the joint capsule and in surrounding muscle tissue. This is a form of myositis ossificans and has been described as a complication of hip surgery (McClure, 1983). In other published series the incidence has been higher than in the present one. Histologically the bone tissue was viable and lamellar in type and there were related adipose marrow spaces. The patient in whom this occurred had survived for 45 weeks after operation. The origin of the cells giving rise to this ectopic bone is a matter of debate. One view holds that they arise from pluripotential marrow stromal cells displaced during the operative procedure (Nade & Burwell, 1977). Another view is that there is metaplastic transformation of ligament cells to chondrocytes which form a cartilaginous nodule which is replaced by bone through a process which recapitulates endochondral ossification (Rooney *et al.*, 1992). In the present case there were caps of cartilage at the margin of the bone nodules, a feature seemingly supporting the second hypothesis. In other studies there is evidence that heterotopic para-articular bone inhibits joint mobility.

The incidence of these local complications is substantial and their effect on patient recovery and mobilisation is also likely to be substantial. Careful enquiry into the clinical situation ante-mortem revealed that the patients were considered to be difficult to mobilise and that the presence, degree and significance of the complications were poorly recognised. Thus it seems important that when difficulties are experienced particular attention should be paid to the exclusion of these local complications.

Fracture of neck of femur and intracerebral lesions

After the accumulation of the cases in the present series it was apparent that there were ten cases in which there were established contralateral intracerebral lesions and there was evidence that these lesions occurred at or before the time at which fracture of the proximal femur was sustained (McClure & Goldsborough, 1986). Clinical and pathological details are given in Table 4.1. The combined median age was 78 years (range 62–91 years) and the median ages of the men and the women were 78 years (range 62–82 years) and 81 years (range 70–91 years), respectively. Death was due to bronchopneumonia in five cases, ischaemic heart disease in four and calcific aortic stenosis

Table 4.1. *Clinical and pathological features in cases of fractured neck of femur and contralateral intracerebral lesions*

Case	Age (years)	Sex	Body weight (kg)	Trabecular bone volume (%)	Fracture	Intracerebral lesion
1	62	M	68	22.9	Subcapital fracture right femur	Astrocytoma (grade IV) left frontoparietal region
2	77	M	105	20.4	Subcapital fracture left femur	Recent infarct right parieto-occipital region
3	81	M	36	13.4	Intertrochanteric fracture left femur	Old infarct right basal ganglia
4	82	M	54	11.9	Intertrochanteric fracture right femur	Recent infarct left parieto-occipital region
5	76	F	49	11.8	Intertrochanteric fracture right femur	Old infarct left tempero-occipital region
6	70	F	55	6.1	Intertrochanteric fracture right femur	Recent infarct left cerebellar and left occipital lobes
7	91	F	34	5.8	Intertrochanteric fracture right femur	Old infarct left internal capsule
8	80	M	46	11.0	Intertrochanteric fracture right femur	Old infarct left parietal region
9	86	F	54	6.3	Intertrochanteric fracture right femur	Established haemorrhage left parietal region
10	76	M	47	15.0	Intertrochanteric fracture left femur	Recent infarct right parietal region

in one. From a consideration of the available pathological and clinical evidence it was concluded that loss of muscle tone and a tendency to fall onto the affected side were significant risk factors in fractures of the proximal femur. In this subgroup there were two men with bone trabecular volumes in the normal range (22.9% and 20.4%) and it was concluded that their body weights acted through the proximal femur on the side which had lost protective muscle tone due to the contralateral intracerebral lesion.

Fracture of neck of femur and metabolic bone disease

Within this group of ten cases the trabecular bone volumes as measured in the iliac crest had a mean value of 12.4% (range 5.8–22.9%) and this leads into a discussion about the relevance of osteopenia to the pathogenesis of fractured neck of femur. Not every osteopenic subject suffers a fracture nor are all patients with fractures osteopenic and this is amply illustrated by the two cases described above. Published reports dealing with the question of patients with fractures being more osteopenic than age-matched controls have been dealt with by Cummings (1985). It was concluded that in most series the differences from controls were small. Aitken (1984) has reported that a series of 200 women with a fracture of the femoral neck after minor trauma had bone mass measurements similar to those of a control population of normal women and 16% were not osteoporotic. In the present series the trabecular bone volumes as measured in the iliac crest were not significantly lower than in the published series of normal controls. There did seem to be a relation between low bone volumes and intertrochanteric fractures and between low bone volumes and the local complication of cutting-out. It is interesting to note that there was no correlation between iliac crest trabecular bone volume and lumbar vertebral trabecular bone volume.

Another metabolic bone disorder which has been implicated in the aetiopathogenesis of fractured neck of femur is osteomalacia (Chalmers *et al.*, 1967; Sokoloff, 1978). More recent Australian studies have not supported this view (Evans *et al.*, 1981; Wicks *et al.*, 1982). The histological diagnosis of osteomalacia has become more precise. Not only must there be an increase in the volume of osteoid (namely uncalcified matrix) but also there must be a demonstrable defect in the rate of mineralisation. In the present series there was no evidence of osteomalacia in femoral, iliac or lumbar vertebral bone tissues. It therefore seems unlikely that a defect in mineralisation resulting in excess osteoid volume is a significant feature in fractured neck of femur. In addition there was no evidence of osteitis fibrosa (hyperparathyroidism) and no evidence of metastatic tumour in any of the material studied.

The idea that diminished bone volume or any other metabolic bone disease is a major determinant of femoral neck fracture cannot be sustained. It has been recognised that postural instability leading to a fall is a common event in relation to the fracture. It may be the major factor in that the presence of osteopenia dictates the anatomical type of the fracture (usually intertrochanteric) that occurs.

Conclusion

In conclusion, it may be said that fracture of the proximal femur in the elderly is a serious disorder with high risks of death and significant morbidity. Meticulous necropsy examinations confirm pulmonary disorders (bronchopneumonia and pulmonary embolism) as the important mechanisms of death and, in addition, there is a high incidence of local complications which have important contributions to the morbidity of the condition and its treatment. It is particularly important to appreciate that these local complications were insufficiently recognised in life. Finally, metabolic bone disease is not an important feature in the aetiopathogenesis of proximal femoral fracture.

References

Aitken, J. M. (1984). Relevance of osteoporosis in women with fracture of the femoral neck. *Br Med J*, **288**, 597–601.

Chalmers, J., Conacher, W. D. H., Gardner, D. L. & Scolt, P. J. (1967). Osteomalacia: a common disease in elderly women. *J Bone Joint Surg*, **49B**, 403–23.

Cummings, S. R. (1985). Are patients with hip fractures more osteoporotic? *Am J Med*, **78**, 487–94.

Evans, R. A., Ashwell, J. R. & Dunstan, C. R. (1981). Lack of metabolic bone disease in patients with fracture of the femoral neck. *Aust NZ J Med*, **11**, 158–61.

Jensen, J. S. & Tøndevold, E. (1979). Mortality after hip fractures. *Acta Orthop Scand*, **50**, 161–7.

Katz, S., Harple, K. G., Downs, T. D. *et al.* (1967). Long-term course of 147 patients with fracture of the hip. *Surg Gynecol Obstet*, **124**, 1219–30.

Lewis, A. F. (1981). Fracture of the neck of femur: changing incidence. *Br Med J*, **283**, 1217–20.

McClure, J. (1982). The demonstration of calcification fronts by *in vivo* and *in vitro* tetracycline labelling. *J Clin Pathol*, **35**, 1278–82.

McClure, J. (1983). The effect of diphosphonates on heterotopic ossification in regenerating Achilles tendon of the mouse. *J Pathol*, **139**, 419–30.

McClure, J. & Goldsborough, S. (1986). Fractured neck of femur and contralateral intracerebral lesions. *J Clin Pathol*, **39**, 920–2.

Nade, S. M. L. & Burwell, R. G. (1977). Decalcified bone as a substrate for osteogenesis. An appraisal of the inter-relation of bone and marrow in combined grafts. *J Bone Joint Surg*, **59B**, 189–95.

Rooney, P., Grant, M. E. & McClure, J. (1992). Endochondral ossification and de novo collagen synthesis during repair of the rat Achilles tendon. *Matrix*, **12**, 274–81.

Sokoloff, L. (1978). Occult osteomalacia in American (USA) patients with fractures of the hip. *Am J Surg Pathol*, **2**, 21–9.

Weiss, N. S., Liff, J. M., Ure, C. L., Ballard, J. H., Abott, C. H. & Daling, J. R. (1983). Mortality in women following hip fracture. *J Chron Dis*, **36**, 879–82.

Wicks, M., Garrett, R., Vernon-Roberts, B. & Fazzalari, N. (1982). Absence of metabolic bone disease in the proximal femur in patients with fracture of the femoral neck. *J Bone Joint Surg*, **64B**, 319–22.

5

Who falls and why?

J. H. DOWNTON

Introduction

Falls are now recognised to be one of the important problems to which elderly people are prone. A substantial proportion of the elderly population falls each year, and many older people become less active because of fear of falling. The consequences of falls represent much suffering, and are an important economic pressure on health and social services.

Injuries sustained in falls are an important cause of death at all ages, but particularly amongst the elderly, although the frequency may in fact be underestimated because of inaccuracies in death certification. National mortality statistics show that about three-quarters of deaths due to falls occur in those over 65 years of age (Eddy, 1973). Approximately 0.2% per year of those over 65 years of age die from accidental falls, with the majority of deaths following fractured neck of femur (Sattin et al., 1990).

Falls are a marker of increasing frailty and risk of dying, and clustering of falls prior to death has been shown in institutionalised subjects (Gryfe et al., 1977). Old people who have fallen become more dependent, need more hospital attention and die more frequently than a control non-falling population (Tinetti et al., 1993). Falls were one of several factors found to be significant predictors of mortality in a community population (Campbell et al., 1985). Those who are unable to get up after their fall have much higher morbidity and mortality rates (Tinetti et al., 1993).

Many elderly express fear of falling and this fear may be present even if no falls have actually occurred (Downton & Andrews, 1990). Falls and fear of falling seem to lead to old people restricting their activity, or to their activity being restricted by carers (Tinetti & Powell, 1993), and may be so severe as to produce inability to walk (Murphy & Isaacs, 1982). Fractured neck of femur is recognised to result in increased dependence compared with pre-fracture state, and falling itself can lead to increased dependency (Tinetti et al., 1993).

Who falls?

Estimates of the prevalence of falling have varied widely: from 23% to 59% of old people in hospital or residential care, and from 28% to 60% of old people at home (Downton, 1987). There are a number of problems associated with attempting to determine the frequency of falls which have led to some of the variations in reported figures. The main problems are first, which population is studied, second, how a 'fall' is defined, and third, the reliability of the history.

Subjects who are known to have fallen are a selected group, as less than half of all falls present to medical attention (Downton & Andrews, 1991), and information from this group may therefore not apply to fallers in general. A high proportion of old people presenting with injuries will have suffered their injury as a result of a fall, usually a fall from standing height or less, although a few falls may occur as a result of a fracture (Sloan & Holloway, 1981); however, not all falls result in injuries.

Most of the studies of old people in hospital or residential care are difficult to interpret because the study population is not defined. The populations considered are obviously selected but with characteristics that are likely to vary between countries (and also perhaps within countries) because of different systems of care for old people.

A large majority of old people (approximately 95%) live in the community in their own homes rather than in residential care. This means that the majority of falls and complications of falls will occur in this group, and information from studies of community elderly is therefore most likely to apply to fallers overall.

Defining a fall can be difficult. Looking at accidents in general will include a variable proportion of non-fall events, though a large proportion (perhaps 80%) of accidents in the elderly are falls. Studies of falls have on many occasions excluded specific types of falls such as epilepsy or those caused by acute illness. In some cases only falls in or close to the home are considered, but 40–50% of falls occur outside the home (Prudham & Evans, 1981; Downton & Andrews, 1991).

Any retrospective study will depend on the subjects' memory of falls that have occurred. As subjects with cognitive impairment are more likely to fall (Morris *et al.*, 1987), those who are most at risk of falling may be those least likely to remember their falls. Even cognitively intact elderly may not remember falling (Cummings *et al.*, 1988).

Epidemiology of falling

There have now been a number of studies of the frequency of falls in more or less randomly selected community populations. They have all produced similar annual prevalence rates: 29–39% for subjects aged 65+ years of age (Blake *et al.*, 1988; O'Loughlin *et al.*, 1993; Lord *et al.*, 1994), 35% for those aged 70+ (Campbell *et al.*, 1989) and 32–42% for those aged 75+ (Tinetti *et al.*, 1988; Downton & Andrews,

1991). The 'healthy elderly' are less likely to fall (Gabell *et al.*, 1985), but those who have already fallen are more likely to fall again. Of those who have fallen in the previous year, 60–70% are likely to fall during the following 12 months (Nevitt *et al.*, 1989).

It is very difficult to draw conclusions about the incidence or prevalence of falls in the elderly in institutional care, because populations are not necessarily comparable, and because some studies look at falls specifically while others look at 'accidents'. Falls among these groups of elderly are very common, however, and are probably commoner than among the elderly in the community.

Virtually all studies have shown increasing risk of falling with increasing age, and most have shown women to be more likely to fall than men, although the reverse seems true in hospital (Berry *et al.*, 1981). In some studies the very elderly have a lower incidence, perhaps because of selective survival of a particularly fit cohort (Woodhouse *et al.*, 1983). Among those in institutional care, the 'young elderly' (those under 75 years) seem to be more prone to fall (Haga *et al.*, 1986).

The rate of injury following falls is a little more difficult to determine as falls are not always brought to medical attention, even if injury has occurred (Downton & Andrews, 1991). Injuries are common reasons for elderly people to attend Accident and Emergency departments (Dove & Dave, 1986) and most serious injuries and the majority of fractures in the elderly are caused by falling (Melton & Riggs, 1987). Old people with fractures commonly give a history of recurrent falls prior to that resulting in their fracture (Johnell & Nilsson, 1985) and are more likely to have fallen in the previous year than controls (Cook *et al.*, 1982).

In general, injury seems to occur in about half of those who fall, but less than 10% of fallers suffer fractures (Campbell *et al.*, 1990). 'Healthy' or 'vigorous' elderly seem at higher risk of injury despite a lower risk of falls (Gabell *et al.*, 1985; Speechley & Tinetti, 1991). People having multiple falls may be less likely to suffer fractures and have a lower fracture rate per fall (Baker & Harvey, 1985).

It has been suggested that impaired neuromuscular responses protecting the skeleton are more important factors in producing fractures in the very elderly than osteoporosis (Cooper *et al.*, 1987). There is evidence that physical activity protects against fracture (Wickham *et al.*, 1989), and that the habitually inactive are at greater risk of fracture (Boyce & Vessey, 1988).

Estimates of population incidence of injuries from falls vary from country to country, perhaps reflecting different systems of medical care. In a poor urban community of black people in the USA, 26 per 1000 of the population aged 65 + years were treated at an Emergency department for injuries following falls. Fall injuries made up almost half of all injuries in this age group, and unlike other injuries, increased in incidence with increasing age (Grisso *et al.*, 1990). A Swedish study of injuries following falls at home found an incidence of 14 per 1000 aged 60 + years (Lucht, 1971). Again incidence increased with age.

Why do old people fall?

Falling at any age is the result of a complex interaction of factors with a common endpoint, and requires both an opportunity and a liability to fall. In young people, opportunity is more important; thus falls in young adults are commonly associated with easily definable environmental risks such as sporting activities. In the elderly, however, liability to fall seems to be dominant, and falls tend to occur with relatively minor stress on balance mechanisms. This may be a reflection of neurological changes with aging, gait and postural changes, medical and psychological ill health, drugs, or in many cases a combination of several such factors.

Physiology of balance

The upright human body is basically unstable, with a very small support base relative to its height, and maintaining this position depends on complex servomechanisms. It is an activity in which muscular corrections are continually made on the basis of proprioceptive information about body position. The afferent limb of the feedback loop consists of sensory input from visual and vestibular pathways and proprioceptive input from muscle spindles, joint proprioceptors, especially lower limb and cervical spine, and skin touch receptors. Central processing occurs in many areas of the brain including cerebellum, brainstem, basal ganglia and the sensorimotor and association cortex, and the efferent limb is the outflow from the brain via spinal cord and peripheral nerves to limb and trunk muscles (Wolfson *et al.*, 1985). Fine control of posture is immensely complex. Minute movements and tiny forces are sensed, and postural reactions anticipate disturbances of posture (Marsden *et al.*, 1981).

Teasing out the contributions of the various factors involved in control of balance is difficult, partly because if one element is impaired, the others can compensate to a greater or lesser degree. This may account for some of the inconsistencies in experimental findings when subjects with postural instability are studied. The complexity of the system is also indicated by the numerous conditions that can cause postural instability (Drachmann & Hart, 1972). There are changes in various parameters of postural control in older adults, but it is not clear whether these are due to pathological changes rather than physiological age changes (Alexander, 1994).

Vision, balance and falls

Of the three main sensory inputs upon which postural control depends (visual, vestibular and muscle and joint proprioceptive) the importance of vision has been most extensively studied. The almost universal finding that sway is greater with eyes closed than with eyes open demonstrates its importance.

Visual input seems to be particularly important in abnormal stance situations (Lee & Lishman, 1975), and also when proprioceptive input is reduced, for example in amputees (Fernie & Holliday, 1978). There does not seem to be an increase in visual dependence with increased age (Fernie *et al.*, 1982). Women, however, seem to be more 'field dependent' (i.e. they rely more on the spatial framework provided by vision) than men (Witkin *et al.*, 1954), and it has been suggested that, in conjunction with the tendency of women to have a narrower walking and standing base than men, this is one factor in the higher frequency of falls in elderly women. Elderly fallers have been shown to be more likely to have errors in visual perception of verticality and horizontality than non-fallers (Tobis *et al.*, 1981).

There does not appear to be any correlation between objective visual impairment and sway (Brocklehurst *et al.*, 1982). Visual impairment has however been found to be associated with falls in several studies (Tobis *et al.*, 1981; Cohn & Lasley, 1985) although in community studies, this has been shown only in subgroups of fallers (Brocklehurst *et al.*, 1978; Campbell *et al.*, 1981). In a healthy elderly group, perceived visual problems were no commoner in fallers than non-fallers but fallers were more likely not to be wearing prescribed glasses (Gabell *et al.*, 1985).

Impaired contrast sensitivity, rather than poor visual acuity, has been shown to be associated with falling, suggesting that risk of falling is related to impairment in the ability to perceive objects under poor contrast conditions rather than a reduced ability to discriminate fine detail (Lord *et al.*, 1991, 1994). This may highlight the importance of discerning edges (e.g. steps, gutters, pavement cracks, etc.). An association has also been found between impaired dark adaptation and falling (McMurdo & Gaskell, 1991).

Vestibular function and balance

The postural disturbance of someone with acute vestibular failure demonstrates the potential importance of vestibular function in the maintenance of balance, but in fact the little evidence available suggests that vestibular impairment is not a major cause of postural disturbance. Abnormalities of vestibular function, measured using a tipping table, have been found significantly more commonly with increasing age (Brocklehurst *et al.*, 1982), but no correlation was shown between vestibular dysfunction and sway measured with a Wright ataxiameter. Sway is greater in elderly than in young subjects with vestibular dysfunction (Norre *et al.*, 1987). Vestibular abnormalities (demonstrated by means of opticokinetic nystagmus and caloric testing) have been found to be an important cause of dizziness (Drachmann & Hart, 1972) but their relation to falls is not clear.

Proprioception and balance

Proprioceptive input seems to be important in maintaining balance. Amputees sway more than normals, although they are able to compensate to some extent with vision (Fernie & Holliday, 1978), and mechanical vibration of the calf muscles, which disturbs somatic proprioception, increases postural sway (Eklund & Lofstedt, 1970), though again the effect of this is most obvious in the absence of visual input. Elderly subjects with poor visual acuity and contrast sensitivity have increased sway only when proprioception is also reduced (Lord *et al.*, 1991).

Cervical spine mechanoreceptors also seem to contribute significantly to static postural sensation and to the awareness of head and neck movement (Wyke, 1979). Local anaesthetic infiltration of the cervical apophyseal joints in normal volunteers produced subjective feelings of unsteadiness while standing and walking (de Jong *et al.*, 1977), and people with cervical spine disorders often complain of similar symptoms.

Relevance of postural control to falls and falling

Postural control as measured by sway seems to be impaired in the elderly (Weiner *et al.*, 1984), but the effects of disease may be more important than those of aging (Wolfson *et al.*, 1985). Subjects with senile dementia of the Alzheimer type have impaired gait and balance compared with age- and sex-matched controls (Visser, 1983), and are more likely to fall.

Impaired postural control in elderly subjects seems to be associated with an increased likelihood of falling (Fernie *et al.*, 1982) although the association may be with falls for reasons other than trips rather than all falls (Overstall *et al.*, 1977). Studies using objective measurements of gait and balance have found some associations between impaired gait and balance and risk of falling, but differences between fallers and non-fallers are small, and are not useful for predicting the risk of falling (Fernie *et al.*, 1982). A more recent study has shown that those suffering multiple falls have significantly poor postural control as demonstrated by sway on a foam rubber surface (Lord *et al.*, 1994).

Changes with aging and their relevance to falling

Neurological changes

There are definite structural changes in the central nervous system in the elderly (reduced cell counts, increase in connective tissue, accumulation of lipofuscin, etc.), and there is some evidence of decrease in nerve conduction rate with age (Dorfman &

Bosley, 1979). There is, however, such wide variability in structural and functional changes found in aging individuals that it is impossible to say that, in the absence of superimposed disease, there is any inevitable change with aging (Creasey & Rapoport, 1985). Ascribing the liability of old people to fall to the neurological changes found with aging is an attractive idea but the little evidence available again suggests that it is neurological disease rather than 'physiological' age change that is associated with falling.

The most consistent finding in studies of the neurological changes with age is loss of vibration sensation in the lower limbs; however, vibration is not a specific modality carried in a specific pathway. It probably travels in both dorsal columns and spinothalamic pathways and is appreciated bilaterally at thalamic level, and its relation to proprioception is not clear. No association has been shown between impairment of proprioception and impaired vibration sensation in elderly subjects (MacLennan *et al.*, 1980; Brocklehurst *et al.*, 1982) and a decline in vibration sense did not have any consistent effect on sway, mobility or the prevalence of falls (MacLennan *et al.*, 1980).

Aging of the eye

There are well recognised structural changes in the eye with ageing – increase in thickness of the crystalline lens (which is so universal that it seems to be 'physiological' rather than 'pathological') and a reduction in pupil size – and these have functional consequences. Presbyopia is an inevitable accompaniment, and impaired dark adaptation also occurs (McMurdo & Gaskell, 1991). A progressive decline in visual acuity with aging has been reported (Milne, 1979) but it is not clear how much of this is related to decreased transparency of the lens and reduction in pupil size, rather than retinal changes. As mentioned above, visual impairment does seem to be associated with poor balance and falls.

Gait changes with age

It has been recognised for many years that changes in gait occur in healthy and diseased elderly. Slower walking speed, shorter step length and smaller swing to support ratios have been reported in healthy elderly men (Murray *et al.*, 1969) and women (Finley *et al.*, 1969) compared with young controls. Slower walking speed in the elderly is more marked in those who are housebound or limited in activity (Imms & Edholm, 1981). Similar gait changes are also more apparent in those who have had falls and in those who are hospitalised, whether because of falls or for other reasons (Guimaraes & Isaacs, 1980), and in subjects with Alzheimer's disease (Visser, 1983).

There seems to be a wide variety of gait abnormalities that may be associated with 'senile gait' (Koller *et al.*, 1985), although many elderly subjects with an abnormal gait have underlying pathological changes and the differential diagnosis of gait disorders is wide (Sabin, 1982). It has been suggested that many of the changes described are not necessarily pathological but are part of a 'cautious gait', also seen in young subjects walking slowly (Berman & O'Reilly, 1995).

It has been shown that elements of gait which are particularly related to balance (stride width and double support time) show much greater variability in both young and elderly subjects than the elements which are related to 'gait patterning' (step time and stride time), suggesting that balance mechanisms are, at all ages, less consistent in their functioning than is the gait patterning mechanism (Gabell & Nayak, 1984). The increase in variability in gait amongst the elderly may therefore not be a true age effect, but related to pathology.

Autonomic dysfunction and postural hypotension

Autonomic dysfunction is recognised to be more common in the elderly. Little is known about age changes in the autonomic nervous system, but some degree of autonomic denervation does seem to occur with increasing age in healthy individuals (Collins *et al.*, 1980), although the functional significance of this is not clear.

A substantial proportion of elderly people have a significant drop in blood pressure on standing (Caird *et al.*, 1973) and old people are more prone to postprandial hypotension (Lipsitz *et al.*, 1983). The mechanism of this drop is probably multifactorial. A number of the neurological diseases that become much commoner with increasing age are associated with postural hypotension, for example autonomic neuropathy, Shy–Drager syndrome, cerebral infarcts and diffuse atherosclerosis, Parkinson's disease, and spinal cord lesions, but there also seem to be age-related changes which lead to a higher risk of postural hypotension, such as atherosclerotic loss of distensibility of large vessels (Robinson *et al.*, 1983), reduced baroreceptor sensitivity (Gribbin *et al.*, 1971) and excessive venous pooling (Caird *et al.*, 1973). Old people with impaired baroreceptor reflexes may also have a failure of cerebral autoregulation (Wollner *et al.*, 1979), increasing their likelihood of symptoms if their blood pressure drops.

Demonstration of a drop in blood pressure on standing, particularly if associated with symptoms of dizziness or light-headedness, in someone who has fallen is assumed to prove the cause of the fall. A study analysing factors contributing to sway, however, did not demonstrate a clear relation between postural hypotension and postural imbalance in the elderly (Overstall *et al.*, 1978). Heart rate response to tilting (as a measure of autonomic function) was not found to be significantly different from healthy controls in a group of fallers with many medical and neurological problems (Kirshen *et al.*, 1984).

Non-posturally related causes of falls

Associated with loss of consciousness

Loss of consciousness will almost invariably result in a fall, unless the subject is already sitting or lying down. The main causes are neurological problems such as epilepsy, or cardiovascular problems such as cardiac arrhythmias, although anything that causes hypotension of sufficient degree may result in a loss of consciousness.

The differential diagnosis of syncope in the elderly is wide (Kapoor *et al.*, 1986), and any event causing cerebral anoxia may be followed by a convulsion; thus the differentiation between epilepsy and cardiac arrhythmia or hypotension in the elderly is a particularly problematic one. Even in an institutionalised population where episodes were witnessed by trained staff, 31% of syncopal events remained unexplained (Lipsitz *et al.*, 1985). Recent work has suggested that carotid sinus hypersensitivity and neurocardiogenic (vasovagal) syncope are significant causes of unexplained syncope, dizziness and falls in the elderly (McIntosh *et al.*, 1993).

There are difficulties in assessing the role of cardiac arrhythmias in falls. Case reports of elderly people with falls who were found to have abnormalities on 24-hour electrocardiograph (ECG) monitoring suggest that cardiac arrhythmias are common causes of falls (Gordon, 1978). Serious episodic arrhythmias seem to be commoner in those with syncope or dizziness than those without (Abdon, 1981). Cardiac arrhythmias are common in asymptomatic elderly (Rodrigues Dos Santos & Lye, 1980) and a study of arrhythmias in fallers compared with well-matched controls demonstrated similar findings in both groups (Rosado *et al.*, 1989).

Not associated with loss of consciousness

Many neurological and neuromuscular problems are likely to predispose to falling. Parkinson's disease is particularly liable to do so because of the gait disturbance and the difficulty in initiating and stopping movement associated with the disease. In addition, postural hypotension is frequent in parkinsonian patients, because of the commonly associated autonomic dysfunction and also the hypotensive effects of drugs used to treat the disease (e.g. L-dopa, bromocriptine). Patients with stroke are also at greater risk of falling (Downton & Andrews, 1991).

Other important factors found to be associated with falls include restriction of joint movement and/or osteoarthritis; lower limb weakness; the presence of multiple illnesses; and foot problems. Diabetics may be at risk of falling because of the development of peripheral or autonomic neuropathy, or hypoglycaemia related to insulin or oral hypoglycaemic drugs.

Drugs and falling

The evidence relating to the role of drugs in the causation of falls is confused, partly because of the difficulty of separating the effects of drugs from the effects of the diseases for which they are prescribed. A large proportion of old people take both prescribed and over-the-counter drugs, and because of changes in pharmacokinetics and pharmacodynamics with aging, the elderly are more liable to suffer side-effects from drug therapy. It seems that consumption of any drug may be associated with an increase in the likelihood of falling, but specific drugs seem to be particularly risky.

Drugs may have an effect on postural stability either because of their central depressant effect (e.g. minor tranquillisers, sedatives, hypnotics), because they tend to cause postural hypotension (e.g. antihypertensives), or both (e.g. tricyclic antidepressants, major tranquillisers). In each of these cases, there has been found to be an association between consumption of such drugs and either falling per se or fractures secondary to falls (Tinker, 1979; Davie *et al.*, 1981; Blake *et al.*, 1988; Sorock & Shimkin, 1988). There also seem to be potential risks with other drugs, for example non-steroidal anti-inflammatory drugs which can produce symptoms of dizziness in elderly people (Goodwin & Regan, 1982). There may also be differences between specific drugs within groups, for instance long and short half-life hypnotics (Ray *et al.*, 1987).

The evidence concerning diuretics is conflicting. There is some evidence that thiazides protect against fracture because of their hypocalciuric effect (Rashiq & Logan, 1986) despite being associated with a high incidence of symptoms of dizziness, fainting and blacking out (Hale *et al.*, 1984). Other studies have found associations between thiazide intake and falls (Prudham & Evans, 1981) or femoral fracture (Muckle, 1976).

The relation of alcohol consumption to falls, particularly in the elderly, has been little studied. Blood alcohol levels above 50 mg/100 ml substantially increase the risk of falling in adults (Honkanen *et al.*, 1983). In elderly fallers, impairment attributable to alcohol is implicated in only a small percentage (less than 10%), commonly in a person with a history of heavy drinking (Svanstrom, 1974; Waller, 1978).

Environment and falls

Environmental factors are important in facilitating and maintaining the independence of older people. Their importance in the causation of falls is also recognised, although separating intrinsic and extrinsic causes of falls is difficult. In general, it seems that for between a third and a half of falls resulting in injury, environmental factors are a sole or major cause (Morfitt, 1983). The proportion is probably less in the very elderly.

The environment and intrinsic factors interact. For example, low lighting levels exacerbate the effects of visual loss (Cullinan *et al.*, 1979), and this may be particularly important for negotiating stairs (Archea, 1985).

Studies of falls in hospitals or residential care institutions mention the importance of staffing levels (Blake & Morfitt, 1986) but very low staffing levels may be associated with fewer falls because activity is discouraged (Morris & Isaacs, 1980). There is a suggestion that environmental temperature affects the risk of falling, at least in women (Campbell *et al.*, 1988), although this may occur only in thin or undernourished women (Bastow *et al.*, 1983), perhaps because of a relation between nutritional state and thermoregulation.

Many factors are implicated in the causation of falls, and it seems likely that combinations of factors are more important than single problems, as is the case for many health problems of the elderly. Although there are statistical associations between many factors and falls it is still very difficult to disentangle the relative risk of any particular factor. The number of potential causes of falls, however, means that there are always some factors amenable to change to reduce the risk of falling in every elderly faller.

References

Abdon, N. J. (1981). Frequency and distribution of long-term ECG-recorded cardiac arrhythmias in an elderly population. *Acta Med Scand*, **209**, 175–83.
Alexander, N. B. (1994). Postural control in older adults. *J Am Geriatr Soc*, **42**, 93–108.
Archea, J. C. (1985). Environmental factors associated with stair accidents by the elderly. *Clin Geriatr Med*, **1**, 555–68.
Baker, S. P. & Harvey, A. H. (1985). Fall injuries in the elderly. *Clin Geriatr Med*, **1**, 501–8.
Bastow, M. D., Rawlings, J. & Allison, S. P. (1983). Undernutrition, hypothermia, and injury in elderly women with fractured femur: an injury response to altered metabolism? *Lancet*, **1**, 143–6.
Berman, P. & O'Reilly, S. C. (1995). Clinical aspects of gait disturbance in the elderly. *Rev Clin Gerontol*, **5**, 83–8.
Berry, G., Fisher, R. H. & Lang, S. (1981). Detrimental incidents, including falls, in an elderly institutional population. *J Am Geriatr Soc*, **29**, 322–4.
Blake, A. J., Morgan, K., Bendall, M. J., Dallosso, H., Ebrahim, S. B. J., Arie, T. H. D., Fentem, P. H. & Bassey, E. J. (1988). Falls by elderly people at home: prevalence and associated factors. *Age Ageing*, **17**, 365–72.
Blake, C. & Morfitt, J. M. (1986). Falls and staffing in a residential home for elderly people. *Public Health*, **100**, 385–91.
Boyce, W. J. & Vessey, M. P. (1988). Habitual physical inertia and other factors in relation to risk of fracture of the proximal femur. *Age Ageing*, **17**, 319–27.
Brocklehurst, J. C., Carty, M. H., Leeming, J. T. & Robinson, J. M. (1978). Medical screening of old people accepted for residential care. *Lancet*, **2**, 141–3.
Brocklehurst, J. C., Robertson, D. & James-Groom, P. (1982). Clinical correlates of sway in old age – sensory modalities. *Age Ageing*, **11**, 1–10.
Caird, F. I., Andrews, G. R. & Kennedy, R. D. (1973). Effect of posture on blood pressure in the elderly. *Br Heart J*, **35**, 527–30.

Campbell, A. J., Borrie, M. J. & Spears, G. F. (1989). Risk factors for falls in a community-based prospective study of people 70 years and older. *J Gerontol*, **44**, M112–M117.

Campbell, A. J., Borrie, M. J., Spears, G. F., Jackson, S. L., Brown, J. S. & Fitzgerald, J. L. (1990). Circumstances and consequences of falls experienced by a community population 70 years and over during a prospective study. *Age Ageing*, **19**, 136–41.

Campbell, A. J., Diep, C., Reinken, J. & McCosh, L. (1985). Factors predicting mortality in a total population sample of the elderly. *J Epidemiol Comm Health*, **39**, 337–42.

Campbell, A. J., Reinken, J., Allan, B. C. & Martinez, G. S. (1981). Falls in old age: a study of frequency and related clinical factors. *Age Ageing*, **10**, 264–70.

Campbell, A. J., Spears, G. F. S., Borrie, M. J. & Fitzgerald, J. L. (1988). Falls, elderly women and the cold. *Gerontology*, **34**, 205–8.

Cohn, T. E. & Lasley, D. J. (1985). Visual depth illusion and falls in the elderly. *Clin Geriatr Med*, **1**, 601–15.

Collins, K. J., Exton-Smith, A. N., James, M. H. & Oliver, D. J. (1980). Functional changes in autonomic nervous responses with ageing. *Age Ageing*, **9**, 17–24.

Cook, P. J., Exton-Smith, A. N., Brocklehurst, J. C. & Lempert-Barber, S. M. (1982). Fractured femurs, falls and bone disorders. *J R Coll Phys Lond*, **16**, 45–9.

Cooper, C., Barker, D. J., Morris, J. & Briggs, R. S. (1987). Osteoporosis, falls and age in fracture of the proximal femur. *Br Med J*, **295**, 13–15.

Creasey, H. & Rapoport, S. I. (1985). The aging human brain. *Ann Neurol*, **17**, 2–10.

Cullinan, T. R., Silver, J. H., Gould, E. S. & Irvine, D. (1979). Visual disability and home lighting. *Lancet*, **1**, 642–4.

Cummings, S. R., Nevitt, M. C. & Kidd, S. (1988). Forgetting falls. The limited accuracy of recall of falls in the elderly. *J Am Geriatr Soc*, **36**, 613–16.

Davie, J. W., Blumenthal, M. D. & Robinson-Hawkins, S. (1981). A model of risk of falling for psychogeriatric patients. *Arch Gen Psychiatry*, **38**, 463–7.

de Jong, P. T. V. M., de Jong, J. M. B. V., Cohen, B. & Jongkees, L. B. W. (1977). Ataxia and nystagmus induced by injection of local anaesthetics in the neck. *Ann Neurol*, **1**, 240–6.

Dorfman, L. J. & Bosley, T. M. (1979). Age-related changes in peripheral and central nerve conduction in man. *Neurology*, **29**, 38–44.

Dove, A. F. & Dave, S. H. (1986). Elderly patients in the accident department and their problems. *Br Med J*, **292**, 807–09.

Downton, J. (1987). The problems of epidemiological studies of falls. *Clin Rehab*, **1**, 243–6.

Downton, J. H. & Andrews, K. (1990). Postural disturbance and psychological symptoms amongst elderly people living at home. *Int J Geriatr Psychiatry*, **5**, 93–8.

Downton, J. H. & Andrews, K. (1991). Prevalence, characteristics and factors associated with falls among the elderly living at home. *Aging*, **3**, 219–28.

Drachmann, D. A. & Hart, C. W. (1972). An approach to the dizzy patient. *Neurology*, **22**, 323–34.

Eddy, T. P. (1973). Deaths from falls and fractures. Comparison of mortality in Scotland and United States with that in England and Wales. *Br J Prev Soc Med*, **27**, 247–54.

Eklund, G. & Lofstedt, L. (1970). Biomechanical analysis of balance. *Biomed Eng*, **5**, 333–7.

Fernie, G. R. & Holliday, P. J. (1978). Postural sway in amputees and normal subjects. *J Bone Joint Surg*, **60A**, 895–8.

Fernie, G. R., Gryfe, C. I., Holliday, P. J. & Llewellyn, A. (1982). The relationship of postural sway in standing to the incidence of falls in geriatric subjects. *Age Ageing*, **11**, 11–16.

Finley, F. R., Cody, K. A. & Finizie, R. A. (1969). Locomotion patterns in elderly women. *Arch Phys Med Rehab*, **50**, 140–6.

Gabell, A. & Nayak, U. S. L. (1984). The effect of age on variability of gait. *J Gerontol*, **39**, 662–6.

Gabell, A., Simons, M. A. & Nayak, U. S. L. (1985). Falls in the healthy elderly: predisposing causes. *Ergonomics*, **28**, 965–75.

Goodwin, J. S. & Regan, M. (1982). Cognitive dysfunction associated with naproxen and ibuprofen in the elderly. *Arthritis Rheum*, **25**, 1013–14.

Gordon, M. (1978). Occult cardiac arrhythmias associated with falls and dizziness in the elderly: detection by Holter monitoring. *J Am Geriatr Soc*, **26**, 418–23.

Gribbin, B., Pickering, T. G., Sleight, P. & Peto, R. (1971). Effect of age and high blood pressure on baroreflex sensitivity in man. *Circ Res*, **29**, 424–31.

Grisso, J. A., Schwarz, D. F., Wishner, A. R., Weene, B., Holmes, J. H. & Sutton, R. L. (1990). Injuries in an elderly inner-city population. *J Am Geriatrics Soc*, **38**, 1326–31.

Gryfe, C. I., Amies, A. & Ashley, M. J. (1977). A longitudinal study of falls in an elderly population. I Incidence and morbidity. *Age Ageing*, **6**, 201–10.

Guimaraes, R. M. & Isaacs, B. (1980). Characteristics of the gait in old people who fall. *Int Rehab Med*, **2**, 177–80.

Haga, H., Shibata, H., Shichita, K., Matsuzaki, T. & Hatano, S. (1986). Falls in the institutionalised elderly in Japan. *Arch Gerontol Geriatr*, **5**, 1–9.

Hale, W. E., Stewart, R. B. & Marks, R. G. (1984). Central nervous system symptoms of elderly subjects using antihypertensive drugs. *J Am Geriatr Soc*, **32**, 5–10.

Honkanen, R., Ertama, L., Kuosmanen, P., Linnoila, M., Alha, A. & Visuri, T. (1983). The role of alcohol in accidental falls. *J Stud Alchol*, **44**, 331–54.

Imms, F. J. & Edholm, O. G. (1981). Studies of gait and mobility in the elderly. *Age Ageing*, **10**, 147–56.

Johnell, O. & Nilsson, B. E. (1985). Hip fracture and accident disposition. *Acta Orthop Scand*, **56**, 302–4.

Kapoor, W., Snustad, D., Peterson, J., Wieand, H. S., Cha, R. & Karpf, M. (1986). Syncope in the elderly. *Am J Med*, **80**, 419–27.

Kirshen, A. J., Cape, R. D. T., Hayes, H. C. & Spencer, J. D. (1984). Postural sway and cardiovascular parameters associated with falls in the elderly. *J Clin Exp Gerontol*, **6**, 291–307.

Koller, W. C., Glatt, S. L. & Fox, J. H. (1985). Senile gait. A distinct neurological entity. *Clin Geriat Med*, **1**, 661–8.

Lee, D. N. & Lishman, J. R. (1975). Visual proprioceptive control of stance. *J Hum Move Stud*, **1**, 87–95.

Lipsitz, L. A., Nyquist, R. P., Wei, J. Y. & Rowe, J. W. (1983). Postprandial reduction in blood pressure in the elderly. *New Engl J Med*, **309**, 81–3.

Lipsitz, L. A., Wei, J. Y. & Rowe, J. W. (1985). Syncope in an elderly institutionalised population: prevalence, incidence and associated risk. *Am J Med*, **55**, 45–54.

Lord, S. R., Clark, R. D. & Webster, I. W. (1991). Visual acuity and contrast sensitivity in relation to falls in an elderly population. *Age Ageing*, **20**, 175–81.

Lord, S. R., Ward, J. A., Williams, P. & Anstey, K. J. (1994). Physiological factors associated with falls in older community-dwelling women. *J Am Geriatr Soc*, **42**, 1110–17.

Lucht, U. (1971). A prospective study of accidental falls and resulting injuries in the home among elderly people. *Acta Socio-Med Scand*, **3**, 105–20.

MacLennan, W. J., Timothy, J. I. & Hall, M. R. P. (1980). Vibration sense, proprioception and ankles reflexes in old age. *J Clin Exp Gerontol*, **2**, 159–71.

Marsden, C. D., Merton, P. A. & Morton, H. B. (1981). Human postural responses. *Brain*, **104**, 513–534.

McIntosh, S., Da Costa, D. & Kenny, R. A. (1993). Outcome of an integrated approach to the investigation of dizziness, falls and syncope in elderly patients referred to a 'Syncope' clinic. *Age Ageing*, **22**, 53–8.

McMurdo, M. E. T. & Gaskell, A. (1991). Dark adaptation and falls in the elderly. *Gerontology*, **37**, 221–4.

Melton, L. J. III & Riggs, B. L. (1987). Epidemiology of age-related fractures. In *The Osteoporotic Syndrome*, ed. L. V. Alvioli. New York: Grune & Stratton.

Milne, J. S. (1979). Longitudinal studies of vision in older people. *Age Ageing*, **8**, 160–6.

Morfitt, J. M. (1983). Falls in old people at home: intrinsic versus environmental factors in causation. *Public Health*, **97**, 115–20.

Morris, E. V. & Isaacs, B. (1980). The prevention of falls in a geriatric hospital. *Age Ageing*, **9**, 181–5.

Morris, J. C., Rubin, E. H., Morris, E. J. & Mandel, S. A. (1987). Senile dementia of the Alzheimer's type: an important risk factor for serious falls. *J Gerontol*, **42**, 412–17.

Muckle, D. S. (1976). Iatrogenic factors in femoral neck fractures. *Injury*, **8**, 98–101.

Murphy, J. & Isaacs, B. (1982). The post-fall syndrome. A study of 36 elderly patients. *Gerontology*, **28**, 265–70.

Murray, M. P., Kory, R. C. & Clarkson, B. H. (1969). Walking patterns in healthy old men. *J Gerontol*, **24**, 169–78.

Nevitt, M. C., Cummings, S. R., Kidd, S. & Black, D. (1989). Risk factors for recurrent non-syncopal falls. A prospective study. *JAMA*, **261**, 2663–8.

Norre, M. E., Forrez, G. & Beckers, A. (1987). Posturography measuring instability in vestibular dysfunction in the elderly. *Age Ageing*, **16**, 89–93.

O'Loughlin, J. L., Robitaille, Y., Boivin, J.-F. & Suissa, S. (1993). Incidence of and risk factors for falls and injurious falls among the community-dwelling elderly. *Am J Epidemiol*, **137**, 342–54.

Overstall, P. W., Exton-Smith, A. N., Imms, F. J. & Johnson, A. L. (1977). Falls in the elderly related to postural imbalance. *Br Med J*, **1**, 261–4.

Overstall, P. W., Johnson, A. L. & Exton-Smith, A. N. (1978). Instability and falls in the elderly. *Age Ageing*, **7** (Suppl.): 92–6.

Prudham, D. & Evans, J. G. (1981). Factors associated with falls in the elderly: a community study. *Age Ageing*, **10**, 141–6.

Rashiq, S. & Logan, R. F. A. (1986). Role of drugs in fractures of the femoral neck. *Br Med J*, **292**, 861–3.

Ray, W. A., Griffin, M. R., Shaffner, W., Baugh, D. K. & Melton, L. J. (1987). Psychotropic drug use and the risk of hip fracture. *New Engl J Med*, **316**, 363–9.

Robinson, B. J., Johnson, R. H., Lambie, D. G. & Palmer, K. T. (1983). Do elderly patients with an excessive fall in blood pressure on standing have evidence of autonomic failure? *Clin Sci*, **64**, 587–91.

Rodrigues Dos Santos, A. G. & Lye, M. (1980). Transient cardiac arrhythmias in healthy elderly individuals: how relevant are they? *J Clin Exp Gerontol*, **2**, 245–58.

Rosado, J. A., Rubenstein, L. Z., Robbins, A. S., Heng, M. K., Schulman, B. L. & Josephson, K. R. (1989). The value of Holter monitoring in evaluating the elderly patient who falls. *J Am Geriatr Soc*, **37**, 430–4.

Sabin, T. D. (1982). Biologic aspects of falls and mobility limitations in the elderly. *J Am Geriatr Soc*, **30**, 51–58.

Sattin, R. W., Lambert Huber, D. A., DeVito, C. A., Rodriguez, J. G., Ros, A., Bacchelli, S., Stevens, J. A. & Waxweiler, R. J. (1990). The incidence of fall injury events among the elderly in a defined population. *Am J Epidemiol*, **131**, 1028–37.

Sloan, J. & Holloway, G. (1981). Fractured neck of the femur: the cause of the fall? *Injury*, **13**, 230–2.

Sorock, G. S. & Shimkin, E. E. (1988). Benzodiazepine sedatives and the risk of falling in a community-dwelling elderly cohort. *Arch Intern Med*, **148**, 2441–4.

Speechley, M. & Tinetti, M. (1991). Falls and injuries in frail and vigorous community elderly persons. *J Am Geriatr Soc*, **39**, 46–52.

Svanstrom, L. (1974). Falls on stairs: an epidemiological accident study. *Scand J Soc Med*, **2**, 113–20.

Tinetti, M. E. & Powell, L. (1993). Fear of falling and low self-efficacy: a cause of dependence in elderly persons. *J Gerontol*, **48**, 35–8.

Tinetti, M. E., Liu, W.-L. & Claus, E. B. (1993). Predictors and prognosis of inability to get up after falls among elderly persons. *JAMA*, **269**, 65–70.

Tinetti, M. E., Speechley, M. & Ginter, S. F. (1988). Risk factors for falls among elderly persons living in the community. *New Engl J Med*, **319**, 1701–7.

Tinker, G. M. (1979). Accidents in a geriatric department. *Age Ageing*, **8**, 196–8.

Tobis, J. S., Nayak, U. S. L. & Hoehler, F. (1981). Visual perception of verticality and horizontality among elderly fallers. *Arch Phys Med Rehab*, **62**, 619–22.

Visser, H. (1983). Gait and balance in senile dementia of Alzheimer's type. *Age Ageing*, **12**, 296–301.

Waller, J. A. (1978). Falls among the elderly – human and environmental factors. *Accid Anal Prev*, **10**, 21–33.

Weiner, W. J., Nora, L. M. & Glantz, R. H. (1984). Elderly in-patients: postural reflex impairment. *Neurology*, **34**, 945–7.

Wickham, C. A. C., Walsh, K., Cooper, C., Barker, D. J. P., Margetts, B. M., Morris, J. & Bruce, S. A. (1989). Dietary calcium, physical activity, and risk of hip fracture: a prospective study. *Br Med J*, **299**, 889–92.

Witkin, H. A., Lewis, H. B., Herzman, M., Machover, K., Meissner, P., Bretnall, P. & Wapner, S. (1954). *Personality Through Perception: an Experimental and Clinical Study*. New York: Harper.

Wolfson, L. I., Whipple, R., Amerman, P., Kaplan, J. & Kleinberg, A. (1985). Gait and balance in the elderly. Two functional capacities that link sensory and motor ability to falls. *Clin Geriatr Med*, **1**, 649–55.

Wollner, L., McCarthy, S. T., Soper, N. D. W. & Macy, D. J. (1979). Failure of cerebral autoregulation as a cause of brain dysfunction in the elderly. *Br Med J*, **1**, 1117–18.

Woodhouse, P. R., Briggs, R. S. & Ward, D. (1983). Falls and disability in old peoples homes. *J Clin Exp Gerontol*, **5**, 309–21.

Wyke, B. (1979). Cervical articular contributions to posture and gait: their relation to senile disequilibrium. *Age Ageing*, **8**, 251–8.

6

Bone

R. M. FRANCIS and A. M. SUTCLIFFE

Bone remodelling

Bone is a living tissue which continuously remodels throughout life. This allows the skeleton to increase in size during growth, respond to the physical stresses placed on it and repair structural damage due to fatigue, failure or trauma. The skeleton comprises cortical and trabecular bone. Cortical bone is predominantly found in the shafts of the long bones, while trabecular bone is mainly located in the vertebrae, pelvis and the ends of long bones. Trabecular bone has a larger surface area, undergoes greater remodelling and is therefore more responsive to metabolic changes than cortical bone. The relative proportion of cortical and trabecular bone varies throughout the body, but overall the skeleton is composed of 80% cortical and 20% trabecular bone.

The major cells involved in bone remodelling are osteoclasts, osteoblasts and osteocytes. Osteoclasts are multinucleate cells derived from macrophage–monocyte precursors which resorb bone and remove degraded organic material. Osteoblasts are derived from fibroblast precursors and synthesise bone matrix or osteoid, which is subsequently mineralised around foci of crystal formation known as matrix vesicles. Osteocytes are mature osteoblasts trapped within calcified bone which are interconnected by long dendritic processes. This may provide a communication network to transmit information about mechanical forces, which can then be used to modify bone resorption and formation.

Bone remodelling is initiated by a period of resorption lasting about 2 weeks, when osteoclasts erode an area of bone. Osteoblasts are then attracted to the resorption cavity, where over the subsequent 3 months, new bone matrix is deposited and mineralised. The processes of bone resorption and bone formation are usually closely coupled, probably through local humoral factors, although bone formation exceeds resorption during skeletal growth and resorption outstrips bone formation after involutional bone loss starts. Bone remodelling may be influenced by mechanical forces applied to the skeleton, by local humoral factors and by circulating hormones such as oestrogens, testosterone, calcitonin, parathyroid hormone (PTH) and 1,25-dihydroxyvitamin D (1,25(OH)$_2$D).

Bone mass throughout life

Bone mass changes throughout life in the three major phases of skeletal growth, consolidation and involution. About 90% of the ultimate bone mass is deposited during skeletal growth, which lasts until the closure of the epiphyses. This is then followed by a phase of skeletal consolidation lasting for up to 15 years, when bone mass increases further until the peak bone mass is achieved in the midthirties. Involutional bone loss starts between the ages of 35 and 40 years. Cortical and trabecular bone is lost with advancing age in both sexes, although the rate of bone loss varies according to bone type and anatomical site. Overall, women lose 35–50% of trabecular and 25–30% of cortical bone mass with age, while men lose 15–45% of trabecular and 5–15% of cortical bone (Francis, 1990).

The potential determinants of peak bone mass include race, sex, heredity, exercise, diet, smoking, alcohol consumption and hormonal factors. Negroid populations have a higher bone mass than Caucasians or Asians, and men have bigger, denser skeletons than women (Cohn et al., 1977; Mazess, 1982). Hereditary factors also influence peak bone mass as there is a greater concordance of bone mass between monozygotic than dizygotic twins, while the daughters of osteoporotic women have a lower than expected bone density (Smith et al., 1973; Seeman et al., 1989). Furthermore, recent work suggests that polymorphism of the vitamin D receptor gene may have an important effect on bone density in women (Morrison et al., 1994). Bone mass is also higher in young adults who exercise regularly than in more sedentary individuals, emphasising the importance of mechanical factors in the determination of bone mass (Nilson & Westlin, 1971). Another potential determinant of peak bone mass is dietary calcium intake, as several studies suggest that a high dietary calcium intake during skeletal growth and consolidation may also be beneficial to the skeleton (Kanders et al., 1988; Johnston et al., 1992). The combination of regular exercise and high dietary calcium intake may act together to produce an optimal peak bone mass (Kanders et al., 1988). In contrast, smoking and alcohol consumption during adolescence and early adult life have an adverse effect on peak bone mass (Stevenson et al., 1989). Endocrine factors also affect peak bone mass as early menarche, pregnancy and the use of the oral contraceptive pill are associated with higher bone mass (Goldsmith & Johnston, 1975).

The onset of bone loss between the ages of 35 and 40 years is likely to be genetically predetermined. This may be related to impaired new bone formation, due to declining osteoblast function. Other causes of age-related bone loss include the menopause, low body weight, smoking, excess alcohol consumption, physical inactivity, nutritional factors and declining calcium absorption (Compston, 1992; Scane & Francis, 1993).

There is a marked reduction in the circulating concentrations of oestradiol and progesterone at the menopause, associated with increased bone resorption and an accelerated rate of bone loss. After the menopause the major circulating oestrogen is oestrone, produced by the conversion of the adrenal androgen androstenedione in fat.

Body weight is an important determinant of bone mass, as bone loss is more rapid in women with low body weight and osteoporotic subjects are lighter than expected. The protective effects of high body weight on bone loss may be due to the mechanical effects of body weight on bone formation and the increased production of oestrone in fat (Davidson *et al.*, 1982; Christiansen *et al.*, 1987).

Smoking may increase bone loss by bringing forward the menopause by several years, decreasing plasma oestrogen levels subsequently by increasing their metabolism, and possibly by depressing osteoblast function (Jick *et al.*, 1977; De Vernejoul *et al.*, 1983; Jensen *et al.*, 1985). The deleterious effect of smoking on the skeleton may also be due in part to the association with low body weight.

The decline in physical activity with advancing age is also likely to cause further bone loss. Physical activity is important to the skeleton, as the associated weight-bearing and muscular activity stimulates bone formation and increases bone mass, while immobilisation leads to rapid bone loss (Krolner & Toft, 1983; Krolner *et al.*, 1983). The importance of physical activity is underlined by several case control studies, which show that patients with femoral fracture are habitually less physically active than control subjects (Cooper *et al.*, 1988; Lau *et al.*, 1988).

The role of dietary calcium intake in the pathogenesis of bone loss remains controversial. Metabolic balance studies suggest that the dietary requirement for calcium increases at the menopause from 1000 to 1500 mg/day (Heaney *et al.*, 1978). There is little relation, however, between dietary calcium intake and bone mass or bone loss at this time of life (Riggs *et al.*, 1987, Stevenson *et al.*, 1988).

The efficiency of calcium absorption from the bowel declines with age in both sexes, which if uncompensated may cause further bone loss (Bullamore, 1970). The reduction in calcium absorption appears to be due to the fall in plasma 25-hydroxyvitamin D (25OHD) with age secondary to reduced sunlight exposure, and to impaired metabolism of 25OHD to $1,25(OH)_2D$ because of declining renal function (Baker *et al.*, 1980; Francis *et al.*, 1984).

Osteoporosis

Osteoporosis is characterised by a reduction in the amount of bone in the skeleton, associated with increased fragility and risk of failure. The mechanical properties of bone are closely related to its mineral content and architectural structure, so a reduction in bone mass is inevitably associated with an increased propensity to fracture. The major osteoporotic fractures are those of the forearm, vertebral body and femoral neck. The lifetime risk of fracture for a 50–year-old white woman in the USA has been estimated at 16.0% for the forearm, 15.6% for the vertebrae and 17.5% for the proximal femur, while the corresponding figures for a 50–year-old man are 2.5%, 5.0% and 6.0% (Melton et al., 1992).

Any factor which adversely affects peak bone mass, hastens the onset of bone loss or increases the rate of bone loss predisposes to the development of osteoporosis. A number of such risk factors have been implicated including women of Caucasian or Asian races, premature menopause, positive family history, short stature, low body weight, low calcium intake or absorption, inactivity, nulliparity, smoking and high alcohol consumption (Riggs & Melton, 1986). Underlying secondary causes of osteoporosis are present in up to 35% of women and 55% of men with vertebral crush fractures (Baillie et al., 1992; Caplan et al., 1994). Common causes of secondary osteoporosis include steroid therapy, male hypogonadism, myeloma, skeletal metastases, thyrotoxicosis and immobilisation (Baillie et al., 1992; Caplan et al., 1994).

Steroid therapy is the commonest cause of secondary osteoporosis, occurring in 10–20% of patients with vertebral crush fractures. Steroids decrease calcium absorption by a direct effect on the bowel mucosa, thereby increasing circulating PTH and $1,25(OH)_2D$, both of which are potential bone resorbing agents. They also suppress the adrenal production of androgens, leading to low plasma oestrone levels. These changes increase bone resorption, but steroids also suppress bone formation and collagen production. Steroid therapy therefore leads to an uncoupling of the processes of bone resorption and formation, causing rapid bone loss and the early development of osteoporotic fractures (Reid, 1990).

Hypogonadism is a common cause of osteoporosis in men, occurring in up to 20% of men with vertebral crush fractures, although the diagnosis may not always be clinically apparent. The pathogenesis of bone loss in hypogonadal men remains uncertain, although histological studies show evidence of increased resorption and decreased bone formation, which has been attributed to androgen or oestrogen deficiency, low plasma $1,25(OH)_2D$ concentration, malabsorption of calcium or reduced calcitonin levels. Treatment with androgens decreases bone resorption and stimulates bone formation, thereby increasing bone mass (Scane & Francis, 1993).

Myeloma causes diffuse osteopenia, with or without multiple lytic lesions, and is commonly associated with vertebral crush fractures and pathological fractures elsewhere. The myeloma cells stimulate bone resorption by secreting osteoclast activating factors. Tumours commonly metastasise to bone, most frequently to the spine, femur, pelvis, ribs, sternum and humerus. Bone destruction associated with metastases may be due to the resorption of bone by tumour cells or to stimulation of osteoclasts by local humoral factors released by the metastatic cells (Francis, 1990).

Thyrotoxicosis is a well established cause of osteoporosis, although the diagnosis may not always be apparent in elderly osteoporotic patients, as the other clinical features of thyrotoxicosis may be absent. Thyrotoxicosis stimulates both bone formation and resorption, although resorption exceeds formation, so that bone is lost from the skeleton. Increased bone resorption in thyrotoxicosis suppresses PTH production, leading to low plasma $1,25(OH)_2D$ and malabsorption of calcium, all of which are reversed when the patient is rendered euthyroid by treatment. Treatment may also increase bone formation further, and the parallel increase in bone formation and plasma $1,25(OH)_2D$ suggests that the initial disparity between bone formation and resorption may be due to low plasma $1,25(OH)_2D$ levels. The apparent uncoupling of bone formation and resorption during treatment of thyrotoxicosis may persist for up to a year, and might be expected to increase bone mass (Francis, 1990).

Immobilisation leads to rapid bone loss of about 1% per week, which then stabilises after about 6 months when a new steady state is reached. Bone loss in immobilisation is due to a stimulation of bone resorption and a decrease in bone formation, and the more rapid loss in weight bearing bones suggests that bone loss is due to mechanical factors rather than changes in circulating PTH, $1,25(OH)_2D$, thyroxine or cortisol. Where practical, remobilisation should be encouraged, as this appears to increase trabecular bone mass by 0.25% per week and may partially replace lost bone (Francis, 1990).

Clinical features of osteoporosis

Osteoporosis is generally considered to be asymptomatic until fractures occur. Fractures of the forearm and femur are usually easy to diagnose, but vertebral crush fractures are more difficult to detect clinically. While crush fractures may cause back pain, this is not always the case, and there are many other causes of this symptom. Classically, however, a crush fracture is associated with an acute episode of pain lasting for 6–8 weeks before settling to a more chronic backache. The pain may radiate anteriorly but rarely radiates to the hips or legs. Osteoporotic subjects may also be aware of a loss of height of several inches and the development of a kyphosis.

Investigation of osteoporosis

Patients with osteoporosis usually present with fractures of the forearm, spine and femur. In patients with suspected fracture of the forearm or femur, radiographs should be taken to confirm the clinical diagnosis prior to subsequent fixation. As vertebral crush fractures are more difficult to diagnose, spine radiographs should be taken in patients with acute back pain, loss of height or kyphosis. These may demonstrate vertebral deformation or other causes of back pain. Such radiographs may also show lytic or sclerotic lesions, which suggest the possibility of neoplastic disease. Although plasma alkaline phosphatase may rise transiently after a fracture, other investigations are generally normal in primary osteoporosis, although they may indicate the presence of a secondary cause of osteoporosis. Secondary osteoporosis is common in individuals with vertebral crush fractures and specific treatment of the underlying condition may prevent or reduce further bone loss in many cases. It is therefore worthwhile performing full blood count, erythrocyte sedimentation rate (ESR), plasma biochemical profile, thyroid function tests and serum and urine electrophoresis in all such patients, together with serum testosterone and gonadotrophins in the males (Baillie *et al.*, 1992; Caplan *et al.*, 1994). Anaemia, raised ESR, persistent elevation of alkaline phosphatase or hypercalcaemia suggests the possibility of myeloma or skeletal metastases. Thyroid function tests, serum testosterone and gonadotrophins may also reveal unsuspected thyrotoxicosis and hypogonadism, respectively. Serum and urine immunoelectrophoresis should probably be performed in all patients with vertebral crush fractures, as myeloma may be present even in the absence of other abnormal laboratory findings (Baillie *et al.*, 1992; Caplan *et al.*, 1994).

Prevention of osteoporosis

Ideally the prevention of osteoporosis should include the promotion of an optimal peak bone mass, the delay of the onset of bone loss and the retardation of the subsequent rate of bone loss. Although the extent to which the attainment of peak bone mass can be modified is uncertain, it seems prudent to encourage children and young adults to eat a balanced diet containing at least 800 mg calcium/day. Excessive dieting should be avoided because of the association between low body weight and osteoporosis. Regular exercise should also be encouraged, although females should avoid exercising to the point where they become amenorrhoeic, as this has a deleterious effect on bone mass because of the associated oestrogen deficiency. Secondary amenorrhoea due to other causes is also common in young women, and should be investigated and treated as rapidly as possible, to avoid the adverse effects of the associated oestrogen deficiency on the skeleton.

The most effective way of delaying the onset of bone loss is by the use of hormone replacement therapy (HRT) at the time of the menopause. HRT reduces bone resorption and prevents bone loss from the lumbar spine and femoral neck (Stevenson *et al.*, 1990). When given for 5–10 years at the time of the menopause, HRT substantially reduces the risk of osteoporotic fractures (Weiss *et al.*, 1980; Kiel *et al.*, 1987). Nevertheless, there is some concern that the benefits of HRT may be lost with advancing age, as women over the age of 75 years who have previously taken HRT for at least 7 years have only 3.2% higher bone density than those who have never taken such treatment (Felson *et al.*, 1993). In addition to the benefits on the skeleton, HRT controls menopausal symptoms such as hot flushes, nocturnal sweats, vaginal dryness and dyspareunia. It also improves the lipid profile and reduces the risk of cardiovascular disease (Stampfer *et al.*, 1991).

There is little relation between dietary calcium intake and bone loss at the menopause, suggesting that increasing dietary calcium alone is unlikely to produce a major effect on bone loss. Nevertheless, the combination of calcium supplementation and regular exercise appears to reduce bone loss, although not as effectively as HRT (Prince *et al.*, 1991). Furthermore, the reduction in calcium absorption later in life may increase the dietary calcium requirements further, so it seems wise to advise post-menopausal women to take a diet rich in calcium. Stopping smoking and reducing alcohol consumption might also be expected to reduce bone loss, although there is no definite evidence to confirm this. In view of the deleterious effects of immobilisation on the skeleton, and the benefits of weight bearing and exercise on bone mass, regular physical activity should be encouraged in later life. As the decline in calcium absorption is in part due to decreased plasma 25OHD concentrations, efforts should be made to ensure that the elderly are vitamin D replete, by encouraging adequate sunlight exposure and considering vitamin D supplementation in housebound individuals.

Screening for osteoporosis

Much interest has revolved around the early detection of asymptomatic osteoporosis, because of the potential importance of hormone replacement therapy in preventing further bone loss. As the correlation between bone mass at different sites is relatively poor, it appears that in order to identify subjects most at risk of vertebral and femoral fractures, techniques capable of measuring bone mass in the lumbar spine and femoral neck should be used. Dual energy X-ray absorptiometry (DEXA) is the most suitable method of measuring bone density at these sites, as it is rapid, has a high precision and involves low radiation exposure. Population-based bone density screening cannot be advocated because of uncertainties about the acceptance of such screening and the uptake, compliance and efficacy of prolonged HRT. Nevertheless, bone density measurement may be helpful in the management of individuals likely to have osteoporosis, because of a past history of fractures after minimal trauma, early menopause or steroid therapy.

Treatment of established osteoporosis

Treatments for osteoporosis may be classified into antiresorptive agents, such as oestrogens, progesterone, calcium supplements, calcitonin and bisphosphonates, which reduce or prevent further bone loss and anabolic agents like sodium fluoride and anabolic steroids which increase bone mass. Antiresorptive agents cause a transient uncoupling of bone resorption and formation, leading to a small increase in bone mass before a new equilibrium is reached. Although anabolic agents lead to a larger increase in bone mass, they do not necessarily improve bone strength, particularly when the trabecular architecture has been disrupted by the osteoporotic process.

Oestrogens

Oestrogen treatment increases spine bone density by 5% in older postmenopausal women with established osteoporosis (Lindsay & Tohme, 1990; Lufkin *et al.*, 1992). One of these small studies has also shown a 60% reduction in the number of further vertebral fractures (Lufkin *et al.*, 1992). Oestrogen treatment should be given with cyclical progestogen in a woman with an intact uterus, to prevent the development of endometrial hyperplasia or carcinoma. Although the effect of oestrogen treatment on bone loss is particularly marked within 5 years of the menopause, when bone loss is at its most rapid, it may still be effective later in life. Nevertheless, oestrogen treatment appears to be less well tolerated with advancing age because of an increased incidence of side-effects and the inconvenience of withdrawal bleeds if the uterus is still present. It is therefore a particularly suitable treatment for the younger postmenopausal woman with osteoporosis.

Calcium supplements

Although calcium supplements were previously used alone in the treatment of osteoporosis, this is probably no longer appropriate as a number of more effective treatments are now available. Calcium supplements decrease bone loss, but not to the same extent as other antiresorptive agents (Prince *et al.*, 1991; Reid *et al.*, 1993). There is no convincing evidence that calcium supplements alone decrease the risk of vertebral or hip fractures.

Vitamin D

With advancing age there is a reduction in cutaneous production and subsequent metabolism of vitamin D. This leads to a decrease in calcium absorption and parathyroid hormone (PTH) mediated bone resorption. A French study in nursing homes and apartment blocks for the elderly showed that 800 IU of vitamin D_3 and 1.2 g of elemental calcium daily reduces the risk of hip fracture by 43% (Chapuy *et al.*, 1992). It is unclear if the benefits of treatment seen in this study were due to vitamin D, calcium or the combination of both, but a Finnish study showed that an annual injection of 150000–300000 IU vitamin D decreases the risk of long bone fractures in elderly people (Heikinheimo *et al.*, 1992). Nevertheless, there is no evidence that vitamin D and calcium supplementation decreases spine bone loss or the incidence of vertebral fractures.

Vitamin D supplementation is therefore most appropriate in frail and housebound elderly people, who are at high risk of vitamin D deficiency and hip fractures.

Vitamin D metabolites

Calcium absorption is lower in osteoporotic individuals than age-matched control subjects, but it is unclear if this is due to an intrinsic defect in the absorption mechanism or low plasma $1,25(OH)_2D$ concentrations (Francis, 1990). Treatment with low dose calcitriol or alfacalcidol improves calcium absorption, and appears to decrease bone loss and the risk of vertebral fractures in women with established osteoporosis (Francis *et al.*, 1990; Tilyard *et al.*, 1992; Orimo *et al.*, 1994). If these findings are confirmed, then the vitamin D metabolites may prove useful in the management of the older woman with osteoporosis.

Calcitonin

Calcitonin is a potent antiresorptive agent, which prevents bone loss in normal postmenopausal and osteoporotic women (Mazzuoli *et al.*, 1986; Reginster *et al.*, 1987). Recent work suggests that calcitonin treatment may also reduce the risk of further vertebral deformation (Rico *et al.*, 1992). Although resistance to calcitonin treatment appears to develop during prolonged treatment, it is uncertain if this is due to the development of antibodies against calcitonin or to the downregulation of calcitonin receptors. Calcitonin may be administered by injection or intranasally, but is expensive and associated with side-effects such as flushing, nausea and vomiting. The role of calcitonin in the treatment of established osteoporosis is therefore still uncertain.

Bisphosphonates

Bisphosphonates are powerful antiresorptive agents, which reduce osteoclast number and function. Although poorly absorbed by mouth, they localise preferentially in bone, where they bind to hydroxyapatite crystals. As they persist in the skeleton for many months, their duration of action is prolonged beyond the period of administration. Two studies have shown that intermittent cyclical etidronate therapy increases spine bone density by about 5% and reduces the risk of further vertebral fractures in older osteoporotic women (Storm *et al.*, 1990; Watts *et al.*, 1990). Alendronate has recently been shown to increase bone density in the spine, forearm and femoral neck and reduce the risk of vertebral and non-vertebral fractures in women with osteoporosis (Liberman *et al.*, 1995).

Anabolic steroids

Anabolic steroids such as stanozolol and nandrolone increase bone mass by 5–10%, presumably by stimulating bone formation, although there may also be an effect on bone resorption (Chesnut *et al.*, 1987). Their use may be associated with androgenic side-effects and fluid retention, and prolonged administration may lead to abnormal liver function tests and even hepatocellular tumours.

Sodium fluoride

Early studies of sodium fluoride treatment in osteoporotic women showed increases in lumbar spine bone density of 35%, but there was no reduction in vertebral fracture incidence, whilst the number of non-vertebral fractures increased with fluoride (Riggs *et al.*, 1990; Kleerekoper *et al.*, 1991). More recent work with low dose slow release sodium fluoride shows smaller increases in spine and hip bone density and a reduction in vertebral fracture incidence, without the adverse effects seen with higher dose treatment (Pak *et al.*, 1995). Nevertheless, the therapeutic window for fluoride appears narrow and this agent cannot yet be advocated for the management of osteoporosis.

Osteomalacia

Osteomalacia is a generalised bone disorder characterised by an impairment of mineralisation leading to accumulation of unmineralised matrix or osteoid in the skeleton. Vitamin D deficiency is the commonest cause of osteomalacia in the elderly, with renal failure a smaller but significant cause in this age group. There is a reduction in plasma 25OHD with advancing age, mainly due to reduced sunlight exposure, although decreased capacity for cutaneous production, low dietary intake, poor absorption and impaired hepatic hydroxylation of vitamin D may contribute to this (Baker *et al.*, 1980). The reduction in renal function with age is associated with decreased plasma $1,25(OH)_2D$ concentrations, which may contribute to the development of osteomalacia in the elderly (Francis *et al.*, 1984).

Osteomalacia is essentially a histological diagnosis, so there is little information on its overall prevalence in the elderly. Nevertheless, low circulating 25OHD concentrations are common in the elderly, particularly in subjects who are housebound (Dunnigan *et al.*, 1982). As about 10% of the elderly are housebound, a significant proportion of the elderly are at risk of developing osteomalacia, and several investigators have shown that osteomalacia occurs in about 4% of elderly people admitted to hospital (Anderson *et al.*, 1966). Histological data from Leeds suggest that 12–20% of elderly patients with femoral fracture have evidence of osteomalacia, although other studies show a much lower prevalence (Aaron *et al.*, 1974; Hordon & Peacock, 1990; Compston *et al.*, 1991).

The presentation of osteomalacia may be variable, and the diagnosis may be easily missed in the early stages of the disease because of the vague nature of the symptoms.

The patient may complain of aches and pains, aggravated by muscular contraction, but tending to persist after rest. Although there is a propensity for fracture in osteomalacia, the soft elastic bone also deforms easily leading to kyphosis, scoliosis and deformity of the rib cage, pelvis and long bones. The patient may also develop a proximal myopathy, causing a waddling gait and difficulty rising from a chair or climbing stairs.

The classical radiological appearances of osteomalacia are relatively rare and may not be found in the early stages of the disease. These include cod-fish vertebrae, deformity of the rib cage, pelvis and long bones, and Looser's zones or pseudofractures. The latter are large areas of osteoid seen particularly in the proximal femur, humeral neck, pubic rami, metatarsals and the outer border of the scapula. There may also be radiological evidence of secondary hyperparathyroidism, with subperiosteal erosions in the metacarpals or phalanges.

The typical biochemical findings in vitamin D deficiency osteomalacia are hypocalcaemia, hypophosphataemia and elevation of the alkaline phosphatase. These abnormalities lack specificity in the diagnosis of osteomalacia in the elderly, as they may occur individually with intercurrent illness.

The only definite way of diagnosing osteomalacia is by bone histology, but this is only required in the minority of cases. In patients with a classical history of bone pain and muscle weakness, with radiological evidence of Looser's zones or typical biochemical changes, there is little indication for bone biopsy. When the diagnosis is less clear cut, measurement of plasma 25OHD and serum PTH may be useful, as the combination of a low 25OHD and elevated PTH is a strong indicator of the presence of osteomalacia (Peacock, 1984).

Vitamin D deficiency osteomalacia will heal with ultraviolent irradiation or vitamin D treatment. Vitamin D treatment is more practical and can either be given orally in a regular daily dose of 25 μg (1000 units) or as a single intramuscular (IM) injection of 7.5 mg (300000 units), which should be repeated every 6–12 months to prevent recurrence. In patients with osteomalacia associated with malabsorption or renal impairment, the metabolites of vitamin D may be required.

Fractures in the elderly

The mechanical properties of an individual bone are determined by the amount of bone present, skeletal architecture and bone quality. Aging is associated with a reduction in bone mass, disruption of trabecular architecture and increased prevalence of disorders such as osteomalacia and Paget's disease which adversely affect the quality of bone. Nevertheless, the risk of fracture is determined not only by skeletal factors but by the incidence of falls and by the presence or absence of protective mechanisms such as extending the arm on falling. It is therefore not surprising that the incidence of fractures increases with advancing age. While fractures in young adults usually occur after extensive trauma, fractures in the elderly may result from minimal trauma, such as falling from standing height. The major fractures occurring in the elderly are those of the forearm, vertebral body, humerus, pelvis and femoral neck. The incidence of these fractures increases with advancing age and is higher in women than men because of their lower peak bone mass, more rapid bone loss and greater risk of falls.

The absolute number of fractures in the elderly is rising rapidly, due in part to the increasing numbers of elderly people and a rising age-specific incidence of fractures (Francis & Sutcliffe, 1990). If present demographic trends continue in the UK the number of young elderly will remain reasonably constant over the next few decades, while the number of people over the age of 85 years will increase considerably. Many of these elderly people will be frail, and therefore particularly at risk of fracture. There is also evidence of a rising age-specific incidence of fractures of the forearm, vertebral body, humerus and femur, which has been attributed to the increased survival of frail individuals and secular changes in smoking, alcohol consumption, diet and physical activity.

Forearm fractures

These are the commonest fractures before the age of 75 years. The incidence rises steeply at the menopause in women and then stabilises above the age of 65 years, while the low incidence changes little with age in men. It has been suggested that the rise in incidence at the menopause is due to an increase in postural instability in women at this time, and the absence of a further increase in forearm fractures after the age of 65 years may be because the arm is less likely to be used to break a fall in the elderly. About 5% of women in the UK will have sustained a forearm fracture at the age of 70 years, rising to 15% at the age of 80 years, compared with 2 and 4%, respectively, for men (Francis & Sutcliffe, 1990).

Vertebral fractures

The incidence and prevalence of vertebral fractures is difficult to quantify as many patients with this fracture do not seek medical attention. A Swedish study suggests that the prevalence of vertebral crush fractures in women is 1% in the seventh decade, 4% in the eighth decade and 13% in the ninth decade, whilst the prevalence in men is 4% in the eighth decade and 7% in the ninth decade (Obrant *et al.*, 1989). Nevertheless, data from the European Vertebral Osteoporosis Study suggest that the prevalence of vertebral deformity may be higher in men than women, possibly due to trauma earlier in life. There is also a large variation in the incidence of vertebral and femoral neck fractures in men across Europe, which may reflect differences in physical activity and other lifestyle factors.

Femoral fractures

This is the most important fracture in the elderly as it causes greater mortality, higher morbidity and more expenditure than all other fractures combined. The incidence of this fracture rises steeply with age in both sexes, but is considerably higher in women than men. Using current age-specific incidence rates for England and Wales, it has been estimated that 12% of women and 5% of men will have sustained a femoral fracture by the age of 85 years. A number of risk factors have been identified for femoral fractures, including reduced bone mass, falls, low body weight, physical inactivity, muscle weakness and the presence of osteomalacia.

Femoral fractures are associated with a considerable mortality, particularly in older more dependent individuals. There has been a reduction in mortality over the past two decades, with Evans reporting a fall in 6 month mortality from 40% in 1975 to 28% in 1985, while Greatorex showed a reduction in mortality from 35% in 1968 to 15% in 1982 (Greatorex, 1986; Evans, 1987). This reduction in mortality may be due to improvements in surgical management and rehabilitation after this fracture.

In addition to the substantial mortality, femoral fractures are associated with considerable morbidity, with many patients becoming more immobile and more dependent. Between 25 and 50% of individuals are more dependent after fracture, with deterioration occurring more often in women over the age of 75 years, those with a poor clinical result and those who were already dependent before fracture (Beals, 1972; Thomas & Stevens, 1974; Jensen & Bagger, 1982).

There are few estimates of the total cost of femoral fracture, but early work suggested that the hospital costs alone of this fracture in England and Wales exceed £165 million/year (Wallace, 1987). This takes no account of the cost of general practitioner or district nursing services, the expense incurred by social service departments in providing home helps and places in day centres and residential homes or the cost to the Department of Social Security of attendance allowance, invalid care allowance and benefit payments to support private nursing home placement.

References

Aaron, J. E., Gallagher, J. C., Anderson, J. *et al.* (1974). Frequency of osteomalacia and osteoporosis in fractures of the proximal femur. *Lancet*, **1**, 229–33.

Anderson, I., Campbell, A. E. R., Dunn, A. & Runciman, J. B. M. (1966). Osteomalacia in elderly women. *Scott Med J*, **2**, 429–36.

Baillie, S. P., Davison, C. E., Johnson, F. J. & Francis, R. M. (1992). Pathogenesis of vertebral crush fractures in men. *Age Ageing*, **21**, 139–41.

Baker, M. R., Peacock, M. & Nordin, B. E. C. (1980). The decline in vitamin D status with age. *Age Ageing*, **9**, 249–52.

Beals, R. K. (1972). Survival following hip fracture: long follow up of 607 patients. *J Chron Dis*, **25**, 235–44.

Bullamore, J. R., Gallagher, J. C., Wilkinson, R., Nordin, B. E. C. & Marshall, D. H. (1970). Effect of age on calcium absorption. *Lancet*, **2**, 535–7.

Caplan, G. A., Scane, A. C. & Francis, R. M. (1994). Pathogenesis of vertebral crush fractures in women. *J R Soc Med*, **87**, 200–2.

Chapuy, M. C., Arlot, M. E., Duboeuf, F., Brun, J., Crouzet, B., Arnaud, S. *et al.* (1992). Vitamin D_3 and calcium to prevent hip fractures in elderly women. *New Engl J Med*, **327**, 1637–42.

Chesnut, C. H., Ivey, J. L., Gruber, H. E. *et al.* (1987). Stanozolol in postmenopausal osteoporosis: therapeutic efficacy and possible mechanisms of action. *Metabolism*, **29**, 559–62.

Christiansen, C., Riis, B. J. & Rodbro, P. (1987). Prediction of rapid bone loss in postmenopausal women. *Lancet*, **1**, 1105–8.

Cohn, S. H., Abesamis, C., Yasumura, S., Aloia, J. F., Sanzi, I. & Ellis, K. J. (1977). Comparative skeletal mass and radial bone mineral content in black and white women. *Metabolism*, **26**, 171–8.

Compston, J. E., Vedi, S. & Croucher, P. I. (1991). Low prevalence of osteomalacia in elderly patients with hip fracture. *Age Ageing*, **20**, 132–4.

Compston, J. E. (1992). Risk factors for osteoporosis. *Clin Endocrinol*, **36**, 223–4.

Cooper, C., Barker, D. J. P. & Wickham, C. (1988). Physical activity, muscle strength, and calcium intake in fracture of the proximal femur in Britain. *Br Med J*, **297**, 1443–6.

Davidson, B. J., Ross, R. K., Paganini-Hill, A., Hammond, G. D., Siiteri, P. K. & Judd, H. L. (1982). Total and free estrogens and androgens in postmenopausal women with hip fractures. *J Clin Endocrinol Metab*, **54**, 115–20.

De Vernejoul, M. C., Bielakoff, J., Herve, M. *et al.* (1983). Evidence for defective osteoblastic function. A role for alcohol and tobacco consumption in osteoporosis in middle-aged men. *Clin Orthop*, **179**, 107–15.

Dunnigan, M. C., McIntosh, W. B., Ford, J. A. & Robertson, I. (1982). Acquired disorders of vitamin D metabolism. In *Clinical Endocrinology 2: Calcium Disorders*, ed. D. A. Heath & S. J. Marx, pp. 125–50. London, Boston, Sydney, Wellington, Durban, Toronto: Butterworths.

Evans, J. G. (1987). Epidemiology of osteoporosis and fractures of the femoral neck. *Int Med*, (Suppl. 12): 4–6.

Felson, D. T., Zhang, Y., Hannon, M. T., Kiel, D. P., Wilson, P. W. F. & Anderson, J. J. (1993). The effect of postmenopausal estrogen therapy on bone density in elderly women. *New Engl J Med*, **329**, 1141–6.

Francis, R. M. (1990). The pathogenesis of osteoporosis. In *Osteoporosis: Pathogenesis and Management*, ed. R. M. Francis, pp. 51–80. Lancaster: Kluwer.

Francis, R. M., Peacock, M. & Barkworth, S. A. (1984). Renal impairment and its effects on calcium metabolism in elderly women. *Age Ageing*, **13**, 14–20.

Francis, R. M., Selby, P. L., Rodgers, A. & Davison, C. E. (1990). The management of osteoporosis. In *Osteoporosis: Pathogenesis and Management*, ed. R. M. Francis, pp. 145–79. Lancaster: Kluwer.

Francis, R. M. & Sutcliffe, A. M. (1990). Implications of osteoporotic fractures in the elderly. In *HRT and Osteoporosis*, ed. J.O. Studd & J. W. W., pp. 87–99. Berlin: Springer-Verlag.

Goldsmith, N. F. & Johnston, J. O. (1975). Bone mineral: effects of oral contraceptives, pregnancy and lactation. *J Bone Joint Surg*, **57A**, 657–68.

Greatorex, I. F. (1986). Femoral neck fractures: improving efficiency in the case of elderly women. *Commun Med*, **8**, 185–90.

Heaney, R. P., Recker, R. R. & Saville, P. D. (1978). Menopausal changes in calcium balance performance. *J Lab Clin Med*, **92**, 953–63.

Heikinheimo, R. J., Inkovaara, J. A., Harju, E. J., Haavisto, M. V., Kaarela, R. H., Kataja, J. M. *et al.* (1992). Annual injection of Vitamin D and fractures of aged bones. *Calcif Tissue Int*, **51**, 105–10.

Hordon, L. D. & Peacock, M. (1990). Osteomalacia and osteoporosis in femoral neck fracture. *Bone Mineral*, **11**, 247–59.

Jensen, J., Christiansen, C. & Rodbro, P. (1985). Cigarette smoking, serum estrogens and bone loss during hormone-replacement therapy early after menopause. *New Engl J Med*, **313**, 973–5.

Jensen, J. S. & Bagger, J. (1982). Long-term social prognosis after hip fractures. *Acta Orthop Scand*, **53**, 97–101.

Jick, H., Porter, J. & Morrison, A. S. (1977). Relation between smoking and the age of natural menopause. *Lancet*, **1**, 1354–5.

Johnston, C. C. Jr, Miller, J. Z. Slemenda, C. W., Reister, T. K., Hui, S., Christian, J. C. & Peacock, M. (1992). Calcium supplementation and increases in bone mineral density in children. *New Engl J Med*, **327**, 82–7.

Kanders, B., Dempster, D. W. & Lindsay, R. (1988). Interaction of calcium nutrition and physical activity on bone mass in young women. *J Bone Min Res*, **3**, 145–9.

Kiel, D. P., Felson, D. T., Anderson, J. J., Wilson, P. W. F. & Moskovitz, M. A. (1987). Hip fractures and the use of estrogen in postmenopausal women. *New Engl J Med*, **317**, 1169–74.

Kleerekoper, M., Peterson, E. L., Nelson, D. A. *et al.* (1991). A randomized trial of sodium fluoride as a treatment for postmenopausal osteoporosis. *Osteoporosis Int*, **1**, 155–61.

Krolner, B. & Toft, B. (1983). Vertebral bone loss: an unheeded effect of therapeutic bed rest. *Clin Sci*, **64**, 537–40.

Krolner, B., Toft, B., Pors Nielsen, S. & Tondevold, E. (1983). Physical exercise as prophylaxis against involutional bone loss: a controlled trial. *Clin Sci*, **64**, 541–6.

Lau, E., Donnan, S., Barker, D. J. P. & Cooper, C. (1988). Physical activity and calcium intake in fracture of the proximal femur in Hong Kong. *Br Med J*, **297**, 1441–3.

Liberman, U. A., Weiss, S. R., Broll, J. *et al.* (1995). Effect of oral alendronate on bone mineral density and the incidence of fractures in postmenopausal osteoporosis. *New Engl J Med*, **333**, 1437–43.

Lindsay, R. & Tohme, J. (1990). Estrogen treatment of patients with established postmenopausal osteoporosis. *Obstet Gynecol*, **76**, 1–6.

Lufkin, E. G., Wahner, H. W., O'Fallon, W. M. *et al.* (1992). Treatment of postmenopausal osteoporosis with transdermal estrogen. *Ann Intern Med*, **117**, 1–9.

Mazess, R. B. (1982). On aging bone loss. *Clin Orthop*, **165**, 239–52.

Mazzuoli, G. F., Passeri, M., Gennari, C. *et al.* (1986). Effects of salmon calcitonin in postmenopausal osteoporosis: a controlled double-blind clinical study. *Calif Tissue Int*, **38**, 3–8.

Melton, L. J. III, Chrischilles, E. A., Cooper, C., Lane, A. W. & Riggs, B. L. (1992). Perspective: how many women have osteoporosis? *J Bone Min Res*, **9**, 1005–10.

Morrison, N. A., Qi, J. C., Tokita, A., Kelly, P. J., Crofts, L., Nguyen, T. V., Sambrook, P. N. & Eisman, J. A. (1994). Prediction of bone density from vitamin D receptor alleles. *Nature*, **367**, 284–7.

Nilson, B. E. & Westlin, N. E. (1971). Bone density in athletes. *Clin Orthop*, **77**, 179–82.

Nordin, B. E. C., Horsman, A., Crilly, R. G., Marshall, D. H. & Simpson, M. (1980). Treatment of spinal osteoporosis in postmenopausal woman. *Br Med J*, **280**, 451–4.

Obrant, K. J., Bengner, U., Johnell, O., Nillson, B. E. & Sernbo, I. (1989). Increasing age-adjusted risk of fragility fractures: a sign of increasing osteoporosis in successive generations? *Calcif Tissue Int*, **44**, 157–67.

Orimo, H., Shiraki, M., Hayashi, Y. *et al.* (1994). Effects of 1α-Hydoxyvitamin D$_3$ on lumbar bone mineral density and vertebral fractures in patients with postmenopausal osteoporosis. *Calcif Tissue Int*, **54**, 370–6.

Pak, C. Y. C., Sakhaee, K., Adams-Huet, B., Piziak, V., Peterson, R. D. & Poindexter, J. R. (1995). Treatment of postmenopausal osteoporosis with slow-release sodium fluoride. Final report of a randomized controlled trial. *Ann Int Med*, **123**, 401–8.

Peacock, M. (1984). Osteomalacia. In *Metabolic Bone and Stone Disease*. 2nd edn, ed. B. E. C. Nordin, pp. 71–111. Edinburgh, London, Melbourne, New York: Churchill Livingstone.

Prince, R. L., Smith, M., Dick, I. M. *et al.* (1991). Prevention of postmenopausal osteoporosis, a comparative study of exercise, calcium supplementation and hormone-replacement therapy. *New Engl J Med*, **325**, 1189–95.

Reginster, J. Y., Denis, J. D., Albert, A. *et al.* (1987). 1-Year controlled randomised trial of prevention of early postmenopausal bone loss by intranasal calcitonin. *Lancet*, **2**, 1481–83.

Reid, D. M. (1990). Corticosteroid osteoporosis. In *Osteoporosis: Parthogenesis and Management*, ed. R. M. Francis, pp. 103–44. Lancaster: Kluwer.

Reid, I. R., Ames, R. W., Evans, M. C. *et al.* (1993). Effect of calcium supplementation on bone loss in postmenopausal women. *New Engl J Med*, **328**, 460–4.

Rico, H., Henandez, E. R., Revilla, M. & Gomez-Castresana, F. (1992). Salmon calcitonin reduces vertebral fracture rate in postmenopausal crush fracture syndrome. *Bone Mineral*, **16**, 131–8.

Riggs, B. L., Hodgson, S. F., O'Fallon, W. M. *et al.* (1990). Effect of fluoride treatment on the fracture rate in postmenopausal women with osteoporosis. *New Engl J Med*, **322**, 802–9.

Riggs, B. L. & Melton, L. J. III. (1986). Involutional osteoporosis. *New Engl J Med*, **314**, 1676–86.

Riggs, B. L., Wahner, H. W., Melton, L. J. III, Richelson, L. S., Judd, H. L. & O'Fallon, W. M. (1987). Dietary calcium intake and rates of bone loss in women. *Clin Invest*, **80**, 979–82.

Scane, A. C. & Francis, R. M. (1993). Risk factors for osteoporosis in men. *Clin Endocrinol*, **38**, 15–16.

Seeman, E., Hopper, J. L., Bach, L. A. *et al.* (1989). Reduced bone mass in daughters of women with osteoporosis. *New Engl J Med*, **320**, 554–8.

Smith, D. M., Nance, W. E., Kang, K. W., Christian, J. C., Johnston, C. C. Jr. (1973). Genetic factors in determining bone mass. *J Clin Invest*, **52**, 2800–8.

Stampfer, M. J., Colditz, G. A., Willett, W. C. *et al.* (1991). Postmenopausal estrogen therapy and cardiovascular disease. Ten-years follow up from the Nurses' Health Study. *New Engl J Med*, **325**, 756–62.

Stevenson, J. C., Cust, M. P., Gangar, K. F., Hillard, T. C., Lees, B. & Whitehead, M. I. (1990). Effects of transdermal versus oral hormone replacement therapy on bone density in spine and proximal femur in postmenopausal women. *Lancet*, **336**, 265–9.

Stevenson, J. C., Lees, B., Devenport, M., Cust, M. P. & Ganger, K. F. (1989). Determinants of bone density in normal women: risk factors for future osteoporosis. *Br Med J*, **298**, 924–8.

Stevenson, J. C., Whitehead, M. I., Padwick, M. *et al.* (1988). Dietary intake of calcium and postmenopausal bone loss. *Br Med J*, **297**, 15–17.

Storm, T., Thamsborg, G., Steiniche, T., Genant, H. K. & Sorensen, O. H. (1990). Effect of intermittent cyclical etidronate therapy on bone mass and fracture rate in women with post-menopausal osteoporosis. *New Engl J Med*, **322**, 1265–71.

Thomas, T. G. & Stevens, R. S. (1974). Social effects of fractures of the neck of femur. *Br Med J*, **3**, 456–8.

Tilyard, M. W., Spears, G. F. S., Thomson, J. & Dovey, S. (1992). Treatment of postmenopausal osteoporosis with calcitriol or calcium. *New Engl J Med*, **326**, 357–62.

Wallace, W. A. (1987). The scale and financial implications of osteoporosis. *Int Med*, (Suppl. **12**), 3–43.

Watts, N. B., Harris, S. T., Genant, H. K. *et al.* (1990). Intermittent cyclical etidronate treatment of postmenopausal osteoporosis. *New Engl J Med*, **323**, 73–9.

Weiss, N. S., Ure, C. L., Ballard, J. H., Williams, A. R. & Darling, J. R. (1980). Decreased risk of fracture of the hip and lower forearm with postmenopausal use of estrogen. *New Engl J Med*, **303**, 1195–8.

7
Thermoregulation, nutrition and injury in the elderly

S. P. ALLISON

Introduction

Each winter, the media report the plight of the elderly in the cold weather, and we are assailed by generalisations on the subject and by slogans such as 'The old and the cold'. This chapter attempts a more precise definition of the problem with particular reference to the interrelations between thermoregulation, nutrition and injury among those over the age of 65 years. The reported number of cases and deaths (600 per annum) from environmentally induced hypothermia per se in the UK is remarkably small even in the coldest winters, and many of these may be caused by other significant clinical conditions (Keatinge, 1986; Collins, 1987). A study of all new patients entering a London casualty department during January and February 1986 also failed to show a widespread incidence of hypothermia, defined as a core temperature of less than 35 °C (Coleshaw et al., 1986; Keatinge, 1986). Only three patients (0.04% of all admissions) were identified as suffering from hypothermia, one with a stroke, one with dementia and another with a fractured femur. Frank hypothermia (less than 35 °C) may be rare, but it is possible that quite minor falls in core temperature in the 35–37 °C range may significantly impair function and be clinically important. During the extra-ordinarily cold winter of 1981 when the outdoor temperature in the UK reached a nadir of −15 °C, Bastow and colleagues studied the elderly population admitted with fractured femur in Nottingham within 4 hours of injury. Using the aural thermistor technique, they found, among 100 patients, 37 with a core temperature of more than 36 °C, 38 with a temperature of 35–36 °C and 25 who were below 35 °C. Furthermore, they found the thinnest or most undernourished patients to be most heavily represented among those with the lowest core temperatures. They postulated a relation between nutritional state and thermoregulation and that small drops in core temperature, by causing impairment of mental function and physical coordination, might be an aetiological factor in domestic accidents. The majority (80%) of the thinnest patients suffered their injuries indoors. The reported incidence of hypothermia may well vary according to: (1) the cut-off point used, i.e. less than 35 °C, less than 36 °C or simply small reductions in the 36–37 °C range, (2) the method used to measure core temperature, (3) the population studied, and (4) the prevailing weather conditions. In this chapter I set out first the arguments for regarding small changes in core temperature as clinically significant. Second, I outline the normal mechanisms by which the normal body temperature is maintained, and third, I address the ways in which these mechanisms may be impaired among the elderly, with particular reference to the effects of nutrition and injury. I focus largely on the clinical consequences of changes in core temperature, rather than problems such as the increased winter incidence of acute cardiovascular or respiratory disease which may be related to cold stimuli to the peripheries and may be unrelated to changes in core temperature.

Potential significance of small reductions in core temperature

Formal studies have been conducted largely on young, fit subjects, for obvious reasons; but if impaired physiological function can be demonstrated in such subjects, how much more may the elderly be affected?

Following concern over the excessive numbers of apparently accidental deaths among deep sea divers, Keatinge and colleagues explored the possibilities that such accidents might have been caused by a loss of judgement secondary to minor degrees of hypothermia (Hayward & Keatinge, 1979; Keatinge *et al.*, 1980; Coleshaw *et al.*, 1983; Keatinge, 1986). He found that when body temperatures of volunteers were lowered experimentally by immersion in cold water, at 36 °C or below memory was impaired and there was a marked slowing of the speed at which complex reasoning tasks could be performed. When Pugh and Edholm (1955) studied swimmers crossing the Channel, they found that despite a water temperature of 15 °C, most were able to maintain a normal core temperature. The two major factors responsible for this were a thick layer of fat, preventing heat loss, and the increased heat production from exercise. When they examined those who failed to complete the race, they found less fat and a body temperature of 35–35.5 °C. This small drop in temperature was sufficient to cause confusion, loss of judgement and hallucinations. Similar observations have been made on hill walkers suffering from exposure and on motor cyclists wearing insufficient clothing to prevent heat loss due to the chill factor of wind. Other studies have shown muscle strength and function to be impaired when limbs are cooled (Bergh & Ekblom, 1979; Davies & Young, 1983). Berg and Ekblom, relating peak torque during knee extensions, maximal speed during bicycling and height of the vertical jump at different vastus lateralis temperatures, found a linear relation with significant decline in muscle function in the range of 37–35 °C and lower. These limb temperatures can easily be achieved by the elderly in a cold environment. When muscle strength and mobility are marginal this may result in falls. There are, therefore, sound theoretical reasons for suggesting that small changes in body temperature may have significant effects, particularly in the elderly, where the margin between coping and collapse may be small. There is a clear need for further research in this area.

Normal physiology

Response to cold

Changes in the heat content and hence the temperature of the body depend on the balance between heat production and heat loss. Normally, humans control heat loss by appropriate behavioural responses such as wearing more or fewer clothes or turning the central heating up or down. Increased heat production can also be stimulated by exercise. Such responses depend on being able to sense the need to respond and having the mental capacity to do so. Elderly people, however, are often slow to react appropriately in order to counteract changes in their thermal environment (Wagner *et al.*, 1974; Collins *et al.*, 1981; Collins and Exton-Smith, 1983; Collins, 1986, 1987). When behavioural responses are insufficient, we become dependent on physiological responses to increase heat production and decrease heat loss. Cold sensors in the exposed hands and face provide afferent stimuli to the autonomic centre in the hypothalamus to increase thermogenesis and to cause vasoconstriction to conserve heat in the core rather than losing it from the skin by the physical processes of radiation, convection, conduction and latent heat of evaporation. An adequate covering of fat provides additional insulation and protection against hypothermia as shown in studies on divers and swimmers. The most obvious example of a relation between nutritional status and thermoregulation is seen when one compares a small thin old lady of 40 kg with a taller and fatter one of 80 kg. The latter is not only better insulated but has a much greater volume to surface ratio, which, by the laws of physics, diminishes the rate of change of core temperature in response to the environment.

The last bastion of thermoregulatory defence is provided by the temperature sensors in the carotid artery territory. A fall in core temperature of only 0.1 °C can cause increased thermogenesis and vasoconstriction. To understand thermogenesis, it is necessary to analyse its components. Resting metabolic expenditure, which declines by approximately 10% with age, as measured by oxygen consumption (normally 100 kJ/kg per day = 24 kcal/kg per day), is determined by intrinsic metabolic activity, by the thyroid and other hormones, and by sympathetic nervous tone. Both exercise and sympathetic stimulation increase thermogenesis, as does exposure to cold or to infection and inflammation. The response to cold may be divided into shivering and non-shivering thermogenesis. The former can cause a fivefold increase in thermogenesis from muscle. Non-shivering thermogenesis in animals and infants is dependent on sympathetic nervous stimulation of brown fat, but this can only account for 5% of the response in adult humans, where it may be related to increased metabolic activity in liver and muscle.

Response to food

Apart from exercise and exposure to cold, the other important stimulus to increased thermogenesis is that of food (Elia *et al.*, 1988). The response to oral ingestion or intravenous infusion of food substrates has been divided into obligatory and facultative components.

Obligatory thermogenesis (sometimes known as the specific dynamic action of food) results from the energy expended in the digestion, assimilation and storage of substrates taken by mouth or the transport and storage of intravenously administered substrates such as glucose. Ingestion of a mixed meal is associated with a 15% increase in metabolic rate. Approximately 5% of the energy content of the ingested meal is used up for obligatory purposes.

Facultative thermogenesis describes the increment in food-induced thermogenesis not accounted for by obligatory costs. It may represent an element of inefficiency or burning off of excess, or it may be a necessary increase in metabolism to supply substrates, e.g. for cell replication and growth. The idea that this excess consumption is mediated by sympathetic drive has recently been challenged, and it may well be a complex product of intrinsic metabolic and hormonal mechanisms.

Thermogenesis in humans is therefore determined by the daily metabolic rate which is approximately 1.4 times the resting level, the difference being due to the thermic effects of food and exercise. Heat loss is limited by the insulation provided by clothing, subcutaneous fat and cutaneous vasoconstrictor responses. Changes in both behavioural and physiological responses may therefore affect thermoregulation and be of particular relevance to the elderly.

Methods of measurement

Metabolic rate and heat production are usually measured by indirect calorimetry; gas exchange from a canopy hood can be measured at frequent intervals and the response to different stimuli, e.g. cold or food, can be measured with considerable accuracy. Oral or underarm measurements clearly underestimate the core temperature. Oesophageal temperature probes provide an accurate picture but are not practical for routine use.

The most reliable practical methods are either a thermoelectric rectal probe placed at an adequate depth (>80 mm) or the aural thermistor method devised by Keatinge & Sloan (1975). This latter arrangement, looking like a pair of ear muffs, correlates well with oesophageal temperatures. The technique of measuring the temperature of urine, just voided, has been useful in epidemiological surveys of large numbers. Reports of changes in body temperature or thermoregulation must be assessed with these methodological differences in mind.

Effects on thermoregulation of ageing

This controversial subject has been well reviewed by Keatinge (1986) and Collins (1987). Reports have differed on whether aging per se, in the absence of disease, prolonged fasting or nutritional depletion, is associated with defects in thermoregulation. The balance of evidence is that some of the elderly population at least have age-related impairment in their physiological responses to protect them against the effects of cold. Basal metabolic rate falls by about 10% between the ages of 20 and 70 years. Evidence also suggests that shivering responses are reduced and that cold adaptation is also impaired. Diminished activity and body mass may also lower daily heat production. For these reasons, the World Health Organisation (WHO, 1987) has recommended a minimum indoor temperature of 18 °C for most of the population, but a temperature 2–3 °C warmer for rooms occupied by elderly persons. Surveys in the UK during the 1970s (Fox et al., 1973; Hunt & Gidman, 1981) found that houses occupied by elderly people were colder than average. Extremely cold winters or intercurrent illness, e.g. stroke, may be necessary to induce significant hypothermia. An increased incidence of illnesses such as respiratory tract infections may, however, be induced when indoor temperatures fall below 20 °C. An analysis of death rates and environmental temperatures in the UK and the USA (Bull & Moreton, 1975; WHO, 1987) has shown that deaths from heart attacks, strokes and respiratory infections increase linearly as the outdoor temperature falls from 20 to 10 °C. There is, therefore, ample scope for improving health and diminishing demand on hospital services by better insulation and heating of houses.

Effects on thermoregulation of nutritional state

Two observations stimulated our interest in this field. The first was the observation by Gale et al. (1981) that thermogenesis could be inhibited by a fall in blood glucose levels, and second that of Bastow et al. (1983), described above, of the relation between thinness, low body temperature and increased admission rate with fractured femur during cold weather. Protocols were devised to explore the separate influences of weight loss or thinness on the one hand and the effect of short and long periods of fasting in normal weight subjects. The thermoregulatory responses to cold, adrenaline infusion and food were measured under these two different circumstances. Thermogenesis was measured by indirect calorimetry, and vasoconstriction in the forearm and hand was measured separately by the venous occlusion plethysmography and strain gauge techniques. A cold stimulus was applied to the body using a water perfused suit. In other studies adrenaline was infused to achieve elevated blood levels within the normal range. The response to food was measured in some studies using a mixed meal by mouth and in others by infusing glucose intravenously using the insulin-glucose clamp technique.

Elderly women recovering from fractured femur, of average age 82 years and a body weight, mid-arm circumference and triceps skinfold thickness within one standard deviation of the reference range, in response to a drop in suit temperature from 35 to 23 °C, had an increase in thermogenesis and vasoconstriction indistinguishable from that seen in young medical students. On the other hand, those who were more than one standard deviation below the mean of the anthropometric reference range showed impaired thermogenesis, even in the face of a small fall (0.1 °C) in core temperature (Fellows *et al.*, 1985). Their vasoconstrictor responses were unimpaired. Weight loss in younger subjects induces the same effect. This means that not only are such changes in thermoregulation related to nutritional status rather than age, but the mechanisms involved can be elucidated by studies on younger subjects with fewer ethical problems. A series of investigations carried out in the physiology laboratory in Nottingham (Fellows *et al.*, 1985; Mansell *et al.*, 1988a,b) showed the following. (1) Even in very thin individuals who had lost their thermogenic response to cold, the thermogenic response to adrenaline was intact, which suggests that changes had occurred in central control mechanisms rather than in peripheral tissue responsiveness. (2) The thermogenic response to cold could be restored by weight gain towards normal. (3) Starvation for 48 hours or more in normal weight individuals caused loss of vasoconstrictor or heat retaining responses to cold, but had only a small effect on thermogenic response. Weight loss and short-term food deprivation, therefore, produce defects in thermoregulation by different mechanisms which may summate in the sick elderly to produce an even greater disposition to develop hypothermia which, although mild in degree, may be of clinical significance.

Effects on thermoregulation of injury, anaesthesia and surgery

Little & Stoner (1981) measured core and skin temperatures in 82 patients shortly after accidental injuries of differing severity and found falls in these parameters commensurate with the severity of injury. They proposed that the initial fall in skin temperature was caused by vasoconstrictor responses to injury and were unrelated to treatment. Decreases in core temperature appeared to be a feature of particularly severe injury and to be related to interference with central control mechanisms causing inhibition of thermogenesis. Despite falls in core temperature, severely ill patients failed to shiver, which suggests a raised threshold for this response in such patients. In a series of studies, Carli and his colleagues (1986, 1989, 1991) described the tendency of patients to become mildly hypothermic during surgery, confirming earlier findings by Brock (1975).

Summary and conclusions

Among the elderly, frank hypothermia (less than 35 °C) may be infrequent, but minor degrees of hypothermia in the range 35–37 °C are more common and may be clinically significant. Minor falls in core temperature are associated with deterioration in cerebral and neuromuscular function which may predispose to accident and acute illness. Ambient indoor temperatures below 20 °C are also associated with an increase in cardiorespiratory disorders among the elderly. Aging per se, low body weight, starvation for more than 48 hours and injury all have deleterious effects on thermoregulatory mechanisms and predispose to a fall in core temperature in the face of low ambient temperatures. As well as being a possible aetiological factor in some injuries, mild hypothermia may complicate illness as the injured elderly patient may be exposed to a number of thermal strains during treatment, i.e. prolonged periods on couches or trolleys in the casualty department, anaesthesia, inadequate thermal protection during and after surgery, opening of body cavities and infusion with cold fluids. Those caring for such patients should be aware of the problem, have adequate monitoring facilities and take appropriate precautions.

References

Bastow, M. D., Rawlings, J. & Allison, S. P. (1983). Undernutrition, hypothermia and injury in elderly women with fractured femur: an injury response to altered metabolism? *Lancet*, **1**, 143–6.

Berg, U. & Ekblom, B. (1979). Influence of muscle temperature on maximal muscle strength and power output in human skeletal muscles. *Acta Physiol Scand*, **1078**, 33–7.

Lord Brock (1975). The importance of environmental conditions, especially temperature, in the operating room and intensive care ward. *Br J Surg*, **62**, 253–8.

Bull, G. M. & Moreton, J. (1975). Relationships of temperature with death rates from all causes and from certain respiratory and arteriosclerotic diseases in different age groups. *Age Ageing*, **4**, 432–46.

Carli, F., Emery, P. W. & Freemantle, C. A. J. (1989). Effect of perioperative normothermia on postoperative protein metabolism in elderly patients undergoing hip arthroplasty. *Br J*

Anaesth, **63**, 276–82.

Carli, F., Gabrielczyk, M., Clark, M. M. & Aber, V. R. (1986). An investigation of factors affecting post-operative re-warming of adult patients. *Anaesthesia*, **41**, 363–9.

Carli, F., Webster, J., Pearson, M., Forrest, J., Venkatesan, S., Wenham, D. & Halliday, D. (1991). Postoperative protein metabolism: effect of nursing elderly patients for 24 hours after abdominal surgery in a thermoneutral environment. *Br J Anaesth*, **66**, 292–9.

Coleshaw, S. R. K., Easton, J. C., Keatinge, W. R., Floyer, M. A. & Garrard, J. (1986). Hypothermia in emergency admissions in cold weather. *Clin Sci*, **70** (Suppl. 13), 93.

Coleshaw, S. R. K., van Someren, R. N. M., Wolff, A. H., Davis, H. M. & Keatinge, W. R. (1983). Imparied memory registration and speed of reasoning caused by low body temperature. *J Appl Physiol*, **55**, 27–31.

Collins, K. J. (1986). Low indoor temperatures and morbidity in the elderly. *Age Ageing*, **15**, 212–20.

Collins, K. J. (1987). Effects of cold on old people. *Br J Hosp Med*, **38**, 506–14.

Collins, K. J. & Exton-Smith, A. N. (1983). Thermal homeostasis in old age. *J Am Geriatr Soc*, **31**, 519–24.

Collins, K. J., Exton-Smith, A. N. & Doré, C. (1981). Urban hypothermia: preferred temperature and thermal perception in old age. *Br Med J*, **282**, 175–7.

Davies, C. T. M. & Young, K. (1983). Effect of temperature on the contractile properties and muscle power of triceps surae in humans. *J Appl Physiol*, **55**, 191–5.

Elia, M., Folmer, P., Schlatman, A., Goren, A. & Austin, S. (1988). Carbohydrate, fat and protein metabolism in muscle and in the whole body after mixed meal ingestion. *Metabolism*, **37**, 547–51.

Fellows, I. W., Macdonald, I. A., Bennett, T. & Allison, S. P. (1985). The effect of undernutrition on thermoregulation in the elderly. *Clin Sci*, **69**, 525–32.

Fox, R. H., Woodward, P. M., Exton-Smith, A. N., Green, M. F., Donnison, D. V. & Wicks, M. H. (1973). Body temperatures in the elderly: a national study of physiological, social and environmental conditions. *Br Med J*, **1**, 200–6.

Gale, E. A. M., Bennett, T., Green, H. J. & Macdonald, I. A. (1981). Hypothermia, hypoglycaemia and shivering in man. *Clin Sci*, **61**, 463–9.

Hayward, M. G. & Keatinge, W. R. (1979). Progressive symptomless hypothermia in water. Possible cause of diving accident. *Br Med J*, **1**, 1182.

Hunt, D. R. G. & Gidman, M. I. (1981). A national field survey of house temperatures. *Build Environ*, **17**, 175–7.

Keatinge, W. R. (1986). Medical problems of cold weather. *J R Coll Phys*, **20**, 283–7.

Keatinge, W. R., Hayward, M. G. & McIver, N. K. I. (1980). Hypothermia during saturation diving in the North Sea. *Br Med J*, **1**, 280–91.

Keatinge, W. R. & Sloan, R. E. G. (1975). Deep body temperature from the aural canal with servo-controlled heating to the outer ear. *J Appl Physiol*, **38**, 919–21.

Little, R. A. & Stoner, H. B. (1981). Body temperature after accidental injury. *Br J Surg*, **68**, 221–4.

Mansell, P. I. (1988a). Undernutrition, refeeding and thermogenesis. In *Clinical Progress in Nutritional Research*, ed. A. Sitges-Serra, A. Sitges-Creus & S. Schwartz-Riera, pp. 280–1. Basel: Karger.

Mansell, P. I., Fellows, I. W., Macdonald, I. A. & Allison, S. P. (1988b). The syndrome of undernutrition and hypothermia: its pathophysiology and clinical importance. *Q J Med*, **69**, 842–3.

Pugh, L. G. C. & Edholm, O. G. (1955). The physiology of Channel swimmers. *Lancet*, **2**, 761–8.

Wagner, J. A., Robinson, S. & Marino, R. P. (1974). Age and temperature regulation of humans in neutral and cold environments. *J Appl Physiol*, **37**, 562–5.

WHO Environmental Health Series. (1987). *Health Impact of Low Indoor Temperatures.* World Health Organization. Regional Office for Europe, Copenhagen.

8

Aging and the febrile response

P. J. L. M. STRIJBOS, N. J. ROTHWELL and
M. A. HORAN

Introduction

The association between an increased body temperature and disease has been known since antiquity and this 'febrile response' remains an important diagnostic sign. The suggestion that the 'febrile response' is attenuated in old age can also be traced to ancient times. Hippocrates in his 'Aphorisms' states 'old men have little innate heat, and for this reason they need but little fuel; too much fuel puts it out. For this reason too, the fevers of old men are less acute than others, for the body is cold'. Although our knowledge of the existence and diagnostic importance of fever has a long history, our understanding of the underlying mechanisms has made little progress until the last decade or so. Furthermore, it remains a matter of conjecture whether fever is a beneficial or harmful host response. Older texts have almost uniformly considered it harmful and have recommended the use of antipyretic drugs; however, in the pre-antibiotic era, the same books would recommend fever therapy (achieved with malaria-carrying mosquitos) as an effective cure for syphilis. The balance of current evidence is heavily weighted in favour of benefit (Mackowiak, 1994).

In this chapter, we provide a summary of current thinking on the pathogenesis of fever, to discuss the evidence about whether fever may be beneficial or harmful and discuss how the ability to mount a fever response might be modified during aging.

Definition and mechanisms of fever

Fever may be defined as a condition in which the thermoregulatory set-point is acutely elevated, thus distinguishing it from passive hyperthermia due to heat gain from the environment or an increased heat loss (Szekely et al., 1973), and from the cyclical changes in thermoregulatory set-point that occur through the menstrual cycle. The definition is important because many experimental studies have recorded fever simply by measuring body temperature without trying to distinguish regulated increases in temperature from passive ones.

Mechanisms of heat gain

The increase in temperature that characterises fever may result from reducing heat loss and/or increasing heat production. Heat loss may be reduced by behavioural means (huddling together, wearing extra clothes, turning up the heating, etc.), vasoconstriction (particularly at peripheral sites) and piloerection. Increased heat production (thermogenesis) results from shivering or from sympathetic nervous system-mediated, non-shivering thermogenesis. Shivering is an inefficient and uncomfortable means of raising body temperature and non-shivering thermogenesis seems to predominate, especially in small or young animals, including children (Girardier, 1983). Extensive studies in experimental animals have indicated that increased rates of heat production resulting from infection, injury, inflammation, brain ischaemia or endotoxin infusion are caused by activation of the sympathetic nervous system (SNS) and thermogenesis in brown adipose tissue (BAT) (Coombes *et al.*, 1987; Cooper *et al.*, 1989a,b; Rothwell, 1991a). This tissue is also responsible for thermogenic responses to cold exposure or dietary modification (Himms-Hagen, 1986; Rothwell & Stock, 1986). Local release of noradrenaline from nerves supplying BAT interacts with a β_3-adrenoreceptor resulting in controlled uncoupling of oxidative phosphorylation by a unique mitochondrial proton conductance pathway (Arch *et al.*, 1984; Nicholls & Locke, 1984). The contribution of BAT to thermogenesis in humans is still debatable. Significant amounts are found in neonates and infants, but the amount declines through adult life (Lean *et al.*, 1986); however, functional BAT has been detected at least up to the age of 80 years.

Afferent signals

The concept that exogenous pyrogens (e.g. microorganisms) caused fever through an indirect mechanism involving an endogenous pyrogen (i.e. an agent produced by the host) was first suggested by Welch (1888). The first contender for the role of endogenous pyrogen was interleukin 1 (IL-1), a cytokine produced by mononuclear phagocytes and many other cell types, including glial cells in the brain (Fontana *et al.*, 1984; Guilian *et al.*, 1986; Higgins & Olschwowka, 1991; Dinarello, 1994; Hopkins & Rothwell, 1995). Several other cytokines (IL-2, IL-6, IL-8, tumour necrosis factor-α (TNF-α), interferons -α and -γ) can also induce fever and have been proposed as endogenous pyrogens (Rothwell, 1990; Kluger, 1991; Rothwell & Hopkins, 1995). These molecules may enter the general circulation and act on or enter the brain (probably at sites that lack a significant blood–brain barrier) to induce synthesis of eicosanoids (Bernheim & Dinarello, 1985; Morimoto *et al.*, 1987; Morimoto *et al.*, 1988a,b; Nakashima *et al.*, 1988). The relative importance of these cytokines and the means by which they signal to the brain to induce fever remain speculative (Coceani *et al.*, 1988; Kluger, 1991; Rothwell & Hopkins, 1995). Interleukin 1 in the circulation is usually undetectable or present in a low concentration, while IL-6 concentrations increase markedly and are strongly associated with the increase in body temperature (Nijsten *et al.*, 1987; LeMay *et al.*, 1990a,b; Miller *et al.*, 1995a,b). Experiments using neutralising antibodies to various cytokines suggest only IL-1β and IL-6 play physiological roles in the generation of fever (Rothwell, 1990; Kluger, 1991; Rothwell & Hopkins, 1995), thus supporting the suggestion by Neta *et al.* (1988) that IL-1 acts locally in the periphery to induce IL-6 as an endogenous circulating pyrogen. There is evidence that TNF-α may act as an endogenous antipyretic agent (Long *et al.*, 1990), although this is controversial, as several other reports indicate that both exogenous and endogenous TNF-α cause fever (e.g. Cooper *et al.*, 1994). Furthermore, early in the inflammatory response to exogenous agents or tissue damage, numerous other factors are generated (e.g. eicosanoids, platelet activating factor, substance P, histamine, etc.) and may modulate the complex pattern of cytokine production. Neural afferent signals can also signal from the periphery to the brain during systemic inflammation, as early febrile responses to localised hind limb inflammation in the rat are inhibited by destruction of c-fibre afferents and there is now considerable evidence that vagal afferents mediate diverse responses to systemic cytokines or lipopolysaccharides (LPS), including fever (Hopkins & Rothwell, 1995).

Central nervous system mechanisms

The pyrogenic cytokines described above can all act directly within the brain to induce fever and several have been shown to alter the firing rate of thermosensitive neurons in the preoptic anterior hypothalamus (POAH) (Hori *et al.*, 1984; Rothwell, 1990). Although the POAH is undoubtedly involved in temperature regulation and the development of fever, numerous other brain areas (ventromedial and paraventricular hypothalamus, organum vasculosum of the lamina terminalis, pons, medulla) are responsive to pyrogens (Blatteis & Hunter, 1987; Morimoto *et al.*, 1988a,b).

The synthesis of eicosanoids, particularly prostaglandins, is essential for the development of most forms of fever. Cyclooxygenase inhibitors attenuate experimentally-induced fever and are in wide clinical use as antipyretics. The pyrogenic actions of most cytokines (with the exception of IL-8 and MIP-1) are also inhibited by prior administration of cyclooxygenase inhibitors and local prostaglandin synthesis occurs in the brain during experimentally-induced fever in animals (Coceani *et al.*, 1983; Kluger, 1991; Rothwell & Luheshi, 1994; Rothwell & Hopkins, 1995).

Aminergic systems (serotonergic, noradrenergic, dopaminergic) and several brain pathways (e.g. corticotrophin releasing factor, β-endorphin, thyrotrophin releasing factor) have been considered to be central mediators of fever (Rothwell & Hopkins, 1995). Experimental manipulation of these systems alters febrile responses, and central injections of 5–hydroxytryptamine (5HT, serotonin), corticotrophin releasing factor (CRF), β-endorphin or thyrotrophin releasing hormone (TRH) all stimulate SNS activity and thermogenesis and raise body temperature (Rothwell, 1991a,c). Impairment in the synthesis, release or action of any one of these factors could therefore explain the apparent age-related changes in the febrile response.

Endogenous antipyretics

As with many biological systems, there appear to be feedback mechanisms that attenuate the development of fever. Glucocorticoids from the adrenal cortex are potent anti-inflammatory agents released during an acute phase response (Baxter & Rousseau, 1979). Natural and synthetic glucocorticoids are also antipyretic, acting centrally to inhibit eicosanoid synthesis and/or CRF release (Abul et al., 1987; Rothwell, 1990; Coelho et al., 1995), probably by release of the peptide lipocortin 1 (annexin-1). Lipocortin 1 is present in glia and neurons in the CNS (Strijbos et al., 1991), and administration of recombinant lipocortin inhibits pyrogenic and thermogenic responses to specific cytokines, whereas injection of neutralising antibodies to lipocortin 1 largely reverses the inhibitory actions of glucocorticoids on the fever response (Carey et al., 1990). Alpha-melanocyte stimulating hormone (α-MSH) and vasopressin also attenuate fever in experimental animals and the time-course of their synthesis follows that of fever (Kasting, 1989; Lipton, 1990).

Several natural and specific inhibitors of cytokine action have recently been identified, e.g. soluble receptors (Arend et al., 1991) or, in the case of IL-1, an endogenous receptor antagonist (Carter et al., 1990; Dinarello, 1994). The IL-1 receptor antagonist is produced by macrophages and its circulating concentration increases dramatically after endotoxin administration (Matsushima et al., 1991).

Mechanisms of fever in humans

Most research on fever in humans has been undertaken on patients with naturally occurring infections, inflammatory disorders or injury, so that the determination of the onset and magnitude of the initial stimulus is impossible to ascertain. Nevertheless, these studies have shown an increased concentration of cytokines (IL-1β, TNFα, IL-8, interferon-γ, IL-6) in the circulation or cerebrospinal fluid during fever and the pattern of their appearance follows the change in temperature (e.g. Dinarello, 1984; Nijsten et al., 1987; Girardin et al., 1988).

Experimental febrile responses have been induced in humans by the administration of bacterial endotoxin or typhoid vaccine. Both methods result in increases in body temperature and metabolic rate which are associated with SNS activation and increases in the concentration of circulating cytokines (Michie *et al.*, 1988; Horan *et al.*, 1989; Cooper *et al.*, 1992). Thus, from the limited data available it seems the mechanisms responsible for pyrogenesis in humans are similar, if not identical, to those in experimental animals.

Evidence for altered fever responses during aging

Human studies

As we have already stated, the notion that fever is attenuated or absent in old age can be traced back to antiquity. The advent of clinical thermometry in the latter half of the nineteenth century further enshrined this concept so that most textbooks of geriatric medicine confidently assert that afebrile infections are characteristic of old age. Such assertions are based largely on uncontrolled clinical observations in ill-defined patient populations rather than on carefully controlled studies. Thus, Gleckman & Hibert (1982) reported on 25 elderly people with no fever in the presence of proven bacteraemia. Finkelstein *et al.* (1983) reported similar findings in pneumococcal bacteraemia, as did Bryant *et al.* (1971) for a variety of bacteraemias and fungaemias, and Weinstein *et al.* (1983) for Gram-negative bacteraemias. Generalised conclusions about aging and the pathogenesis of fever cannot be drawn from such studies for various reasons: inadequate or absent control groups, the effects of co-morbidity and malnutrition, etc. Moreover, methods for the measurement of body temperature were suboptimal or inadequately specified.

Body temperature has usually been measured using a mercury-in-glass thermometer at the mouth or axilla, thus reflecting usual clinical practice. It is unusual in clinical practice to allow sufficient time for the thermometer to reach equilibrium (up to 9 minutes for mercury-in-glass thermometers and 3 minutes for electronic digital devices, and much longer when the respiratory rate is elevated or the subject is mouth breathing) (Nicholls *et al.*, 1966, 1969; Tandberg & Sklar, 1983). Even when the instruments are used correctly, to make measurements at sites of heat loss as a proxy for core temperature measurement is illogical. The production of heat inside the body creates a temperature gradient between the interior and the superficial layers (radial temperature gradient). At the extremities the temperature also decreases in a longitudinal fashion (axial temperature gradient). As a result of the irregular geometry of the body, a complicated spatial temperature field is created which can be characterised by a series of isotherms (lines jointing points of equal temperature). Thus, from the point of view of temperature, the body may be considered to comprise a series of layers, rather like an onion. The temperature of the inner layers (core) is carefully regulated (i.e. the core is homoeothermic) while that of the outer layers is highly dependent on ambient temperature (i.e. the outer layers are effectively poikilothermic). Regardless of ambient temperature, it has been suggested that the temperature gradient from core to periphery is much steeper in old age (Downton *et al.*, 1987), thus making axillary temperature measurements even less reliable as a proxy for core temperature.

The highly regulated core temperature does not remain static but exhibits distinct fluctuations over the course of a day with a peak around 22.00 h and a trough at about 03.00 h. The amplitude of this fluctuation in healthy young people is about 1 °C. In several rat and mouse strains, the amplitude of this diurnal variation is diminished in old age (Brock, 1985), but there are few comparable data for humans. A well-designed recent study comparing healthy old and young people of both sexes showed no age-related decline in amplitude of the diurnal rhythm, although there was some evidence of a phase shift in old men (Monk *et al.*, 1995). Notwithstanding, it has been suggested that old people thermoregulate around a lower set point than young people (Howell, 1948; Fox *et al.*, 1973; Primrose & Smith, 1982), but more recent studies suggest this is not generally the case (Darowski *et al.*, 1991a; Marion *et al.*, 1991).

It is therefore clear that the detection of fever presents a number of problems with elderly patients. One thing that is clear is that the only reliable method for routine measurement of core temperature is to do so rectally. Even then, an arbitrary defini- tion of fever based on a temperature threshold may be misleading as core temperature can vary by around 1 °C over the day, and the subject may normally thermoregulate around an unusually low core temperature. An upwards re-setting of the 'hy- pothalamic thermostat' may bring the core temperature into a conventionally defined normal range (with the conclusion that fever is absent) when, for that subject, fever is clearly present. These difficulties apart, a number of authors have studied fever in old age using appropriate methods at the rectal site and an arbitrary definition of fever (rectal temperature > 37.5 °C) and have found that fewer than 10% of old people with proven infections fail to become febrile (Berman & Fox, 1985; McAlpine *et al.*, 1986; Darowski *et al.*, 1991a,b). Furthermore, even if body temperature is not raised on admission to hospital, in almost all of those with infections it will rise over the next 24 hours. Presumably, these subjects were either at a very early stage during the develop- ment of fever or were unable to increase heat production/prevent heat loss sufficiently to raise body temperature until they were in an environment with a high enough ambient temperature. One may therefore conclude that afebrile infections are not especially common in older people provided core temperature is determined at an appropriate site and allowing sufficient time for the thermometer to reach equilibrium. More subtle defects, however, might well be present that cannot be uncovered in the rather uncontrolled setting of routine clinical practice.

Animal studies

Studies in the rat have demonstrated that the febrile responses to peripherally or intracerebroventricularly (ICV) injected live bacteria or lipopolysaccharide (isolated from the cell wall of the bacteria) are reduced in the aged rat when compared with the febrile responses of their young counterparts (Tocco-Bradley *et al.*, 1985a; Maitland *et al.*, 1986; Bradley & Kauffman, 1990). Dose–response curves to lipopolysaccharide have not been constructed, and it is therefore possible that the aged rats show reduced sensitivity to pyrogens and respond normally at higher doses. It is not clear whether these altered febrile responses are due to a defect in one of the early events of the pyrogenic pathway, i.e. the phagocytosis of bacterial endotoxin by cells of the mononuclear phagocytic system and their concomitant production and release of cytokines (Dinarello, 1988), as *in vitro* incubations of monocytes or macrophages from young and aged rats with bacterial endotoxin have yielded conflicting data (Bruley-Rosset & Vergnon, 1984; Jones *et al.*, 1984; Kauffman, 1986). The febrile response of the aged rats to peripheral or ICV injection of 'endogenous pyrogen', a crude preparation of IL-1, has been reported to be intact (Tocco-Bradley *et al.*, 1985b; Maitland *et al.*, 1986). We have recently constructed full dose–response curves to ICV administration of highly purified recombinant IL-1β. It was observed that the aged rat exhibits comparable febrile responses to those of its young counterparts at higher doses, 250–500 ng per rat, but exhibited significantly reduced fevers over the lower dose range, 2.5–50 ng per rat (Strijbos, 1991). This indicates that the aged rat exhibits a reduced sensitivity to the central effects of IL-1β, although its maximal capacity to respond remains intact. A recent study also reported reduced febrile responses to IL-6 in aged mice (Miller *et al.*, 1995a). In addition, it has been reported that the febrile response of aged rats to ICV injection of prostaglandin E$_2$ is intact (Maitland *et al.*, 1986; Strijbos *et al.*, unpublished results), suggesting that the impairment in the febrile response occurs at a stage prior to prostaglandin action.

In addition to alterations in the action and production of cytokines in the aged rat, it has also been reported that the central concentrations and actions of several neurotransmitters involved in body temperature regulation are modified with senescence. It appears that brain concentrations of noradrenaline and dopamine increase with age (Estes & Simpkins, 1980; Cox *et al.*, 1981). Furthermore, a reduced sensitivity to the central actions of these compounds has been reported, and has been associated with an age-related decrease in the ability to tolerate heat and cold stress (Cox *et al.*, 1981). It is not known, however, whether the changes in central sensitivity to neurotransmitters with age are due to alterations in receptor number or populations, or in their binding characteristics, although a decrease in neuron density and total neuron number has been reported (Hsu & Peng, 1978).

In mice up to 24 months of age, peripheral injection of bacterial endotoxin triggers similar fevers to those observed in their young counterparts (Habicht, 1981; Strijbos *et al.*, 1993). We have recently observed that mice of 36 months of age exhibit significantly reduced febrile responses to peripheral injection of bacterial endotoxin, indicating an age-related impairment (Strijbos *et al.*, 1993). Interestingly, the febrile response of these aged mice to systemic administration of IL-1β was also reduced. This suggests that their impaired responses to endotoxin may be due to a reduced induction of IL-1β following endotoxin administration or a blunted response to IL-1β (Strijbos *et al.*, 1993). In addition, we have recently observed that these aged mice exhibit intact febrile responses to peripheral injection of prostaglandin E$_2$ (Strijbos *et al.*, 1993). This suggests that in the aged mouse, as in the rat, the impairment in fever occurs at a stage prior to prostaglandin action.

Experiments performed on rabbits have indicated that aging blunts the febrile responses to peripherally injected live bacteria or bacterial endotoxin (Deeter *et al.*, 1989; Ruwe *et al.*, 1988). The aged rabbit also exhibits reduced febrile responses over a full dose range to peripheral or central administration of 'endogenous pyrogen' (Lipton & Ticknor, 1979). In addition, studies on the effects of central injections of IL-1 have revealed that the biphasic fever of the aged rabbit is reduced compared to that of young rabbits (Dao *et al.*, 1988). However, experiments to assess the effects of central injection of prostaglandin E$_2$ have yielded conflicting data (Ruwe *et al.*, 1988; Lipton & Ticknor, 1979). It has been reported that aged rabbits respond to intracerebroventricular injection of prostaglandin E$_2$ in an identical manner and magnitude to young rabbits (Lipton & Ticknor, 1979). However, when it was injected directly into the POAH, aged rabbits showed smaller fevers in response to prostaglandin E$_2$ than their young counterparts (Ruwe *et al.*, 1988). These data indicate that the sensitivity of the POAH of the aged rabbit, unlike that of rats or mice, to PGE$_2$ is reduced. Studies on the febrile responses of aged guinea pigs have not yet been performed. However, peripheral administration of bacterial endotoxin in newborn guinea pigs, provided they are older than eight days, triggers a febrile response, whereas guinea pigs in their first post-natal week do not develop a fever (Blatteis, 1975). Furthermore, injection of leucocytic pyrogen, most likely to contain a large proportion of IL-1, directly into the hypothalami of newborn guinea pigs elicits fevers in only a small number of guinea pigs injected, with increasing numbers responding with increasing age (Blatteis & Smith, 1979). Thus, in the guinea pig, the febrile response depends upon the stage of development, although it is not known whether the guinea pig also demonstrates an age-related decrease in febrile response as observed in many other species (see above).

Investigations into the febrile responses of primates have demonstrated that the development of fever in aged squirrel monkeys, *Saimiri sciureus*, following peripheral or central (icv) administration of bacterial endotoxin is reduced compared to those of their young counterparts (Clark *et al.*, 1980). Interestingly, the reduced fever of aged monkeys to centrally administered endotoxin is restored using an inhibitor of the central inactivation of endogenous pyrogen and PGE_2, probenecid, whereas the reduced febrile response to peripheral endotoxin is not affected (Clark *et al.*, 1980). Therefore, the reduced febrile responses of the aged squirrel monkeys may be due to a reduced central sensitivity to pyrogens.

Peripheral effector mechanisms

Vasomotor responses Although a general reduction in sensitivity to both vasoconstrictor and vasodilator stimuli has been thought to accompany aging, more recent observations suggest that the age-related defect is in the β-adrenergic receptor system and that responsiveness to other stimuli may be only minimally affected during aging (Lakatta, 1993). In a careful study, Pan *et al.* (1986) showed that the ability of phenylephrine (an α-adrenergic agonist) to cause constriction in human superficial hand veins was unimpaired in older people, as was the ability of nitroglycerine to cause dilation; however, there was a marked reduction in β-adrenergic-mediated vascular relaxation. These results are in keeping with the findings of Tsujimoto *et al.* (1986), who examined the ability of nitroglycerine, acetylcholine and isoprenaline to induce dilation in mesenteric artery constricted with serotonin. No age changes were seen with nitroglycerine or acetylcholine but there was a marked impairment in the ability of isoprenaline to induce dilation. This was associated with a lesser accumulation of cyclic AMP in the old vessels, which also showed a reduced sensitivity to exogenous dibutyryl cyclic AMP.

Mechanisms of heat production The reduced febrile response with ageing may be a reflection of a more general disorder in thermoregulation, as highlighted by the impaired capacity of aging humans and rats to regulate body temperatures and to tolerate heat and cold exposure (Collins *et al.*, 1977; Kiang-Ulrich & Horvath, 1985). Moreover, age-related reductions in the amount and thermogenic capacity (assessed from the effect of noradrenergic agonists and the activity of BAT) in the rat and humans are well documented (Bruck, 1973; Lean *et al.*, 1986; Horan *et al.*, 1988). This, together with the twofold decrease in β-adrenergic receptor number observed in BAT in aging rats (Scarpace *et al.*, 1988), may contribute to the impaired ability to thermoregulate in senescence. Although maximal thermogenic capacity is usually diminished in aging animals, they can nevertheless exhibit significant increases in metabolic rate in response to noradrenaline which are usually similar to, or greater than, the responses to pyrogenic stimuli (Strijbos, 1991). Diminished activity of BAT (or other effectors of thermogenesis) is therefore unlikely to contribute significantly to reduced fever in aging rodents although alterations in sympathetic outflow or decreased sensitivity to low concentrations of noradrenaline cannot be excluded.

Altered cytokine production or action

Few studies have reported circulating concentrations of cytokines or their inhibitors, or cytokine receptor density, in aging subjects. Recent investigations have established that aged Fisher 344 rats (24–27 months of age) exhibit significantly elevated plasma concentrations of TNFα (approximately 30–fold) and IL-6 (approximately 15–fold) after endotoxin administration (Foster *et al.*, 1992). These findings are partly supported by studies in the aged mouse (24 months of age) which indicate that caecal ligation and puncture-induced sepsis result in significantly increased concentrations of TNFα (approximately 20–fold) in aged mice compared with their mature (12 months old) counterparts (Hyde & McCallum, 1992). In contrast, *in vitro* analysis of the release of cytokines from macrophages of young and aged donors, performed in the presence of a pyrogenic stimulus (endotoxin), have yielded variable and conflicting data (Bruley-Rosset & Vergnon, 1984; Jones *et al.*, 1984; Kauffman, 1986).

Alpha-melanocyte stimulating hormone

Alpha-MSH appears to act as a potent endogenous anti-inflammatory and antipyretic peptide (Lipton, 1990), and has thus been implicated in the reduced febrile responses of aging rabbits. To assess whether reduced fever in aged rabbits is due to an increased antipyretic activity of αMSH, antiserum to this peptide was administered centrally to neutralise endogenous αMSH, and the febrile responses to IL-1 were investigated (Bell *et al.*, 1987). This treatment resulted in an augmentation of fever in the young rabbits but neither pretreatment nor acute injections of antiserum significantly enhanced febrile response to IL-1 of the aged rabbits (Bell *et al.*, 1987). Synthesis of αMSH appears to be reduced in the brains of aging rats (Barnea *et al.*, 1982; Bell & Lipton, 1987). These findings do not agree with the proposed role of endogenous αMSH in the reduced febrile response of aging rabbits. If endogenous αMSH is indeed responsible for this phenomenon, one would expect an antiserum to αMSH to increase the febrile responses of ageing rabbits and to detect increased concentrations of αMSH in the brains of these animals. The antipyretic effects of exogenous αMSH, however, were greatest in aged rabbits (Bell *et al.*, 1987), indicating that αMSH receptors are still present in the aged brain, and are perhaps hypersensitive to the inhibitory actions of αMSH. Thus, central endogenous αMSH appears not to be primarily responsible for the reduced febrile response to IL-1 in the aged rabbit.

Glucocorticoids

The role of glucocorticoids in aging has been the subject of extensive study. There is increasing evidence that the cumulative, long-term exposure of the brain, and the hippocampal neurons in particular, to glucocorticoids is involved in neuronal degeneration during aging, at least in rodents (McEwen *et al.*, 1986; Sapolsky *et al.*, 1986;

Landfield, 1987; Sapolsky, 1992). This is supported by observations that plasma corticosterone concentrations and adrenal weight correlate with quantitative measures of hippocampal aging (as assessed by astrocyte reactivity) in the rat (Landfield *et al.*, 1978). Moreover, chronic stress and prolonged exposure to corticosterone cause 'premature aging' of the hippocampus (Kerr *et al.*, 1986; Sapolsky *et al.*, 1990). Conversely, adrenalectomy protects rats against the age-related loss of hippocampal neurons and the increase in astrocyte reactivity (Landfield, 1987). This age-related loss in hippocampal neurons seems to be irreversible and is directly proportional to the loss of type 1 and type 2 corticosteroid receptors in the hippocampus (Roth, 1976; Sapolsky *et al.*, 1983a; Reul *et al.*, 1988), although the loss of type 1 receptors appears to be reversible by the use of a synthetic $ACTH_{4-9}$-analogue ORG2766 (Reul *et al.*, 1988).

Corticosteroid receptors play a key role in mediating the inhibitory effects of glucocorticoids on the activated HPA-axis during stress. Therefore, any loss of receptors eventually results in impairments in the feedback inhibition of the activated HPA-axis (Sapolsky *et al.*, 1986; Meites *et al.*, 1987). CRF concentrations in aged rats have not been reported, but increased plasma concentrations of ACTH (Tang & Philips, 1978; Issa *et al.*, 1989; van Eekelen *et al.*, 1990) and corticosterone (Serio *et al.*, 1970; Landfield *et al.*, 1978, 1980; Tang & Phillips, 1978; Sapolsky *et al.*, 1983b; DeKosky *et al.*, 1984; van Eekelen *et al.*, 1992) have been observed in the aged laboratory rodent. Several workers have been unable to confirm the elevation in basal plasma corticosterone concentrations with increasing age, and this remains a controversial issue (Phillips Brett *et al.*, 1983; Sonntag *et al.*, 1987; Lorens *et al.*, 1990). Basal corticosterone secretion is subject to a diurnal rhythm which appears to be intact in the aged rat (Sapolsky *et al.*, 1983b). Plasma concentrations of corticosterone are therefore dependent upon the time of sampling, and this could be partially responsible for the observed discrepancy.

While the aged laboratory rat is reportedly capable of initiating corticosterone secretion in response to stress, there is probably an impairment in terminating its secretion during the recovery period (Sapolsky *et al.*, 1983b). Aged rats show significantly higher peak plasma corticosterone concentrations to immobilisation stress than their young counterparts, although these concentrations peak at similar time points (Sapolsky *et al.*, 1983b). Moreover, plasma corticosterone concentrations of young rats return to pre-stress values within 60 minutes, while those of aged rats remain elevated 24 hours after stress (Sapolsky *et al.*, 1983b). Clearly, an impairment in feedback inhibition on the HPA-axis in the aged rat could explain this phenomenon.

There is an apparent paradox associated with the involvement of glucocorticoids in brain aging, in that age-related changes in the hippocampus appear to accelerate with increasing age, whereas hippocampal glucocorticoid receptor number has been reported to decline with advancing age. If these hippocampal degenerative changes depend upon corticosterone activation, it is not clear why the rate of hippocampal aging does not decrease as the hippocampal receptor population declines, as this should confer a protective effect. This paradox is apparent only if there is a direct quantitative correlation between receptor number and corticosterone impact, and factors other than receptor density may be significant. This incongruity has only recently been resolved with the observation that the affinity of the type 2 receptor, which is involved in mediating the effects of corticosterone during stress on feedback inhibition of the HPA-axis, is significantly increased in aged rats (Landfield & Eldridge, 1989). This finding has important physiological implications for aged animals under stress conditions, as it has been reported that activation of the type 2 receptor induces the expression of a range of mRNA sequences (Nichols *et al.*, 1988). As 90–95% of the type 2 receptors appear to be occupied during stress or peak diurnal concentrations of corticosterone, an increase in the affinity of these receptors, in conjunction with the potentially elevated basal corticosterone concentrations, could lead to excessive and inappropriate mRNA and protein expression in the aged.

Support for the involvement of glucocorticoids in the impaired pyrogenesis of aging rats and mice is derived from the finding that administration of the glucocorticoid type 2 receptor antagonist (RU38486) markedly enhances the pyrogenic and thermogenic responses to central and peripheral administration of IL-1β in aging rats and mice respectively (Figure 8.1; Strijbos *et al.*, 1993). Young animals of the same species exhibit significant responses to IL-1β, which are not significantly affected by the glucocorticoid antagonist. It is of interest to note that both species exhibit elevated plasma concentrations of glucocorticoids and that this treatment did not affect the pyrogenic or thermogenic response of their young counterparts.

Lipocortin 1

We have demonstrated that lipocortin 1 is a potent antipyretic agent, and proposed that it mediates the antipyretic and antithermogenic actions of glucocorticoids (Carey *et al.*, 1990; Strijbos *et al.*, 1992). Neutralisation of endogenous lipocortin 1 by peripheral or central injection of a neutralising antiserum to lipocortin 1, or its purified IgG fraction, in aged mice or aged rats has actions which are almost identical to those of the glucocorticoid receptor antagonist RU38486, i.e. complete restoration of the pyrogenic and thermogenic responses to IL-1β (Strijbos *et al.*, 1993; Figure 8.2). In contrast, lipocortin antiserum treatment does not affect fever in young animals. Analysis of the lipocortin 1 content of the brains of these rats by immunohistochemical techniques revealed an increased lipocortin 1 staining in the hippocampi of these aged rats compared with their young counterparts (P. J. L. M. Strijbos *et al.*, unpublished results). These data suggest that increased synthesis or sensitivity to the antipyretic actions of lipocortin 1 is involved in the impairment of fever in aging rats and mice although its site or mechanism of action is unknown.

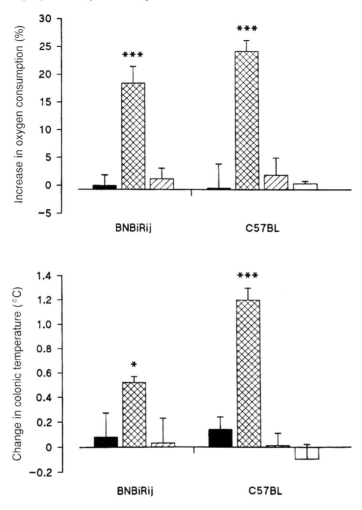

Figure 8.1. Effects of injection of IL-1β in 27 to 36-month-old C57BL/Icrf a^t mice (10 μg/kg, intraperitoneally) or 32 to 38-month-old BNBiRij rats (5 ng, intracerebroventricularly) on (a) oxygen consumption and (b) colonic temperature, and the modification of the effects by subcutaneous injection of RU38486 (10 mg/kg) (▨) or vehicle (□).*,*** $P < 0.05$ and $P < 0.001$, respectively, for IL-1β plus RU38486 (▦) versus IL-1β treated animals (■), ANOVA and Scheffe's *post hoc* test. Mean values $\pm$ SEM for $n = 8$–9.

Summary and conclusions

In spite of numerous casual observations and the widely held belief that fever is impaired in old people, few carefully controlled studies have been undertaken in humans. Research on experimental animals has reported impaired febrile responses to a number of stimuli which may be associated with altered synthesis or actions of endogenous pyrogens (cytokines). Experimental data vary somewhat between species but generally indicate that reduced fevers are due to some impairment at a stage prior to prostaglandin synthesis. Recent studies indicate that overactivity of endogenous antipyretic agents may be responsible, at least in part, for changes in pyrogenesis with aging.

Impaired fever in aging has several important implications. First, because of its general diagnostic value, an apparent afebrile state may mask infection. Second, because of the similarities between actions of cytokines on body temperature on other parameters (e.g. behaviour, neuroendocrine status), changes associated with aging may be indicative of alterations in other responses to injury and infections. Finally, perhaps most controversial is the consideration of whether fever has biological value and thus whether impairments in the elderly represent an advantageous adaptation which

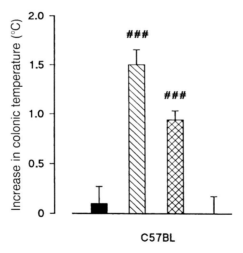

Figure 8.2. Effects of intraperitoneal injection of Il-1β (10 μg/kg; ■); on colonic temperature of 27- to 36-month-old C57BL/Icrf a^t mice, and modification of the effects of IL-1β by intravenous injection of polyclonal lipocortin 1 antiserum (50 μl; ▨), purified anti-lipocortin 1 IgG fraction (50 μl; ▧) or control IgG fraction (50 μl; ☐).### $P < 0.001$; IL-1β in 27- to 36-month-old mice versus IL-1β treated mice, ANOVA and Scheffe's *post hoc* test. Mean values $\pm$ SEM for $n = 8$–9.

conserves energy reserves, or whether this is detrimental and should be treated. This question remains unsolved, but with the availability of animal models and defined experimental protocols in humans can now be addressed.

References

Abul, H., Davidson, J., Milton, A. S. & Rotondo, D. (1987). Dexamethasone pretreatment is antipyretic toward polyinosinic:polycytidylic acid, lipopolysaccharide and interleukin 1/endogenous pyrogen. *Naunyn Schmiedeberg's Arch Pharmacol*, **335**, 305–9.

Arch, J. R. S., Ainsworth, A., Cawthorne, M. A., Piercy, M. A., Sennit, M. V., Thody, V. E., Wilson, C. & Wilson, S. (1984). A typical β-adrenoreceptor on brown adipocytes: target for anti-obesity drugs. *Nature*, **309**, 163–5.

Arend, W. P., Malyak, M., Bigler, C. F., Smith, M. F. & Janson, R. W. (1991). The biological role of naturally-occurring cytokine inhibitors. *Br J Rheumatol*, **30**, 49–52.

Barnea, A., Cho, G. & Porter, J. C. (1982). A reduction in the concentration of immunoreactive corticotropin, melanotropin and lipotropin in the brain of the aging rat. *Brain Res*, **232**, 345–53.

Baxter, J. D. & Rousseau, G. G. (1979). Glucocorticoid hormone action: an overview. In *Glucocorticoid Hormone Action* (*Monographs on Endocrinology* 12), ed. J. D. Baxter & G. G. Rousseau, pp. 1–24. Berlin: Springer.

Bell, R. C. & Lipton, J. M. (1987). Concentration of melanocyte stimulating hormone (MSH) within specific brain regions in aged squirrel monkeys. *Brain Res Bull*, **18**, 577–9.

Bell, R. C., Feng, J. & Lipton, J. M. (1987). Is the endogenous antipyretic neuropeptide α-MSH responsible for reduced fever in aged rabbits? *Peptides*, **8**, 501–4.

Berman, P. & Fox, R. A. (1985). Fever in the elderly. *Age Ageing*, **14**, 327–32.

Bernheim, H. A. & Dinarello, C. A. (1985). Effects of purified human interleukin 1 on the release of prostaglandin E_2 from fibroblasts. *Br J Rheumatol*, **24**, 122–7.

Blatteis, C. M. (1975). Postnatal development of pyrogenic sensitivity in guinea pigs. *J Appl Physiol*, **39**, 251–7.

Blatteis, C. M. & Hunter, W. S. (1987). Effects of separation of the ventromedial (VMH) from the pre-optic anterior (POAH) hypothalamus on thermoregulation of guinea pigs. *Physiologist*, **30**, 205.

Blatteis, C. M. & Smith, K. A. (1979). Hypothalamic sensitivity to leucocytic pyrogen of adult and newborn guinea pigs. *J Physiol*, **296**, 177–92.

Bradley, S. F. & Kauffman, C. A. (1990). Aging and the response to salmonella infection. *Exp Gerontol*, **25**, 75–80.

Brock, M. A. (1985). Biological clocks and aging. In *Review of Biological Research in Aging*, vol. 2, ed. M. Rothstein, pp. 445–62. New York: Liss.

Bruck, K. (1973). NST and BAT in relation to age and their integration in the thermoregulatory system. In *Brown Adipose Tissue*, ed. A. Lundberg, pp. 117–53. New York: Elsevier.

Bruley-Rosset, M. & Vergnon, I. (1984). Interleukin 1 synthesis and activity in aged mice. *Mech Aging Dev*, **24**, 247–64.

Bryant, R. E., Hood, A. F., Hood, C. E. & Koenig, M. G. (1971). Factors affecting mortality of Gram-negative rod bacteraemia. *Arch Intern Med*, **127**, 120–8.

Carey, F., Forder, R., Edge, M. D., Greene, A. R., Horan, M. A., Strijbos, P. J. L. M. & Rothwell, N. J. (1990). Lipocortin 1 fragment modifies pyrogenic actions of cytokines in rats. *Am J Physiol*, **259**, R266–R269.

Carter, D. B., Deibel, M. R., Dunn, C. J., Tomich, C. S., Laborde, A. L., Slightom, J. L., Berger, A. E., Bienkowski, M. J., Sun, F. F. *et al.* (1990). Purification, cloning, expression and biological characterisation of an interleukin 1 receptor antagonist protein. *Nature*, **344**, 633–8.

Clark, S. M., Gean, J. & Lipton, J. M. (1980). Reduced febrile responses to peripheral and central administration of pyrogen in aged squirrel monkeys. *Neurobiol Aging*, **1**, 175–80.

Coceani, F. (1974). Prostaglandins and the central nervous system. *Arch Intern Med*, **133**, 119–29.

Coceani, F., Bishai, I., Dinarello, C. A. & Fitzpatrick, F. A. (1983). Prostaglandin E_2 and thromboxane B_2 in cerebrospinal fluid of afebrile and febrile cat. *Am J Physiol*, **244**, R785–R793.

Coceani, F., Lees, J. & Dinarello, C. A. (1988). Occurrence of interleukin 1 in cerebrospinal fluid of the conscious cat. *Brain Res*, **446**, 245–50.

Coelho, M. M., Luheshi, G., Hopkins, S. J., Pela, I. R. & Rothwell, N. J. (1995). Multiple mechanisms mediate antipyretic action of glucocorticoids. *Am J Physiol*, **38**, R527–R535.

Collins, K. J., Dore, C., Exton-Smith, A. N., Fox, R., McDonald, I. C. & Woodward, P. M. (1977). Accidental hypothermia and impaired temperature homeostasis in the elderly. *Br Med*, **1**, 353–6.

Coombes, R. C., Rothwell, N. J., Shah, P. & Stock, M. J. (1987). Changes in thermogenesis and brown fat activity in response to tumour necrosis factor in the rat. *Biosci Rep*, **7**, 791–9.

Cooper, A. L., Dascombe, M. J., Rothwell, N. J. & Vale, M. J. (1989a). Effects of malaria on O_2 consumption and brown adipose tissue activity in mice. *J Appl Physiol*, **67**, 1020–3.

Cooper, A. L., Fitzgeorge, R. B., Baskerville, A., Little, R. A. & Rothwell, N. J. (1989b). Bacterial infection (*Legionella pneumophilia*) stimulates fever, metabolic rate and brown adipose tissue activity in the guinea pig. *Life Sci*, **45**, 843–7.

Cooper, A. L., Horan, M. A., Little, R. A. & Rothwell, N. J. (1992). Metabolic and febrile responses to typhoid vaccine in humans: effect of beta-adrenergic blockade. *J Appl Physiol*, **72**, 2322–8.

Cooper, A. L., Brouwer, S., Turnbull, A. V., Luheshi, G. N., Hopkins, S. J., Kunkel, S. L. & Rothwell, N. J. (1994). *Am J Physiol*, **36**, R1431–R1436.

Cox, B., Lee, T. F. & Pankes, J. (1981). Decreased ability to cope with heat and cold linked to a dysfunction in a central dopaminergic pathway in elderly rat. *Life Sci*, **28**, 2039–44.

Dao, T. K., Bell, R. C., Ferguson, J., Jameson, D. M. & Lipton, J. M. (1988). C-reactive protein, leucocytosis and fever after central IL-1 and α-MSH in aged rats. *Am J Physiol*, **254**, R401–$409.

Darowski, A., Najim, Z., Weinberg, J. R. & Guz, A. (1991b). The increase in body temperature of elderly patients in the first twenty-four hours following admission to hospital. *Age Ageing*, **20**, 107–12.

Darowski, A., Weinberg, J. R. & Guz, A. (1991a). Normal rectal, auditory canal, sublingual and axillary temperatures in elderly afebrile patients in a warm environment. *Age Ageing*, **20**, 113–19.

Deeter, L. B., Martin, L. W. & Lipton, J. M. (1989). Age and sex-related differences in febrile response to peripheral pyrogens in the rabbit. *Gerontology*, **35**, 297–304.

DeKosky, S., Scheff, S. & Cotman, C. (1984). Elevated corticosterone levels: a possible cause of reduced axon sprouting in aged animals. *Neuroendocrinology*, **38**, 33–8.

Dinarello, C. A. (1984). Interleukin 1. *Rev Infect Dis*, **6**, 51–94.

Dinarello, C. A. (1994). The interleukin 1 family: 10 years of discovery. *FASEB J*, **8**, 1314–25.

Downton, J. H., Andrews, K. & Puxty, J. A. H. (1987). 'Silent' pyrexia in the elderly. *Age Ageing*, **16**, 41–4.

Estes, K. S. & Simpkins, J. W. (1980). Age-related alterations in catecholamine concentrations in discrete preoptic and hypothalamic regions in the male rat. *Brain Res*, **194**, 556–60.

Finkelstein, M. S., Petkun, W. M., Freedman, M. L. & Antopol, S. C. (1983) Pneumococcal bacteremia in adults: age-dependent differences in presentation and in outcome. *J Amer Geriatr Soc*, **31**, 19–27.

Fontana, A., Weber, E. & Dayer, J.-M. (1984). Synthesis of interleukin 1/ endogenous pyrogen in the brain of endotoxin-treated mice: a step in fever induction? *J Exp Med*, **133**, 1696–8.

Foster, K. D., Conn, C. A. & Kluger, M. J. (1992). Fever, tumor necrosis factor, and interleukin 1 in young, mature and aged Fischer 344 rats. *Am J Physiol*, **262** (31), R211–$215.

Fox, R. H., Woodward, P. M., Exton-Smith, A. N., Green, M. F., Donnison, D. V. & Wicks, M. H. (1973). Body temperatures in the elderly: a national study of physiological, social and environmental conditions. *Br Med J*, **1**, 200–6.

Girardier, L. (1983). Brown fat: an energy dissipating issue. In *Mammalian Thermogenesis*, ed. L. Girardier & M. J. Stock, pp. 50–98. London: Chapman and Hall.

Girardin, E., Brau, G. E., Dayer, J.-M., Roux-Lombard, P. & Lambert, P. H. (1988). Tumor necrosis factor and interleukin 1 in the serum of children with severe infectious purpura. *New Eng J Med*, **319**, 397–402.

Gleckman, R. & Hibert, D. (1982). Afebrile bacteraemia: a phenomenon of geriatric patients. *JAMA*, **248**, 1478–81.

Guilian, D., Baker, T. J., Shih, L. N. & Lachman, L. B. (1986). Interleukin 1 of the central nervous system is produced by amoid microglia. *J Exp Med*, **164**, 594–604.

Habicht, G. S. (1981). Body temperature in normal and endotoxin-treated mice of different ages. *Mech Aging Dev*, **16**, 97–204.

Higgins, G. A. & Olschwowka, J. A. (1991). Induction of interleukin 1β mRNA in adult rat brain. *Mol Brain Res*, **9**, 143–8.

Himms-Hagen, J. (1986). Brown adipose tissue and cold acclimation. In *Brown Adipose Tissue*, ed. P. Trayhurn & D. Nicholls, pp. 214–68. London: Arnold.

Hopkins, S. J. & Rothwell, N. J. (1995). Cytokines in the nervous system. I: Expression and recognition. *TINS*, **18**, 83–8.

Horan, M. A., Little, R. A., Rothwell, N. J. & Stock, M. J. (1988). Changes in body composition, brown adipose tissue activity and thermogenic capacity in BN/BiRij rats undergoing senescence. *Exp Gerontol*, **23**, 455–6.

Horan, M. A., Gibbons, L., Hopkins, S. J., Cooper, A., Strijbos, P., Rothwell, N. J. & Little, R. A. (1989). Changes in plasma interleukin 6 during experimentally-induced fever in normal subjects. *Cytokine*, **1**, 393.

Hori, T., Nakashima, T., Koyohara, T. & Shibata, M. (1984). Effects of leukocytic pyrogen and sodium salicylate on hypothalamic thermosensitive neurons in vitro. *Neurosci Lett*, **49**, 313–18.

Howell, T. H. (1948). Normal temperatures in old age. *Lancet*, **1**, 517–18.

Hsu, H. K. & Peng, M. T. (1978). Hypothalamic neuron number of old female rats. *Gerontology*, **24**, 434–40.

Hyde, S. R. & McCallum, R. E. (1992). Lipopolysaccharide-tumor necrosis factor: glucocorticoid interactions during cecal ligation and puncture-induced sepsis in mature versus senescent mice. *Infect Immun*, **60**, 976–82.

Issa, A., Gauthier, S., Rowe, W. & Meanney, M. (1989). Age-related changes in plasma ACTH concentrations in Long Evans rats. *Soc Neurosci Abst*, **429.11**, 1080.

Jones, P. G., Kauffman, C. A., Bergman, A., Hayes, C., Kluger, M. J. & Cannon, J. G. (1984). Fever in the elderly: production of leukocytic pyrogen by monocytes from elderly persons. *Gerontology*, **30**, 182–7.

Kasting, N. W. (1989). Criteria for establishing a physiological role for brain peptides. A case in point: the role of vasopressin in thermoregulation during fever and antipyresis. *Brain Res Rev*, **14**, 143–53.

Kauffman, C. A. (1986). Endogenous pyrogen/interleukin-1 production in aged rats. *Exp Gerontol*, **21**, 75–8.

Kerr, D. S., Applegate, M., Campbell, L. W., Goliszek, A., Brodish, A. & Landfield, P. W. (1986). Chronic stress-induced acceleration of age-related hippocampal neurophysiological changes. *Soc Neurosci Abstr*, **12**, 274.

Kiang-Ulrich, M. & Horvath, M. (1985). Age-related differences in the responses to acute cold challenge ($-10°C$) in male F344 rats. *Exp Gerontol*, **20**, 201–9.

Kluger, M. J. (1986). Is fever beneficial? *Yale J Biol Med*, **59**, 89–96.

Kluger, M. J. (1991). Fever: role of pyrogens and cryogens. *Physiol Rev*, **71**, 93–127.

Lakatta, E. G. (1993). Cardiovascular regulatory mechanisms in advanced age. *Physiol Rev*, **73**, 413–67.

Landfield, P. W. (1987). Modulation of brain aging correlates by long-term alterations of adrenal steroids and neurally-active peptides. In *Progress in Brain Research*, ed. E. R. de Kloet, V. Wiegant & D. de Wied, pp. 279–300. New York: Elsevier.

Landfield, P. W. & Eldridge, J. C. (1989). Increased affinity of type 2 corticosteroid binding in aged rat hippocampus. *Exp Neurol*, **106**, 110–13.

Landfield, P. W., Sundberg, D., Smith, M., Eldridge, J. & Morris, M. (1980). Mammalian brain aging: theoretical implications of changes in brain and endocrine systems during mid and late life. *Peptides*, **1**, 185–96.

Landfield, P. W., Waymire, J. & Lynch, G. S. (1978). Hippocampal aging and adrenocorticoids: quantitative correlations. *Science*, **202**, 1098–102.

Lean, M. E. J., James, W. P., Jennings, G. & Trayhurn, P. (1986). Brown adipose tissue uncoupling protein content in human infants, children and adults. *Clin Sci*, **71**, 291–7.

LeMay, D. R., LeMay, L. G., Kluger, M. J. & D'Alecy, L. G. (1990a). Plasma profiles of IL-6 and TNF with fever-inducing doses of lipopolysaccharide in dogs. *Am J Physiol*, **259**, R126–R132.

LeMay, L. G., Vander, A. J. & Kluger, M. J. (1990b). Role of interleukin-6 in fever in rats. *Am J Physiol*, **258**: R798–R803.

Lipton, J. M. (1990). Modulation of host defense by the neuropeptide α-MSH. *Yale J Biol Med*, **63**, 173–82.

Lipton, J. M. & Ticknor, C. B. (1979). Influence of sex and age on febrile responses to peripheral and central administration of pyrogens in the rabbit. *J Physiol*, **295**, 263–72.

Long, N. C., Otterness, I., Kunkel, S. L., Vander, A. J. & Kluger, M. J. (1990). Roles of interleukin 1β and tumor necrosis factor in lipopolysaccharide fever in rats. *Am J Physiol*, **259**, R724–R728.

Lorens, S., Hata, N., Handa, R., van der Kar, L., Guschwan, M., Goral, J., Lee, J., Hamilton,

M., Bethea, C. & Clancy, J. (1990). Hypothalamo–pituitary–adrenal axis responsiveness in the aged. *Neurobiol Aging*, **11**, 139–50.

Luheshi, G. N., Turnbull, A. V., Brouwer, S., Hopkins, S. J. & Rothwell, N. J. (1994). *Br J Pharmacol*, **113**, 86P.

Mackowiak, P. A. (1994). Fever: blessing or curse? A unifying hypothesis. *Ann Intern Med*, **120**, 1037–40.

Maitland, S. J., Ruwe, W. D. & Veale, W. L. (1986). Characterisation of the febrile response in old and young rats. In *Homeostatsis and Thermal Stress*, ed. Cooper, Lomax, Schonbaum & Veale, pp. 81–83. Sixth International Symposium on Pharmacological Thermoregulation, Jasper, Alta. Basel: Karger.

McAlpine, C. H., Martin, B. J., Lennox, I. M. & Roberts, M. A. (1986). Pyrexia in infection in the elderly. *Age Ageing*, **15**, 230–4.

McEwen, B., de Kloet, E. R. & Rostene, W. (1986). Adrenal steroid receptors and actions in the nervous system. *Physiol Rev*, **66**, 1121–88.

Marion, G. S., McGann, K. P. & Camp, D. L. (1991). Core body temperature in the elderly and factors which influence its measurement. *Gerontology*, **37**, 225–32.

Matsushima, H., Roussel, M. F., Matsushima, K., Hishinuma, A. & Sherr, C. J. (1991). Cloning and expression of murine interleukin-1 receptor antagonist in macrophages stimulated by colony-stimulating factor 1. *Blood*, **78**, 616–23.

Meites, J., Goya, R. & Takahashi, S. (1987). Why the neuroendocrine system is important in aging processes. *Exp Gerontol*, **22**, 1–15.

Michie, H. R., Manogue, K. R., Spriggs, D. R., Revhaug, A., O'Dwyer, S., Dinarello, C. A., Cerami, A., Wolff, S. M. & Wilmore, D. W. (1988). Detection of circulating tumor factor after endotoxin administration. *New Engl J Med*, **318**, 1481–6.

Miller, D. J., Yoshukawa, T. T. & Norman, D. C. (1995a). Effect of age on fever response to recombinant interleukin 6 in a murine model. *J Gerontol*, **50A**, M276–M278.

Miller, A. J., Luheshi, G. N. & Rothwell, N. J. (1995b). Fever and interleukin-6 (IL-6) responses to localised inflammation induced in air pouch in the rat. *Br J Pharmacol*, **114**, 213P.

Monk, T. H., Buysse, D. J., Reynods, C. F., Kupfer, D. J. & Houck, P. R. (1995). Circadian temperature rhythms of older people. *Exp Gerontol*, **30**, 455–74.

Morimoto, A., Murakami, N., Nakamori, T. & Watanabe, T. (1987). Evidence for separate mechanisms of induction of biphasic fever inside and outside the blood-brain barrier. *J Physiol*, **383**, 629–37.

Morimoto, A., Murakami, N., Nakamori, T. & Watanabe, T. (1988a). Multiple control of fever production in the central nervous system. *J Physiol*, **397**, 269–80.

Morimoto, A., Murakami, N. & Watanabe, T. (1988b). Is the arachidonic acid cascade involved in the development of acute phase response in rabbits? *J Physiol*, **397**, 281–9.

Nakashima, T., Hori, T., Kuriyama, K. & Matsuda, T. (1988). Effects of interferon-α on the activity of preoptic thermosensitive neurons in tissue slices. *Brain Res*, **454**, 361–7.

Neta, R., Vogel, S. N., Sipe, J. D., Wong, G. G. & Nordan, R. P. (1988). Comparisons of *in vivo* effects of human recombinant IL-1 and human recombinant IL-6 in mice. *Lymphokine Res*, **7**, 403–7.

Nicholls, D. G. & Locke, R. (1984). Thermogenic mechanisms in brown fat. *Physiol Rev*, **64**, 1–64.

Nichols, G. A., Fielding, J. J., McKevitt, R. K. & Posner, I. (1969). Taking oral temperatures of febrile patients. *Nurs Res*, **18**, 448–50.

Nichols, G. A., Ruskin, M. M., Glor, B. A. K. & Kelly, W. H. (1966). Oral, axillary and rectal temperature determinations and relationships. *Nurs Res*, **15**, 307–10.

Nichols, N. R., Lerner, S. P., Masters, J. N., May, P., Millar, S. L. & Finch, C. E. (1988). Rapid corticosterone-induced changes in gene expression in rat hippocampus display type II glucocorticoid receptor specificity. *Mol Endocrinol*, **2**, 284–90.

Nijsten, M. W. N., de Groot, E. R., Ten Duis, H. J., Klaasen, H. J., Hack, C. E. & Aarden, L. A. (1987). Serum levels of interleukin-6 and acute phase responses. *Lancet*, **85**, 921.

Pan, H. Y.-M., Hoffman, B. B., Pershe, R. A. & Blaschke, T. F. (1986). Decline in beta-adrenergic receptor-mediated vascular relaxation with aging in man. *J Pharmacol Exp Ther*, **239**, 802–7.

Phillips Brett, L., Chong, G. S., Coyle, S. & Levine, S. (1983). Age changes in components of the hypothalamo-pituitary adrenal axis. *Neurobiol Aging*, **4**, 133–8.

Primrose, W. R. & Smith, L. R. N. (1982). Oral and environmental temperatures in a Scottish urban population. *J Clin Exp Gerontol*, **4**, 151–65.

Reul, J. M. H. M., Tonnaer, H. A. D. M. & de Kloet, E. R. (1988). Neurotrophic ACTH analogue promotes plasticity of type 1 corticosteroid receptor in brain of senescent rats. *Neurobiol Aging*, **8**, 253–61.

Roth, G. (1976). Reduced glucocorticoid binding site concentration in cortical neuronal perikarya from senescent rats. *Brain Res*, **107**, 345–54.

Rothwell, N. J. (1990). Mechanisms of the pyrogenic actions of cytokines. *Eur Cytokine Net*, **1**, 211–13.

Rothwell, N. J. (1991a). Thermogenesis in obesity and cachexia. In *Hormones and Nutrition in Obesity and Cachexia*, ed. M. Muller, E. Darforth, A. Burger & U. Siedentopp, pp. 77–85. Berlin: Springer-Verlag.

Rothwell, N. J. (1991b). Functions and mechanisms of interleukin 1 in the brain. *TIPS*, **12**, 430–6.

Rothwell, N. J. (1991c). Central effects of CRF on metabolism and energy balance. *Neurosci Biobehav Rev*, **14**, 263–71.

Rothwell, N. J. & Hopkins, S. J. (1995). Cytokines and the nervous system II: Actions and mechanisms of action. *TINS*, **18**, 130–6.

Rothwell, N. J. & Luheshi, G. N. (1994). Pharmacology of interleukin-1 actions in the brain. *Adv Pharmacol*, **25**, 1–20.

Rothwell, N. J. & Stock, M. J. (1986). Brown adipose tissue and diet-induced thermogenesis. In *Brown Adipose Tissue*, ed. P. Trayhurn & D. Nicholls, pp. 269–98. London: Arnold.

Ruwe, W. D., Naylor, A. M., Dinarello, C. A. & Veale, W. L. (1988). Characteristics of pyrogen fevers are altered in the aged rabbit. *Exp Gerontol*, **23**, 103–13.

Sapolsky, R. M. (1992). *Stress, the Aging Brain, and the Mechanisms of Neuronal Death*. Cambridge, USA: MIT Press.

Sapolsky, R., Krey, L. C. & McEwen, B. S. (1983a). Corticosterone receptors decline in a site-specific manner in the aged brain. *Brain Res*, **289**, 235–40.

Sapolsky, R., Krey, L. C. & McEwen, B. S. (1983b). The adrenocortical stress response in the aged male rat: impaired recovery from stress. *Exp Gerontol*, **18**, 55–61.

Sapolsky, R., Krey, L. C. & McEwen, B. S. (1986). The neuroendocrinology of stress and aging: the glucocorticoid cascade hypothesis. *Endocrine Rev*, **7**, 284–301.

Sapolsky, R., Uno, H., Rebert, C. S. & Finch, C. E. (1990). Hippocampal damage associated with prolonged glucocorticoid exposure in primates. *J Neurosci*, **10**, 2897–902.

Scarpace, P. J., Mooradian, A. D. & Morley, J. E. (1988). Age-associated decrease in beta-adrenergic receptors and adenylate cyclase activity in rat brown adipose tissue. *J Gerontol*, **43**, B65–B70.

Serio, M., Piolanti, P., Romano, S., DeMagistris, L. & Guistri, G. (1970). The circadian rhythm of plasma cortisol in subjects over 70 years of age. *J Gerontol*, **25**, 95–7.

Sonntag, W. E., Goliszek, A. G., Brodish, A. & Eldridge, J. C. (1987). Diminished diurnal secretion of adrenocorticotrophin (ACTH) but not corticosterone in old male rats: possible relation to increased adrenal sensitivity to ACTH *in vivo*. *Endocrinology*, **120**, 2308–15.

Strijbos, P. J. L. M. (1991). *The role of lipocortin 1 in the central control of fever and thermogenesis.* PhD Thesis, University of Manchester, UK.

Strijbos, P. J. L. M., Hardwick, A., Relton, J. K., Carey, F. & N. J. Rothwell (1992). Inhibition of central actions of cytokines on fever and thermogenesis by lipocortin 1 involves CRF. *Am J Physiol*, **263**, E632–E636.

Strijbos, P. J. L. M., Horan, M. A., Carey, F. & Rothwell, N. J. (1993). Impaired febrile responses of aging mice are mediated by endogenous lipocortin-1 (annexin-1). *Am J Physiol*, **265**, E289–297.

Strijbos, P. J. L. M., Tilders, F. J. H., Carey, F., Forder, R. & Rothwell, N. J. (1991). Lipocortin-1 immunoreactivity in normal rat brain. Effects of adrenalectomy, dexamethasone and colchicine treatment. *Brain Res*, **553**, 249–60.

Szekely, M., Szelenyi, Z. & Sumegi, I. (1973). Brown adipose tissue as a source of heat during pyrogen induced fever. *Acta Physiol Acad Sci Hung*, **43**, 265–77.

Tandberg, D. & Sklar. (1983). Effect of tachypnoea on the estimation of body temperature by an oral thermometer. *New Engl J Med*, **308**, 945–6.

Tang, G. & Phillips, R. (1978). Some age-related changes in pituitary-adrenal function in the male laboratory rat. *J Gerontol*, **33**, 377–82.

Tocco-Bradley, R., Kluger, M. J. & Kauffman, C. A. (1985a). Effect of age on fever and acute phase response of rats to endotoxin and *Salmonella typhimurium*. *Infect Immun*, **47**, 106–11.

Tocco-Bradley, R., Singer, R., Kluger, M. J. & Kauffman, C. A. (1985b). Effects of age on the febrile response of rats to endogenous pyrogen. *Gerontology*, **31**, 349–54.

Tsujimoto, G., Lee, C.-H. & Hoffman, B. B. (1986). Age-related decrease in beta adrenergic receptor-mediated vascular smooth muscle relaxation. *J Pharmacol Exp Ther*, **239**, 411–15.

van Eekelen, J. A. M., Rots, N. Y., Sutanto, W. & de Kloet, E. R. (1992). The effect of aging on stress-responsiveness and central corticosteroid receptors in the Brown Norway rat. *Neurobiol Aging*, **13**, 159–70.

Weinstein, M. P., Murphy, J. R. & Reller, L. B. (1983). The clinical significance of positive blood cultures: a comprehensive analysis of 500 episodes of bacteraemia and fungaemia in adults II. Clinical observations with special reference to factors influencing prognosis. *Rev Infect Dis*, **5**, 54–70.

Welch, W. H. (1888). The Cartwright Lectures on the general pathology of fever. *Medical News*, **52**, 365, 393, 397, 539, 565.

9

Infections, aging and the host response

M. A. HORAN and S. G. PARKER

The nature of immunity

Two, interactive immune systems are recognised: innate (natural) immunity and acquired (adoptive or specific) immunity. Innate immunity comprises polymorphonuclear leucocytes, natural killer (NK) cells and mononuclear phagocytes, and utilises the complement cascade as its main soluble protein effector mechanism. It also utilises numerous recognition molecules including C-reactive protein (CRP), serum amyloid protein (SAP) and mannose-binding protein (MBP). These molecules have been selected during evolution to bind carbohydrate structures that do not occur on eukaryotic cells and thus differentiate potentially harmful invaders from innocuous self.

Acquired immunity employs several subtypes of lymphocytes and utilises antibody as its effector protein. Antibody and the T cell receptor (TCR) are the recognition structures. B lymphocytes can recognise protein, carbohydrate and simple chemical structures whereas T lymphocytes appear only to recognise peptides. Clones of lymphocytes with receptors of sufficient affinity are triggered by antigen to proliferate and differentiate into the various effector cells: T-helper cells, cytotoxic T cells, suppressor T cells and plasma cells.

After an immune response subsides, specific antibody often persists in the blood for many years and even decades. This implies that humoral effector cells (plasma cells) persist and continue to secrete antibody. In contrast, the antibody response in the mucosal immune system (see later) is generally short lived (a few months to a year). Effector T cells do not persist long but antigen-specific clones remain expanded as memory lymphocytes which can differentiate into effector cells whenever the antigen is again encountered. In general, memory responses are most effective in protecting against systemic infections (e.g. measles, mumps, yellow fever, poliomyelitis, smallpox). Localised infections at mucosal surfaces (e.g. rotavirus, respiratory syncytial virus, rhinoviruses) can recur before memory lymphocytes can differentiate into effector cells, although these subsequent episodes of disease are usually less severe.

126

The flexible nature of specific immunity poses the problem of differentiating innocuous antigens from harmful ones, a problem that innate immunity does not have. One mechanism to overcome this is to delete potentially self-reactive clones during maturation of the cells (in the thymus for T cells and at an, as yet, unknown site for B cells). Further specificity is ensured by interactions with innate immunity. For T cells antigen presentation is the critical step. Uptake of antigen into antigen-presenting cells (e.g. mononuclear phagocytes, dendritic cells) is determined by the presence of the carbohydrate moieties that are recognised by innate immunity. For B cells, the interaction with innate immunity seems to be their membrane receptors for the C3d component of complement which is found in association with CD19. CD19 is needed for antibody production for T cell-dependent antigens and amplifies signalling after the antigen binds membrane immunoglobulin. This process is facilitated by covalent binding of C3d to microbial carbohydrate structures.

Interferon-induced resistance to viruses

The antiviral state of cells exposed to viruses depends on the 2′,5′-oligoadenylate (2′,5′-A) system which is induced by interferons. A 2′5′-A-dependent ribonuclease (RNase L) that cleaves viral (and cellular) RNA mediates this effect. The activity of this system is decreased in old rats which presumably increases their susceptibility to viruses, especially RNA viruses (Pfeifer *et al.*, 1993). This loss is associated with increased activity of 2′,-3′-exoribonuclease which inactivates 2′,5′- A. Interestingly, older people infected with HIV cannot contain viral replication as well as younger ones and have considerably poorer survival (Ferro & Salit, 1992).

Specific immune response to infectious agents

Different pathogens require different types of response for their elimination. These have come to be called type 1 responses, which are characterised by dependence on macrophages for phagocytosis and intracellular killing, and type 2 responses, which are macrophage-independent (but rely on non-cytotoxic antibodies, mast cells and eosinophils). Helper T lymphocytes are needed for both types of response; however, T lymphocytes occur as at least two subtypes labelled T_H1 and T_H2 cells.

T_H1 cells produce interleukin 2 (IL-2), interleukin 3 (IL-3), tumour necrosis factor-α (TNFα) and interferon-γ (IFNγ), and this pattern of cytokines promotes type 1 responses. Macrophages are activated and B cells are switched to IgG1 production (in humans) which binds macrophage Fc receptors and activates complement, both of which promote phagocytosis. T_H1 cells also express the Fas ligand which induces contact-mediated apoptosis in Fas-positive cells. Activated macrophages produce

IL-12, TNFα and IFNγ. This pattern of cytokines (especially IL-12) induces activation and proliferation of NK cells, differentiation of naive T cells into T_H cells and the expression of the T_H1 phenotype.

T_H2 cells promote type 2 responses to pathogens. T_H2 cells require IL-4 to prime naïf cells. Once activated, they produce IL-3, IL-4, IL-5, IL-6, IL-10 and IL-13. This pattern of cytokines leads to growth and activation of mast cells and eosinophils. It also switches B lymphocytes to IgG4 production and inhibits macrophage activation. This pattern of response is characteristic of helminth infections but it may also have a role in the downregulation of type 1 responses.

The aging immune system

Of all the systems in the body, the immune system is probably the best understood, both in mechanistic terms and in the ways in which it changes during aging. Studies of the aging immune system (immunogerontology) can be traced to the early part of this century (and even earlier) and the literature has burgeoned in the past three decades. Perhaps the first publication was the investigation undertaken by Peter Ludwig Panum (a Danish physician and discoverer of endotoxin) on the outbreak of measles in the Faroes in 1846. The Faroes had been free of measles since the previous epidemic of 1781. The 1846 outbreak affected 75–95% of the population though, 'of the many aged people still living on the Faroes who had had measles in 1781, not one was attacked a second time' (Panum, 1847).

As in most fields of gerontological research, the literature is cluttered with apparent inconsistencies. Among the reasons for them are inappropriate and inadequate characterisation of the people (or animals) studied, failure to control for co-morbid factors, the selection of inappropriate control groups and over-interpretation of the available evidence. Despite these difficulties, a reasonable consensus has emerged so that we have a fair understanding of the broad picture of immune senescence, in humans as well as laboratory animals, even though many of the details remain speculative. It is this broad picture that we present and we do not address those aspects that are controversial. Therefore, we do not intend to cite references to original publications when we present this consensus view: the interested reader will find ample of these in the many excellent review articles (Horan *et al.*, 1990; Ben-Yehuda & Weksler, 1992; Miller, 1995; Pawalec *et al.*, 1995).

The classical view of immune aging (immunosenescence) is of an immunodeficiency state that predisposes the host to infectious diseases and possibly neoplasms, despite the virtual absence of any supporting evidence, particularly in humans. Immunosenescence is generally attributed to involution of the thymus gland and is thought to be characterised by decreased proliferation of T lymphocytes and impaired T-helper activity which lead to impaired cell-mediated and humoral responses to T cell-dependent antigens. Paradoxically, there is an increased incidence of autoantibodies (although these are inevitably of low titre) and of benign monoclonal B lymphocyte proliferations with monoclonal antibody production (Radl, 1985). Interestingly, old people in Japan have a very low incidence of benign monoclonal proliferations (Bowden *et al.*, 1993).

Stem cells

All haemopoietic cells derive from a common pluripotent stem cell in the bone marrow, a tissue that continues to supply precursor cells for the immune systems throughout life. Bone marrow stem cells are little affected by aging (Horan, 1993), although there is evidence of decreased responsiveness to the late-acting unilineage stimulator for neutrophils, G-CSF (Chatta *et al.*, 1993). Normal numbers of myeloid progenitor cells (CD34–positive) are present in the bone marrow of healthy old people but there is a twofold reduction in sensitivity to the proliferative stimulus of G-CSF and normal responsiveness to early multilineage regulators such as GM-CSF and IL-3. This implies that although no defect in granulocyte production is present in the basal state, when increased production is required the aged bone marrow may not always meet the demand.

After lymphoid precursors migrate to systemic lymphoid areas, defective immune responses might reflect intrinsic defects in the cells or downregulating influences within the systemic immune system microenvironment. The available evidence is insufficient to determine the relative contributions from these two possibilities. It is clear that bone marrow from aged mice, while not identical to young bone marrow (Astle & Harrison, 1984; Averill & Wolf, 1985), retains the potential to respond almost normally in a 'young' microenvironment (Zharkhary & Klinman, 1983; Zharkhary, 1986). Likewise, when bone marrow cells from young donors repopulate aged bone marrow, responses come to resemble those of old animals.

Thymus gland

Progenitors of T lymphocytes (prothymocytes) migrate from the bone marrow in the blood and are first located in the subcapsular cortex of the thymus gland. These cells, which lack typical T cell differentiation antigens, give rise to cortical thymocytes, the largest cell population within the gland. Cortical thymocytes express characteristic T lymphocyte differentiation antigens (e.g. CD4 and CD8 in humans), the thymic cortex-specific antigen (CD6) and the enzyme, terminal deoxynucleotidyl transferase (TdT). It has been reported that movement of precursor cells to the thymus ceases before adolescence, at least in long-lived, autoimmune disease-resistant mice, as assessed by chromosomal markers in parabiotic animals.

With further development, CD6 and TdT gradually disappear and two distinct populations emerge, one CD1,3 and 4 positive and the other CD1,3 and 5/8 positive. Studies with circulating T lymphocytes suggest CD4–positive cells are helper cells and CD5/8–positive cells are cytotoxic/suppressor cells. These cells have also become MHC (major histocompatibility complex) restricted in that antigens are only recognisable in the context of class I (HLA – A, B and C) or class II (HLA – DR, Dc, SB) molecules of the major histocompatibility complex. For cytotoxic T lymphocytes, the relevant MHC molecules are class I (present on all cells). For T helper cells, class II molecules are required (present in large numbers only on antigen-presenting cells such as macrophages). Suppressor T lymphocytes are heterogeneous in that some recognise antigens in the context of class I molecules and some in the context of class II molecules.

T cell development in the thymus requires physical contact with thymic epithelial cells mediated by class I and II molecules and classical adhesion molecules (e.g. LFA-3 and ICAM-1) and thymic dendritic cells. There is an age-related decline in the expression of class II molecules. T lymphocyte development is also modulated by the elaboration of soluble factors such as thymic hormones, interleukins (1, 3 and 6), colony-stimulating factors for granulocytes and/or macrophages (GM-CSF) and transforming growth factor-alpha (TGFα).

From the age of about 1 year, there is a decline in thymic epithelial cell mass which appears to progress throughout life. After the age of about 15 years, the lymphocytic perivascular space is replaced by adipose tissue and the lymphocytic cell mass declines. The rate of this involution seems to be slower in women than in men until the time of the menopause, but thereafter, the rates are indistinguishable. Furthermore, the earliest studies were performed using autopsy specimens. This is unfortunate because thymic composition may change rapidly in response to many stressors (e.g. severe illness, surgery, starvation, endocrine changes, pregnancy) and most old people die after a prolonged illness whereas most young people die suddenly. More recent studies (Steinmann & Muller-Hermelink 1984; Steinmann & Hartwig, 1995) have made allowance for this and have shown that the gland maintains a morphologically active cellular compartment throughout life and that the size of this compartment is much greater in biopsy samples than in those obtained at autopsy. Finally, there is considerable interest in the possibility that thymic development can occur in other, yet unidentified, sites (Franceschi *et al.*, 1995).

The changes in the thymus gland described above represent two patterns of involution. One is clearly related to stressful stimuli, is restricted to the lymphocytic compartment and is largely mediated by activation of the hypothalamic–pituitary–adrenal axis. This form of involution occurs quickly and regeneration takes place on resolution of the stressful stimulus. It has been suggested that this form of involution might be purposeful to the extent that it might prevent the induction of toleration to the pathogen concerned (Ritter & Crispe, 1992). The other pattern of involution is related to both development and aging and affects all cell types in the gland and also the extracellular matrix. The stimulus for this form of involution is unknown. Although it is not generally regarded as purposeful, Ritter & Crispe (1992) have suggested that it could minimise the likelihood of developing autoimmune diseases. This suggestion is interesting in the light of evidence provided by Utsuyama *et al.* (1991) that the age-involuted thymus actually produces factors that downregulate peripheral immune functions.

Circulating lymphocytes

There is no consensus on the effects of advancing age on the numbers of circulating lymphocytes and both normal and reduced numbers have been recorded. As well as the factors already mentioned, another possible reason for the inconsistency in the published studies has emerged from the Baltimore Longitudinal Study of Aging (BLSA). Bender *et al.* (1986) report sequential total lymphocyte counts over 16 years in 105 healthy participants in the study. They reported no longitudinal change except in the 3 years leading up to death, during which the lymphocyte count fell. This suggests that the change represents some underlying disease. It was already known that a low preoperative lymphocyte count predicted death and infective complications after operation (Grossbad *et al.*, 1984) and old people with bacterial infections who also had a low lymphocyte count experienced a high death rate (Proust *et al.*, 1985).

Circulating T lymphocytes

Total T lymphocyte numbers decline somewhat with age; the numbers of activated (CD3$^+$, HLA-DR$^+$) T cells increase (Sansoni *et al.*, 1993), but there is a marked decline in most measures of T lymphocyte functions. The proliferative responses to mitogenic lectins, anti-CD3 antibodies and to soluble antigens are all reduced in all species studied. Animal studies have also shown reduced adoptive transfer of helper activity for antibody responses, a reduced graft-versus-host response and reduced rejection of alloantigen-bearing tumour cells. These changes are associated with defective production of IL-2 by CD4–positive cells as well as a reduced responsiveness to exogenous IL-2. Not all old people show this reduced response to mitogenic stimuli but those who do seem to have high circulating concentrations of IL-2 (Huang *et al.*, 1992). Studies with murine T lymphocyte clones have shown that a population remains with normal responses but that there is a much larger population with reduced proliferative activity. This latter group fails to raise the intracellular calcium concentration (thought to be a key factor in activation) in response to appropriate stimuli and it has been proposed that this is due to a failure of G-protein-mediated activation of phospholipase C, a phenomenon that has also been observed in granulocytes and parotid acinar cells. Interestingly, centenarians show only modest declines in T lymphocyte functions (Franceschi *et al.*, 1995) and, like many old people, they have an increased proportion of activated (i.e. expressing HLA-DR molecules) cells and the numbers of naïf T lymphocytes decline little after the age of about 40 years.

Aging is also associated with an increase in suppressor signals, both cellular and humoral (anti-idiotype antibodies). These suppressor signals are largely confined to 'non-self' antigens. Thus, the addition of old murine spleen cells to young ones incubated with either 'non-self' or 'self' antigens results in the suppression only of the response to 'non-self' (Russo *et al.*, 1990). There is also an exaggerated sensitivity to suppressor stimuli from macrophages (prostaglandin E_2, $TGF\beta_2$ and hydrogen peroxide) (Franklin *et al.*, 1993).

In healthy old people, these changes in cellular immunity can only be described as modest and certainly do not approach a severity characteristic of important immunodeficiency disorders such as AIDS. Frailty, chronic illness and malnutrition tend to be associated with much more marked defects of cellular immunity and, indeed, defects in most aspects of the host response. Nutritional supplements with vitamins and trace elements produce significant increases in circulating T cell numbers and in their proliferative responses as well as fewer infective episodes than in comparable old people receiving a placebo (Chandra, 1992).

Circulating B lymphocytes

The numbers of circulating B lymphocytes decline more markedly than T cells during aging (Sansoni *et al.*, 1993) but the aggregated amount of immunoglobulin (which must ultimately represent the activity of the entire B lymphocyte compartment) increases. The levels of natural antibody to blood group antigens and certain ubiquitous microbes declines.

Many studies in both humans and experimental animals have shown that the antibody response to a variety of antigens declines in old age and that in a substantial number, standard immunisation protocols do not confer adequate protection. For example, Shapiro *et al.* (1991) reported a case control study of people with pneumococcal infections and matched controls. This showed that the efficacy of previous immunisation was 93% in those under the age of 55 years but was only 46% in those over the age of 85 years. Furthermore, in the old, the protective effect of vaccine waned over about 5 years, at which time, in the oldest old, protection had been completely lost.

Several studies suggest, however, that it is possible to improve the immunogenicity of vaccine preparations. Ben-Yehuda *et al.* (1993) reported that a genetically engineered vaccinia virus expressing the PR/8 influenza haemagglutinin gene overcomes the impaired antibody response and increased susceptibility of old mice to influenza infection. Gravenstein *et al.* (1994) reported enhanced protection of old people during an influenza outbreak by giving the vaccine conjugated to diphtheria toxoid and Treanor *et al.* (1992) report similar benefits accrue when the standard killed vaccine (given intramuscularly) is given with an attenuated virus (intranasally).

The prevalence of circulating autoantibodies increases during aging but follows a complex pattern, depending on the health state of the individuals concerned. The healthy elderly show an increase in non-organ specific autoantibodies but not organ-specific ones, while the unhealthy elderly tend to show the reverse (Franceschi *et al.*, 1995).

Mucosal immunity

Mucosal surfaces have a specialised immune system, the mucosa-associated lymphoid tissue (MALT) which functions more or less independently of systemic immunity. MALT is characterised by the ability to secrete antibody, mainly IgA, and it also contains all the other cells needed to mount a cellular immune response.

Interest in age-effects on the mucosal immune system was stimulated by reports that, in contrast to systemic immunity, the MALT was little affected by aging, at least in the mouse strains used (Szewczuk *et al.*, 1980; Wade *et al.*, 1988). This conclusion appears to be supported by the results of Fulk *et al.* (1970) who examined IgA in nasal secretions after administration of an influenza vaccine. More recently, Arranz *et al.* (1992) have shown that aging does not reduce the amount of IgA in gut lavage fluid. Quantitative microscopy on jejunal biopsy specimens showed a significant age-related decrease in intraepithelial lymphocytes (exclusively T lymphocytes) and an increase in IgA-secreting plasma cells. Other studies in rats, dogs and subhuman primates have not confirmed this relative sparing of the mucosal immune system during aging (Schmucker and Daniels, 1986). One study with cholera toxin in rats suggested that in the old animals, however, antigen may have reduced access to inductive sites or the microenvironment reduces responsiveness (Daniels *et al.*, 1993). The same investigators have also found an impaired ability of rat hepatocytes from old donors to take up IgA and to secrete it into the bile (Gregoire *et al.*, 1992). This effect is probably mediated by reduced expression of the polymeric immunoglobulin receptor in hepatocyte membranes. Clearly, more detailed studies are needed to elucidate mucosal immune function in the aged and whether oral immunisation might be a more appropriate route of vaccine administration for some common pathogens.

Non-specific immune defences

The natural killer (NK) cell compartment enlarges in old age and these cells are functionally active (Ligthart *et al.*, 1989). Interestingly, both old and young people have greater numbers of NK cells than middle-aged people (Sansoni *et al.*, 1993). There have been few studies of complement activity in old age but they have shown no significant decline; occasional studies have even shown an increase. Aging is not associated with any significant granulocytopenia but the peripheral granulocyte count may be maintained with a hypoplastic marrow by increased proliferation of committed granulopoietic stem cells (Resnitzky *et al.*, 1987). There is controversy over whether there are age-related changes in granulocyte functions, although malnutrition can certainly impair them (Lipschitz & Udupa, 1986) as can co-morbid conditions and their treatments (Laharrague *et al.*, 1983). One interesting study in C57BL/6 mice (Esposito *et al.*, 1990) showed a greater neutrophil influx into the lungs in the older animals, a finding consistent with our own observations on pulmonary injury following the systemic injection of endotoxin into rats (Durham *et al.*, 1989) and our unpublished findings on experimental cutaneous wound healing in both mice and healthy humans. If such observations are confirmed, it may be that old age is a 'pro-inflammatory state' and the old may be particularly susceptible to develop the systemic inflammatory response syndrome after injury or sepsis, an hypothesis that has not been specifically addressed.

Aging, cytokines and the immune system

Cytokines are small proteins or glycoproteins produced by cells in response to appropriate stimuli. Constitutive production is very low excepting some interferons, insulin-like growth factor 1 (IGF-1) and IL-6. Their production is not usually restricted to specific organs (unlike classical peptide hormones) but they are produced in various tissues to act in an autocrine, juxtacrine or paracrine manner. A few cytokines like $TGF\beta_1$, erythropoietin, IGF-1, IL-6 and tumour necrosis factor (TNF) may be carried in the blood to act at distant sites and thus resemble classical hormones.

Cytokines are key mediators of immune and inflammatory responses. Although they play critical regulatory roles in normal, injured and diseased tissues, very few biological effects are mediated by a single cytokine. Gene deletion experiments suggest that few cytokines are absolutely essential for life or particular functions, but deletion of receptors (which are often shared by several cytokines) can have severe effects whose magnitude and precise manifestations depend on the strain of animal used.

Interleukin 1 produced by mononuclear phagocytes is generally considered to be the major stimulus to T and B lymphocyte activation by inducing IL-2 and its receptor. Despite the inevitable studies to the contrary (e.g. Bradley *et al.*, 1990), the consensus view is that IL-1 production does not decline during healthy aging (Rosenberg *et al.*, 1983; Jones *et al.*, 1984; Rudd & Banerjee 1989; Goldberg *et al.*, 1991; Nafziger *et al.*, 1993; Brouwer *et al.*, 1995). One study of IL-1 production by monocytes from old people with nosocomical pneumonia showed less was produced than by monocytes from similarly infected younger people. They also showed that activated T lymphocytes interfere with IL-1 production, possibly by producing other cytokines that inhibit it (e.g. IL-4, IL-10, mainly products of T_H2 cells). Interestingly, IL-10 can be induced by glucocorticoid hormones (Tabardel *et al.*, 1996) which are a major feature of the endocrine response to trauma and whose secretion is unusually prolonged in aged trauma victims (Chapter 16). Furthermore, age effects on the kinetics of IL-1 production (and IL-6 and TNF) may depend on the precise nature of the stimulus. Chen *et al.* (1993) stimulated murine peritoneal exudate cells with killed *Staphylococcus aureus*, *E. coli* or *Candida albicans* and showed that different organisms elicited qualitatively different release of TNF and IL-1 and a tendency to greater IL-6 production in the old.

There are few data about age effects on the production of other cytokines. Gauchat *et al.* (1988) studied the amounts of mRNA for several cytokines in peripheral blood mononuclear cells from young and old healthy donors stimulated with a variety of agents. They found reduced amounts of IL-1, IL-2, IL-6, interferon gamma and GM-CSF as well as reduced amounts of mRNA for the IL-2 receptor. Hobbs *et al.* (1993) conducted more detailed studies in mice using CD4[+] cells stimulated with a monoclonal antibody against CD3 and found no age-related decline for TNF or IL-2 messenger RNA and increased production of IL-3, IL-4, IL-5 and interferon-gamma mRNAs. The same pattern was also observed for the cytokine product. One explanation for these results is an accumulation of memory CD4[+] cells versus naïf ones. This notion that changes in the proportions of cells within a population rather than fundamental cellular defects may explain age-related changes is extremely important and deserving of closer examination in other settings.

Finally, TGFβ is worthy of special mention since it is generally known as an inhibitor of cell proliferation and its receptors are present on many cell types. Zhou *et al.* (1992) have reported a substantial increase in the production of this cytokine by both quiescent and activated CD8[+] lymphocytes from old C57BL/6J mice. Furthermore, lymphocytes from old donor animals exhibit an increased sensitivity to it and incubation with neutralising antibodies to this cytokine increases proliferative responses in animals of all ages, but particularly in the old.

Immunosuppressive effects of injury

The body's response to surgery and trauma is evoked mainly by afferent nerve signals from the site of injury and the release of cytokines and other autacoids from the damaged tissue. TNF, IL-1, IL-6 and IFNγ are among the earliest cytokines to be observed and may be important stimuli for other responses, particularly activation of the HPA axis. The pattern of cytokines produced, together with circulating stress hormones, can have important effects on the immune systems and might well predispose to infective complications.

Infective complications account for most of the delayed deaths after injury, at least in younger people, and such complications are not uncommon after elective surgical procedures. Such observations have prompted many studies of immune function after injury and 'immune deficiency' is now known to complicate traumatic injury, surgery, burns and haemorrhage (Dries, 1992). Cell-mediated immunity is particularly affected. This is associated with reduced expression of HLA-DR antigens on mononuclear phagocytes and seems to be associated with the development of septic complications (Wakefield *et al.*, 1993a). Activation of the HPA axis can induce differentiation of T_H2 cells and inhibit differentiation to T_H1 cells (Root *et al.*, 1994). Decker *et al.* (1996) have reported this pattern of response after cholecystectomy. Circulating polymorphonuclear leucocytes exhibit exaggerated activation and this too is associated with the development of septic complications (Wakefield *et al.*, 1993b). Many other changes have been described, but as very little is known about the immune system following trauma in the aged, it seems inappropriate to describe them in detail here. In fact, the only study we could find examined cellular immunity following the minor injury of herniorrhaphy and this showed a more marked dysfunction in the older people, although anxiety had a greater effect than age (Linn *et al.*, 1983).

Acute phase response

The term 'acute phase response' was first used in the 1940s to describe the properties of sera from patients with febrile infectious diseases. These changes in the blood are now known to form part of an early and non-specific but complex response to a variety of injuries including mechanical tissue injury, burns, ischaemia, malignant growth and bacterial and parasitic infections. These stimuli trigger the synthesis and release of several cytokines which act locally at the site of tissue damage and may also act systemically after entry to, or formation in, the bloodstream. So far, most studies have measured cytokines in the peripheral blood, though some investigators have looked in wounds (Tokunaga *et al.*, 1993) or at the site of surgery (Tsukuda *et al.*, 1993). The concentration of IL-6 in the circulation rises after most types of tissue damage, while that of IL-2 falls. Other cytokines such as IL-1 and TNF are found much less often and their presence usually indicates severe tissue damage. The changes in circulating cytokines are generally felt to be beneficial but, when the response is excessive or prolonged, it is believed to be harmful and may trigger the systemic inflammatory response syndrome and multiple organ failure (Waage *et al.*, 1989; Bone, 1996).

A series of characteristic changes accompany the rise in IL-6 and these form part of 'the acute phase response'. It is thought that IL-6 is the main (but not the sole) regulator of the response, the main features of which are fever, anorexia, somnolence, neutrophilia, increased metabolic rate, characteristic endocrine changes, reduced circulating iron and zinc concentrations and changes in plasma proteins. The changes in plasma proteins include elevations in tissue plasminogen activator (followed by a rise in plasminogen activator inhibitor), complement components, protease inhibitors (e.g. alpha-1-antitrypsin), SAP and C-reactive protein. There are also falls in the concentration of other proteins such as retinol-binding protein, transferrin, pre-albumin and albumin. The fall in the concentration of albumin (and possibly other proteins) is caused, at least in part, by increased vascular permeability (Fleck *et al.*, 1986).

We have used the systemic administration of endotoxin as a model of sepsis in rats of differing ages and we have demonstrated an exaggerated rise in t-PA followed by a particularly exaggerated and prolonged rise in PAI in old rats (Emeis *et al.*, 1992). Similar changes were seen in the response to administered IL-1 and TNF but not IL-6.

The best studied of these plasma protein changes in the context of human aging is the rise in C-reactive protein. This has been shown to be the most sensitive marker of infection and the response to treatment (Kenny *et al.*, 1984, 1985; Cox *et al.*, 1986; Smith *et al.*, 1995). The response is well preserved in most old people, although a few of them with serious infections showed little or no rise.

Local defences

Skin

Owing to its dry, acidic conditions, the skin provides a hostile environment for most potential pathogens which must compete with the resident microflora for colonisation sites. Pores, hair follicles and sweat glands offer a more conducive environment, but one protected by toxic lipids and lysozyme. Although many age-related changes occur in the skin and its associated structures, we do not know if they predispose to infection. Wounds are undoubtedly the major portal of entry, regardless of age.

Mucosal surfaces

The lining of the respiratory, gastrointestinal and urogenital tracts are protected by a mucus layer which immobilises bacteria. It also contains toxic secretions such as lysozyme, lactoperoxidase and sIgA. Sloughing cells remove adherent bacteria and tight junctions prevent invasion. Cell turnover probably declines during aging.

Malnutrition and catabolism impair all these mucosal responses and facilitate micro-bial translocation and possibly sepsis.

Gastrointestinal tract

Gastric acid is a very important defence against enteric organisms. Achlorhydria and the use of antacids, H_2 receptor antagonists and proton pump inhibitors will all undermine this defence and predispose the aged to such infections (Horan *et al.*, 1984).

The proliferating cells occur at the base of the crypts and close to these cells are another cell type: Paneth cells. The precise function of Paneth cells has long been the subject of speculation but it is now known that they secrete lysozyme and toxic peptides known as cryptdins. The effects of aging on Paneth cells are not known.

Respiratory tract

The lungs are protected by the creation of turbulent airflow which causes inhaled particles to impact in the mucus layer, usually at sites of bifurcation (where, inciden-tally, aggregations of lymphoid tissue are also found). This mucus is moved ever upwards, towards the mouth, by a mechanism known as the mucociliary escalator. Larger collections of mucus and other material will be removed by coughing. Both the mucociliary escalator and the cough reflex are believed to be impaired in the aged.

Urogenital tract

The major defence of the urinary tract is the repeated voiding of urine. It is thought that age-related anatomical changes facilitate the ascent of faecal organisms into the bladder, particularly in women, although whether the growth of organisms from a urine sample is sufficient to constitute an infection is debatable (Clague & Horan, 1994; Orr *et al.*, 1996).

In premenopausal women, oestrogens ensure the colonisation of the vagina by lactobacilli which, by creating a very acidic environment, impede the proliferation of potential pathogens. After the menopause, the vagina tends to become colonised by coliforms and other Gram-negative bacteria which sometimes ascend to the uterus where they may cause endometritis or pyometra (Horan *et al.*, 1983).

Aging and infections

Predisposition to infection

Immunogerontologists would like there to be a relation between the reported changes in immune function and predisposition to infectious diseases and such a relation is

asserted in most discussions on infections in the aged. There are two important issues
to be addressed: (1) are the elderly particularly predisposed to infectious diseases?; and
(2) is the putative predisposition explained by immunosenescence?

At the time of writing, there is no reliable evidence that aging per se is an independent risk factor for infectious diseases. What we have is a collection of largely
uncontrolled clinical studies in which the subjects are not well characterised for other,
less controversial, risk factors like frailty, malnutrition, and associated chronic diseases
(reviewed in Horan *et al.*, 1990). In fact, one large community-based study in the USA
showed reduced rates of common respiratory infections in the aged; however, once
acquired, the old are sicker and at a considerably greater risk than the young of dying
as a result. These general conclusions about infections in aged humans are reflected in
studies in aged mice (reviewed in Horan *et al.*, 1990).

Dynamics of infections

Of course, the likelihood of acquiring an infection depends not only on host defences
but also on other important factors. First of all, exposure to any potential pathogen is
a *sine qua non*, and the likelihood of exposure will be modified by environment and
lifestyle. Indeed, this may partly explain why the community-dwelling old are so much
less likely than the young to acquire the common cold or influenza. Once exposed, any
potential pathogen must proliferate at some surface, the success of which will be
modified by the resident microflora. Successful proliferation may lead to colonisation
of the host or progress to invasive infection, a process that will be modified by local and
systemic host factors.

Potential pathogens may display greater or less virulence; the more virulent the
organism, the more likely is tissue invasion and infection. Pathogenic bacteria express
numerous virulence factors such as thick capsules, adhesins, sIgA proteases, C5a
peptidases, toxic proteases and the ability to induce phagocytosis in cells that are not
normally phagocytic.

Hospitals provide an immense reservoir of potential pathogens and, of course, older
people are more likely than the young to require hospitalisation, tend to stay longer
and are more likely than the young to be debilitated and malnourished. Thus, they run
a high risk of exposure to virulent, often antibiotic-resistant, bacteria. It should not be
surprising that they have a high rate of nosocomical (hospital-acquired) infections
(Hussain *et al.*, 1996), about three times higher than occurs with younger patients
(Freeman & McGowan, 1978).

Outcome of infections

Although the evidence for increased susceptibility to infections in old age is complex
and controversial, the evidence for a poorer outcome is hardly disputed, although the

reasons are not clear. For example, in the USA, the elderly have the greatest number and rate of diarrhoeal deaths of any age group (Lew *et al.*, 1991). People with influenza aged over 70 years have been reported to have a 35–fold greater risk of dying than similarly infected children (Couch *et al.*, 1986). Similarly people with bacterial meningitis aged 40–60 years have a threefold greater risk of death than similarly infected teenagers (Finland & Barnes, 1977). We have previously shown old rats to be exquisitely sensitive to the lethal effects of endotoxin (Horan *et al.*, 1991) and a number of experimental infections in mice show a similar phenomenon (Louria *et al.*, 1982). One important study has utilised caecal ligation and puncture as a model of sepsis in aging mice (Hyde & McCallum, 1992). The old animals showed shorter survival despite a smaller bacterial burden than younger animals. They also had higher levels of TNF which were refractory to downregulation by the synthetic glucocorticoid, dexamethasone, unlike in the younger animals. Several studies have reported higher death rates in old people with a variety of infections: Gram-negative septicaemia (McCue, 1987), pneumococcal bacteraemia (Finkelstein *et al.*, 1983), community acquired pneumonia (Macfarlane *et al.*, 1982). The reasons for the high death rates have not been clearly elucidated but appear to be a mixture of late diagnosis, aging changes, co-morbidity and malnutrition. Malnutrition certainly compromises most host defences, including immune defences (Nogues *et al.*, 1995), and the elderly seem to be especially vulnerable to the effects of malnutrition (Lipschitz & Udupa, 1986; Castenada *et al.*, 1995).

Diagnostic difficulty, often attributed to the atypical presentation of disease in old age, has come to be one of the dogmas of geriatric medicine. One interesting study from Aberdeen which was conducted in an infectious diseases unit with an 'open-access' policy showed that only 20% of old people referred with a presumed infection actually had one, whereas the corresponding figure for those under 20 years old was 80% (Ellis *et al.*, 1985). A recent study suggests that a relatively low degree of confidence in diagnosing many kinds of infection may be a more generalised phenomenon and not one restricted to the old (Emmerson *et al.*, 1996). Other recent studies have confirmed the atypical pattern of presentation in old patients with Gram-negative septicaemia (Chassagne *et al.*, 1996) and infective endocarditis (Werner *et al.*, 1996).

Finally, we have suggested that the old may be particularly susceptible to developing the 'malignant systemic inflammation' of the systemic inflammatory response syndrome (SIRS). This syndrome was once thought of as 'the fatal expression of uncontrolled sepsis' but is now known to be inducible by a variety of stimuli. We also know that advancing age is an independent risk factor for developing this syndrome (Sauaia *et al.*, 1994). Furthermore, trauma seems to prime and activate neutrophils, thus sensitising them to a second stimulus which causes release of free radicals and other mediators thought to be involved in SIRS (Botha *et al.*, 1995). If, as we have previously suggested, neutrophils from old people are already primed for a second stimulus, trauma may be the second stimulus that precipitates the SIRS.

Conclusions

In this short chapter we have attempted to sketch the age-related changes in the host response to infections but it is clear that there are large gaps in our knowledge. Changes occur in both specific and non-specific defences but we are still unsure whether these changes predispose to acquiring infections. Until such evidence is forthcoming, it would be better to view immunosenescence as a state of immune dysregulation rather than as an immunodeficiency state. It may be that this issue will never be satisfactorily resolved as it is virtually impossible to control for nutritional status and co-morbidity.

Be that as it may, the injured elderly represent a particularly vulnerable group in whom these aging changes will most likely conspire with the immunosuppressive effects of trauma, undernutrition and co-morbidity to reduce resistance. The hospital environment will be particularly hazardous for these people by markedly increasing their chances of encountering potential pathogens. Once an infection occurs, it will tend to be more severe than in the young and the risk of death will be high. Doctors who look after these patients must be aware of the problem and ensure scrupulous hygiene and infection control procedures. They should also take steps to reduce the risks for all patients by following antibiotic policies aimed at minimising the production of resistant organisms.

We have presented evidence that the diagnosis of infections in older people can be problematic and the doctor must be constantly alert. Infection should always be considered when evaluating a patient whose condition has deteriorated. Although atypical presentations do occur (Chapter 2), their effects can be minimised by ensuring that optimal diagnostic techniques are used including the measurement of rectal temperature before concluding that a patient is truly afebrile. Older patients constantly present challenges to our diagnostic skills and we must ensure that we are up to the task.

References

Arranz, F., O'Mahony, S., Barton, I. R. & Ferguson, A. (1992). Immunosenescence and mucosal immunity: significant effects of old age on secretory IgA concentrations and intraepithelial lymphocyte counts. *Gut*, **33**, 882–6.

Averill, L. E. & Wolf, N. S. (1985). The decline in murine splenic PHA and LPS responsiveness with age is primarily due to an intrinsic mechanism. *J Immunol*, **134**, 3859–63.

Astle, C. M. & Harrison, D. E. (1984). Effect of marrow donor and recipient age on immune responses. *J Immunol*, **132**, 673–7.

Ben-Yehuda, A., Ehleiter, D., Hu, A.-R. & Weksler, M. E. (1993). Recombinant vaccinia virus expressing the PR/8 influenza haemagglutinin gene overcomes the impaired immune response and increased susceptibility of old mice to influenza infection. *J Infect Dis*, **168**,

352–7.

Ben-Yehuda, A. & Weksler, M. E. (1992). Host resistance and the immune system. *Clin Geriatr Med*, **8**, 701–11.

Bender, B. S., Nagel, J. E., Adler, W. H. & Andres, R. (1986). Absolute peripheral blood lymphocyte count and subsequent mortality of elderly men. The Baltimore longitudinal study of aging. *J Am Geriatr Soc*, **34**, 649–54.

Bone, R. C. (1996). Toward a theory regarding the pathogenesis of the systemic inflammatory response syndrome: what we do and do not know about cytokine regulation? *Crit Care Med*, **24**, 163–72.

Botha, A. J., Moore, F. A., Moore, E. E., Kim, F. J., Banerjee, A. & Petersson, V. M. (1995). Postinjury neutrophil priming and activation: an early vulnerable window. *Surgery*, **118**, 358–65.

Bowden, M., Crawford, J., Cohen, H. J. & Noyama, O. (1993). A comparative study of monoclonal gammaopathies and immunoglobulin levels in Japanese and United States elderly. *J Am Geriatr Soc*, **41**, 11–14.

Bradley, S. F., Vibhagool, A., Fabrick, S., Terpenning, M. S. & Kauffman, C. A. (1990). Monokine production by malnourished nursing home patients. *Gerontology*, **36**, 165–70.

Brouwer, A., Parker, S. G., Hendriks, H. F. J., Gibbons, L. & Horan, M. A. (1995). Stimulation of Kupffer cells from young and old rats by endotoxin: 1. Induction of eicosanoids and cytokines. *Clin Sci*, **88**, 211–17.

Castenada, C., Charnley, J. M., Evans, W. J. & Crim, M. C. (1995). Elderly women accommodate to a low-protein diet with losses of body cell mass, muscle function, and immune response. *Am J Clin Nutr*, **62**, 30–9.

Chandra, R. K. (1992). Effect of vitamin and trace-element supplementation on immune responses and infection in elderly subjects. *Lancet*, **340**, 1124–7.

Chassagne, P., Perol, M.-B., Doucet, J., Trivalle, C., Menard, J.-F., Manchai, N.-D., Moynot, Y., Humbert, G., Bourille, J. & Bercoff, G. (1996). Is presentation of bacteraemia in the elderly the same as younger patients? *Am J Med*, **100**, 65–70.

Chatta, G. S., Andrews, R. G., Rodger, E., Schrag, M., Hammond, W. P. & Dale, J. C. (1993). Hematopoietic progenitors and aging: alterations in granulocytic precursors and responsiveness to recombinant human G-CSF, GM-CSF and IL-3. *J Geront*, **48**, M207–M212.

Chen, Y., Ramsey, M. A. & Bradley, S. F. (1993). Differential monokine production by macrophages from aged mice stimulated with various microorganisms. *Aging Immunol Infect Dis*, **4**, 155–67.

Clague, J. E. & Horan, M. A. (1994). Urine culture in the elderly: scientifically dubious and practically useless? *Lancet*, **344**, 1035–6.

Couch, R. B., Kasel, J. A. & Glezen, W. P. (1986). Influenza: its control in persons and populations. *J Infect Dis*, **153**, 431–40.

Cox, M. L., Rudd, A. G., Gallimore, R., Hodkinson, H. M. & Pepys, M. B. (1986). Real-time measurement of serum C-reactive protein in the management of infection in the elderly. *Age Ageing*, **15**, 257–66.

Daniels, C. K., Schmucker, D. L. & Irvin, B. J. (1993). Differential IgA responses in the aging Fischer rat following mucosal stimulation with cholera toxin or B subunit. *Aging Immunol Infect Dis*, **4**, 95–107.

Decker, D., Schondorf, M., Bidlingmaier, F., Hirner, A., von Rueker, A. (1996). Surgical stress induces a shift in the type-1/type-2 T-helper cell balance, suggesting down-regulation of cell-mediated and upregulation of antibody-mediated immunity commensurate to trauma. *Surgery*, **119**, 316–25.

Dries, D. J. (1992). The immune consequences of trauma: an overview. In *Trauma 2000. Strategies for the New Millenium*, ed. R. L. Ganelli & D. J. Dries, pp. 64–73. Austin, Texas, USA: R. G. Landes Company.

Durham, S. K., Horan, M. A., Brouwer, A., Barelds, R. J. & Knook, D. L. (1989). Platelet participation in the increased severity of endotoxin-induced pulmonary injury in aged rats. *J Pathol*, **157**, 339–45.

Ellis, M. E., Burnett, J., McGrath, C. & Smitt, C. C. (1985). An analysis of twelve months admissions to a regional infection unit with an 'open door' admission policy. *J Infect*, **10**, 4–16.

Emeis, J. J., Brouwer, A., Barelds, R. J., Horan, M. A., Durham, S. K. & Kooistra, T. (1992). On the fibrinolytic system in aged rats and its reactivity to endotoxin and cytokines. *Thromb Haemost*, **67**, 697–701.

Emmerson, A. M., Enstone, J. E., Griffin, M., Kelsey, M. C. & Smyth, E. T. M. (1996). The second national prevalence survey of infection in hospitals: overview of the results. *J Hosp Infect*, **32**, 175–90.

Esposito, A. L., Piorier, W. T. & Clark, C. A. (1990). In vitro assessment of chemotaxis by peripheral blood neutrophils from adult and senescent C57BL/6 mice. *Gerontology*, **36**, 2–7.

Ferro, S. & Salit, I. E. (1992). HIV infection in patients over 55 years of age. *J Acq Immune Defic Syndro*, **5**, 348–55.

Finkelstein, M. S., Petkun, W. M., Freedman, M. L. & Antopol, S. C. (1983). Pneumococcal bacteraemia in adults. Age-dependent differences in presentation and outcome. *J Am Geriatr Soc*, **31**, 119–21.

Finland, M. & Barnes, M. W. (1977). Acute bacterial meningitis at Boston City Hospital during twelve selected years, 1935–1972. *J Infect Dis*, **136**, 400–15.

Fleck, A., Rains, G., Hawker, F., Trotter, J., Wallace, P. I., Ledingham, I. McA. & Kalman, K. C. (1986). Increased vascular permeability: a major cause of hypoalbuminaemia in disease and injury. *Lancet*, **1**, 781–4.

Franceschi, C., Monti, D., Sansoni, P. & Cossarizza, A. (1995). The immunology of exceptional individuals: the lesson of centenarians. *Immunol Today*, **16**, 12–16.

Franklin, R. A., Arkins, S., Li, Y. M. & Kelley, K. W. (1993). Macrophages suppress lectin-induced proliferation of lymphocytes from aged rats. *Mech Ageing Devel*, **67**, 33–46.

Freeman, J. & McGowan, J. (1978). Risk factors for nosocomial infections. *J Infect Dis*, **138**, 811–16.

Fulk, R., Fedson, D. & Huber, M. (1970). Antibody responses in serum and nasal secretions according to age of recipient and method of administration of A2/Hong Kong/68 inactivated influenza virus vaccine. *J Immunol*, **104**, 8–13.

Gauchat, J. F., Walker, C., De Weck, A. L. & Staadler, B. M. (1988). Stimulation-dependent lymphokine mRNA levels in human mononuclear cells. *Eur J Immunol*, **18**, 1441–6.

Goldberg, T. H., Baker, D. G. & Schumacher, H. R. (1991). Interleukin-1 and the immunology of aging. *Aging Immunol Infect Dis*, **3**, 81–9.

Gravenstein, S., Drinka, P., Duthie, E. H., Miller, B. A., Brown, C. S., Hensley, M., Circo, R., Langer, E. & Ershler, W. B. (1994). Efficacy of an influenza haemagglutin-diphtheria toxoid conjugate vaccine in elderly nursing home subjects during an influenza outbreak. *J Am Geriat Soc*, **42**, 245–51.

Gregoire, C. D., Zhang, L. & Daniels, C. K. (1992). Expression of the polymeric immunoglobulin receptor by cultured rat hepatocytes. *Gastroenterology*, **103**, 296–301.

Grossbad, L. J., Desai, M. H. & Lemeshow, S. (1984). Lymphocytopenia in the surgical intensive care unit patient. *Am Surg*, **50**, 209–15.

Hobbs, M. V., Weigle, W. O., Noonan, D. J., Torbett, B. E., McEvilly, R. J., Kocj, R. I., Cardenas, G. & Ernst, D. N. (1993). Patterns of cytokine gene expression by CD4[4] T cells from young and old mice. *J Immunol*, **150**, 3602–14.

Horan, M. A. (1993). Immunosenescence and mucosal immunity. *Lancet*, **341**, 793–4.

Horan, M. A., Brouwer, A., Barelds, R. J., Wientjens, R., Durham, S. K. & Knook, D. L. (1991). Changes in endotoxin sensitivity in aging. Absorption, elimination and mortality. *Mech Ageing Devel*, **57**, 145–62.

Horan, M. A., Gulati, R. S., Fox, R. A., Glew, E., Ganguli, L. & Kaeney, M. (1984). Outbreak of *Shigella sonnei* dysentery on a geriatric assessment ward. *J Hosp Infect*, **5**, 210–12.

Horan, M. A., Hendriks, H. F. J. & Brouwer, A. (1990). Systems under stress: infectious agents and their products. In *Gerontology: Approaches to Biomedical and Clinical Research*, ed. M. A. Horan & A. Brouwer, pp. 105–34. London: Edward Arnold.

Horan, M. A., Puxty, J. A. H. & Fox, R. A. (1983). Gynecologic sepsis as a cause of covert infection in old age. *J Am Geriatr Soc*, **31**, 213–15.

Huang, Y.-P., Pechere, J.-C., Michel, M., Gauthey, L., Loreto, M., Curran, J. A. & Michel, J.-P. (1992). In vivo T cell activation, in vitro defective IL-2 secretion, and responses to influenza vaccination in elderly women. *J Immunol*, **48**, 715–22.

Hussain, M., Oppenheim, B. A., O'Neill, P., Trembath, C., Morris, J. & Horan, M. A. (1996). Prospective survey of the incidence, risk factors and outcome of hospital-acquired infections in the elderly. *J Hosp Infect*, **32**, 117–26.

Hyde, S. R. & McCallum, R. E. (1992). LPS-TNF-glucocorticoid interactions during cecal ligation and puncture-induced sepsis in mature versus senescent mice. *Infect Immun*, **60**, 976–82.

Jones, P. G., Kauffman, C. A., Bergman, A. G., Hayes, C. M., Kluger, M. & Cannon, J. G. (1984). Fever in the elderly. Production of leukocytic pyrogen by monocytes from elderly persons. *Gerontology*, **30**, 182–7.

Kenny, R. A., Hodkinson, H. M., Cox, M. L., Caspi, D. & Pepys, M. B. (1984). Acute phase protein response to infections in elderly patients. *Age Ageing*, **13**, 89–94.

Kenny, R. A., Saunders, A. P., Coll, A., Harrington, M. G., Caspi, D., Hodkinson, H. M. & Pepys, M. B. (1985). A comparison of the erythrocyte sedimentation rate and serum C-reactive protein concentration in elderly patients. *Age Ageing*, **14**, 15–20.

Laharrague, P., Corberand, J., Fillola, G., Nguyen, F., Fontanilles, A. M., Gleizes, B., Gyrard, E. & Jean, C. (1983). Impairment of polymorphonuclear functions in hospitalized geriatric patients. *Gerontology*, **29**, 325–31.

Lew, J. F., Glass, R. I., Gangarosa, R. E., Cohen, I. P., Bern, C. & Moe, C. L. (1991). Diarrheal deaths in the United States, 1979 through 1987: a special problem for the elderly. *JAMA*, **265**, 3280–4.

Ligthart, G. J., Schuit, H. R. E. & Hijmans, W. (1989). Natural killer cell function is not diminished in the healthy aged and is proportional to the number of NK cells in the peripheral blood. *Immunology*, **68**, 396–402.

Linn, B. S., Linn, M. W. & Jensen, J. (1983). Surgical stress in the healthy elderly. *J Am Geriatr Soc*, **31**, 544–8.

Lipschitz, D. A. & Udupa, K. B. (1986). Influence of aging and protein deficiency on neutrophil function. *J Gerontol*, **41**, 690–4.

Louria, D. B., Sen, P. & Buse, M. (1982). Age-dependent differences in outcome of infections, with special reference to experiments in mice. *J Am Geriatr Soc*, **30**, 769–73.

Macfarlane, J. T., Ward, M. J., Finch, R. G. & Macrae, A. D. (1982). Hospital study of adult community-acquired pneumonia. *Lancet*, **2**, 255–8.

McCue, J. (1987). Gram-negative bacillary bacteraemia in the elderly: incidence, ecology, etiology, and mortality. *J Am Geriatr Soc*, **35**, 213–18.

Miller, R. A. (1995). Immune system. In *Handbook of Physiology*, Section 11, ed. E. J. Masoro, pp. 555–90. New York: Oxford University Press.

Nafziger, J., Bessage, J. P., Guillosson, J. J., Damais, C. & Lesourd, B. (1993). Decreased capacity of IL-1 production by monocytes of infected elderly patients. *Aging Immunol Infect Dis*, **4**, 25–34.

Nogues, R., Sitges-Seria, A., Sancho, J. J., Sanz, F., Monne, J., Girvent, M. & Gubern, J. M. (1995). Influence of nutrition, thyroid hormones, and rectal temperature on in-hospital mortality of elderly patients with acute illness. *Am J Clin Nut*, **61**, 597–602.

Orr, P. J., Nicolle, L. E., Duckworth, H., Brunka, J., Kennedy, J., Murray, D. & Harding, G. K. (1996). Febrile urinary infection in the institutionalized elderly. *Am J Med*, **100**, 71–7.

Panum, P. L. (1847). *Virchows Arch*, **1**, 492–507. Reprinted in *Medical Classics*, **3**, 829–41.

Pawalec, G., Adibzadeh, M., Pohla, H. & Schaudt, K. (1995). Immunosenescence: aging of the immune system. *Immunol Today*, **16**, 420–2.

Pfeifer, K., Ushijima, H., Lorenz, B., Müller, W. E. G. & Schröder, H. C. (1993). Evidence for age-dependent impairment of antiviral 2′,5′-oligoadenylate synthetase/ribonuclease L-system in tissues of rat. *Mech Ageing Dev*, **67**, 101–14.

Proust, J., Rosenzweig, P., Debouzy, C. & Moulias, R. (1985). Lymphopenia induced by actue bacterial infections in the elderly: a sign of age-related immune dysfunction of major prognostic significance. *Gerontology*, **31**, 178–85.

Radl, J. (1985). Monoclonal gammopathies. An attempt at a new classification. *Netherlands J Med*, **28**, 134–7.

Resnitzky, P., Segal, M., Barak, Y. & Dassa, C. (1987). Granulopoiesis in aged people: inverse correlation between bone marrow cellularity and myeloid progenitor cell numbers. *Gerontology*, **33**, 109–14.

Ritter, M. A. & Crispe, I. N. (1992). *The Thymus*, Oxford: IRL Press, pp. 23–4.

Root, G. A. W., Hernadez-Pando, R. & Lightman, S. L. (1994). Hormones, peripherally activated prohormones and regulation of the TH1/TH2 balance. *Immunol Today*, **15**, 301–3.

Rosenberg, J. S., Gilman, S. C. & Feldman, J. D. (1983). Effect of aging on cell co-operation and lymphocyte responsiveness to cytokines. *J Immunol*, **130**, 1754–9.

Rudd, A. G. & Banerjee, D K. (1989). Interleukin-1 production by human monocytes in ageing and disease. *Age Ageing*, **18**, 43–6.

Russo, C., Schwab, R. & Weksler, M. E. (1990). Immune dysregulation associated with aging. *Aging Immunol Infect Dis*, **2**, 211–16.

Sansoni, P., Cossarizza, A., Brianti, V., Fagnoni, F., Snelli, G., Manti, D., Marcato, A., Passeri, G., Ortolani, C., Forti, E., Fragiolo, U., Passeri, M. & Franceschi, C. (1993). Lymphocyte subsets and natural killer cell activity in healthy old people and centenarians. *Blood*, **82**, 2767–73.

Sauaia, A., Moore, F. A., Moore, E. E., Haenel, J. B., Read, R. A. & Lezotte, D. C. (1994). Early predictors of postinjury multiple organ failure. *Arch Surg*, **129**, 39–45.

Schmucker, D. L. & Daniels, C. K. (1986). Aging, gastrointestinal infections, and mucosal immunity. *J Am Geriatr Soc*, **34**, 377–84.

Shapiro, E. D., Berg, A. T., Austrian, R., Schroeder, D., Parcello, V., Margolis, A., Adair, R. K. & Clemens, J. D. (1991). Protective efficacy of polyvalent pneumococcal polysaccharide vaccine. *New Eng J Med*, **325**, 1453–60.

Smith, R. P., Lipworth, B. J., Cree, I. A., Spiers, E. M. & Winter, J. H. (1995). C-reactive protein. A clinical marker in community-acquired pneumonia. *Chest*, **108**, 1288–91.

Steinmann, G. G. & Hartwig, M. (1995). Immunology of centenarians. *Immunol Today*, **16**, 549.

Steinmann, G. G. & Muller-Hermelink, H.-K. (1984). Lymphocyte differentiation and its microenvironment in the human thymus during aging. *Monogr Devel Biol*, **17**, 142–55.

Szewczuk, M. R., Campbell, R. J. & Jung, L. K. (1980). Lack of age-associated dysfunction in mucosal-associated lymph nodes. *J Immunol*, **126**, 2200–4.

Tabardel, Y., Duchateau, J., Schmartz, D., Marecaux, G., Shahla, M., Barvais, L., Leclerc, J.-L. & Vincent, J.-L. (1996). Corticosteroids increase blood interleukin-10 levels during cardio-pulmonary bypass in men. *Surgery*, **119**, 76–80.

Tokunaga, A., Onda, M., Fujita, I., Okuda, T., Mizutani, T. & Kiyama, T. (1993). Sequential changes in the cell mediators of peritoneal and wound fluids after surgery. *Surg Today*, **23**, 841–4.

Treanor, J. J., Mattison, H. R., Dumyati, G., Yinnon, A., Erb, S., O'Brien, D., Dolin, R. & Betts, R. F. (1992). Protective efficacy of combined live intranasal and inactivated influenza A virus vaccine in the elderly. *Ann Intern Med*, **117**, 625–33.

Tsukuda, K., Katoh, H., Shiojima, M., Suzuki, T., Takenoshita, S. & Nagamachi, Y. (1993). Concentrations of cytokines in peritoneal fluid after abdominal surgery. *Eur J Surg*, **159**, 475–9.

Utsuyama, M., Kesai, M., Kurashima, C. & Hirokawa, K. (1991). Age-influence on the thymic capacity to promote differentiation of T cells: induction of different composition of T cell subsets by aging thymus. *Mech Ageing Dev.* **58**, 267–77.

Waage, A., Brandtzaag, P., Halstensen, A., Kierulf, P. & Espevik, T. (1989). The complex pattern of cytokines in serum from patients with meningococcal septic shock. Association between interleukin-6, interleukin-1 and fatal outcome. *J Exp Med*, **169**, 333–8.

Wade, A. W., Green-Johnson, J. & Szewczuk, M. R. (1988). Functional decline in systemic and mucosal lymphocyte repertoires with age: an update review. *Aging Immunol Infect Dis*, **1**, 65–97.

Wakefield, C. H., Carey, P. D., Foulds, S., Monson, J. R. & Guillou, P. J. (1993a). Polymorphonuclear leukocyte activation. An early marker of the surgical sepsis response. *Arch Surg*, **128**, 390–5.

Wakefield, C. H., Carey, P. D., Foulds, S., Monson, J. R. & Guillou, P. J. (1993b). Changes in the major histocompatibility complex class II expression in monocytes and T cells of patients developing infection after surgery. *Br J Surg*, **80**, 205–9.

Werner, G. S., Schulz, R., Fuchs, J. B., Andreas, S., Prange, H., Ruschewski, W. & Kreuzer, H. (1996). Infective endocarditis in the elderly in the era of transesophageal echocardiography: clinical features and prognosis compared with younger patients. *Am J Med*, **100**, 90–7.

Zharkhary, D. (1986). T cell involvement in the decrease of antigen-responsive B cells in aged mice. *Eur J Immunol*, **16**, 1175–8.

Zharkhary, D. & Klinman, N. R. (1983). Antigen responsiveness of the mature and generative B cell populations of aged mice. *J Exp Med*, **157**, 1300–8.

Zhou, D., Chrest, F. J., Adler, W., Munster, A. & Winchurch, R. A. (1992). Age-related changes in the expression of the TGF-β receptor on CD4$^+$ and CD8$^+$ subsets of T cells. *Aging: Immunol Infect Dis*, **3**, 217–26.

10

Aging and cutaneous wound healing

G. S. ASHCROFT, M. A. HORAN and
M. W. J. FERGUSON

Introduction

The ability to repair tissues is critical for survival and it has long been thought that this ability is impaired in old age (Goodson & Hunt, 1979). Chronic, persistent wounds are certainly common among older people but these are generally associated with systemic illnesses (e.g. vasculitis, atherosclerosis, diabetes mellitus, malnutrition) or local conditions (e.g. venous insufficiency). Furthermore, most studies that report impaired wound healing in the aged have failed to control for the presence of such conditions when making comparisons.

Carrel & DuNouy (1921) studied soldiers wounded in World War I and used a 'cicatrisation index' to assess the rate of wound healing. They found that 30–year-old men healed less well than 20–year-olds and that 40–year-olds healed less well than 30–year-olds. These authors made no attempt to control for the site and nature of the wound, wound depth and infection. In such circumstances, the age effect they described seems intrinsically unlikely. Halasz (1968) reported a cooperative study of 19 Veterans Administration hospitals in the USA in which wound dehiscence was recorded after duodenal ulcer surgery in 3000 patients. Wound dehiscence increased from 1% in 30 to 39–year-old patients to 5% in those over the age of 70 years, a finding confirmed by White & Cook (1977) in a similar group of patients.

In the remainder of this chapter we confine ourselves to cutaneous wound healing as so little is known about age effects on the repair of other tissues that sensible conclusions cannot be drawn.

Skin morphology and aging

A number of time-dependent changes have been described in the skin, but not all are the consequence of aging; environmental factors, particularly exposure to the sun (so-called photoaging), also have important effects. During aging, the epidermis becomes thinner and its barrier function may be impaired because of reduction in sterol esters and triglycerides (Grove, 1986). The dermo-epidermal junction flattens because of the retraction of epidermal papillae and the microprojections of basal cells into the dermis (Kurban & Bhavan, 1990). The dermis becomes less cellular with changes in the collagen and elastin networks which are thought to be caused by a loss of ground substance. There is a reduction in fibrous collagen and elastin, the latter becoming frayed (Smith, 1989). The dermis becomes less vascular and the remaining vessels appear dilated and tortuous (Braverman, 1989).

The healing process

The inflammatory phase

The immediate consequence of skin wounding is disruption of vascular integrity and extravasation of blood. Platelets aggregate when exposed to subendothelial types IV and V collagen, a process involving secretion of von Willebrand factor. Platelets induce haemostasis by (1) aggregation (enhanced by ADP and thromboxane), (2) vasoconstriction (involving ADP and serotonin), and (3) activation of the coagulation cascade (following a rearrangement of membrane phospholipids that facilitates factor V binding). The resultant fibrin gel is an important early component of wound repair as evidenced by impaired wound healing in animals depleted of fibrinogen (Clark, 1988). Local mediators result in the recruitment of more platelets which release fibrin, fibronectin, thrombospondin, von Willebrand factor and a host of other mediators. Fibrin and fibronectin form a provisional matrix for the influx of phagocytic cells.

Platelet products and products of the blood coagulation cascade are chemoattractants for circulating phagocytic cells and upregulate membrane beta-2 integrins which recognise matrix proteins like fibronectin, laminin and collagen as well as cellular adhesion molecules. This facilitates margination of phagocytic cells close to the site of injury, followed by chemotaxis into the wound (Tonneson, 1989). Neutrophils are usually considered to be the first cells to infiltrate a wound within a few hours of injury but mononuclear phagocytes probably migrate at approximately the same time, although the latter cells persist in the wound considerably longer (Clark, 1991). Migration of neutrophils across a vessel wall (diapedesis) is further facilitated by other vasodilating mediators such as serotonin and bradykinin. Both neutrophils and mononuclear phagocytes debride the wound and kill contaminating microbes. Mononuclear phagocytes are also an important source of cytokines such as interleukins IL-1 and IL-6, tumour necrosis factor (TNF), transforming growth factor (TGF) α and β and platelet-derived growth factor (PDGF), thus underlining their crucial role in the regulation of wound healing. PDGF is an especially potent mitogen for mesenchymal cells such as fibroblasts and smooth muscle cells (Ross *et al.*, 1986) as well as being a chemoattractant for these and phagocytic cells. TGFβ stimulates fibroblasts to secrete collagen and fibronectin. Lysed cells produce fibroblast growth factor (FGF) which is mitogenic for fibroblasts and endothelial cells (Gospodarowicz, 1979).

Lymphocytes enter the wound soon after macrophages and they too may play a role in wound healing. Lymphotrophic agents such as IL-2 enhance final wound strength (Barbul, 1988) and lympholytic agents (e.g. cyclosporin A) impair it. Cytokines produced by lymphocytes are likely to be important in this regard. Recombinant IL-2 enhances collagen production in experimental wounds but IFNγ reduces it (Regan & Barbul, 1991).

Aging has been reported to increase the ability of dermal collagen from old rats to aggregate platelets which would theoretically enhance the inflammatory response (Grigorova-Borsos *et al.*, 1988). Acute inflammatory reactions, however, have been shown to be less intense in the skin of old humans when challenged with ammonium chloride (Kligman, 1979). Similarly, cutaneous delayed-type (type IV) hypersensitivity is also markedly attenuated (Makinodan *et al.*, 1991) and this is, at least in part, an intrinsic change in the immune system. There is some evidence that impaired macrophage function may contribute to impaired wound healing in the aged. Young mice injected subcutaneously with antimacrophage serum at the site of a cutaneous punch biopsy wound exhibited similar wound healing kinetics to untreated old mice (Cohen *et al.*, 1987). Furthermore, the addition of peritoneal macrophages to wounds in old mice brought about similar wound healing kinetics to those observed in young mice (Danon *et al.*, 1989).

The proliferation phase

Fibroblasts

Within about 72 hours of injury, fibroblasts, attracted by chemotactic cytokines and guided by the provisional matrix, enter the wound. They are also induced to move from G_0 to G_1 in the cell cycle under the influence of PDGF, FGF and calcium (sometimes referred to as acquiring 'competence'). Progression to DNA synthesis and mitosis is controlled by other cytokines, especially insulin-like growth factor (IGF-1) and epidermal growth factor (EGF). These 'activated' fibroblasts produce IFNβ which acts as an autocrine and paracrine growth inhibitor. Collagen production is largely controlled by TGFβ but other cytokines are likely to be involved (Kulozik *et al.*, 1991). PDGF stimulates fibroblasts to produce TGFβ, thereby enhancing collagen synthesis (Pierce *et al.*, 1989). In the early stages, large quantities of fibronectin are produced together with collagen (types I and III) and hyaluronate. Later, type III collagen is replaced with type I. As well as extracellular matrix production, fibroblasts are involved in wound contraction. Precisely how this takes place is not known but it appears not to depend on fibroblasts within the wound granulation tissue but rather on a rim of densely packed, freshly proliferated fibroblasts around the wound edge (Gross *et al.*, 1995).

It has been reported that young animals form granulation tissue in experimental wounds faster than old ones (Howes & Harvey, 1932; Doberauber, 1963). Fibroblasts from old donors show reduced motility independent of chemotactic gradients (Pienta & Coffey, 1990) and the chemotactic response to fibronectin is diminished in the old (Albini *et al.*, 1988). The proliferative capacity of fibroblasts obtained from old donors is reduced in a number of *in vitro* settings. Confluent monolayers, when 'wounded', have a reduced capacity to restore confluence (Muggleton-Harris *et al.*, 1982) and this may be associated with a reduced ability to respond to a variety of proliferative stimuli such as insulin, IGF-1, FGF, serum and PDGF (Rattan & Derventzi, 1991), although the inhibitory effects of IFNβ are unimpaired (Tamm *et al.*, 1984).

Epithelial cells

The epidermis is a stratified squamous epithelium that, in the unwounded state, is in contact with the basement membrane molecules laminin, heparan sulphate and the bullous pemphigoid antigen. The lamina lucida space separates it from the lamina densa (rich in type IV collagen), below which is a fibrillar zone comprising dermatan and chondroitin sulphate, fibronectin and collagen (types V and VII). Within hours of wounding, epithelial cells (keratinocytes) start to migrate from the wound margins and residual hair follicles (Winter, 1962). Migration is induced by the cytokines TNF (from keratinocytes, lymphocytes and macrophages), IL-1 and TGFβ (from keratinocytes, macrophages and platelets). If the basement membrane has been disrupted, migration is slow as the migrating cells must also construct a new basement membrane. Basement membrane disruption allows contact of keratinocytes with fibronectin, dermatan and chondroitin sulphate and unfamiliar types of collagen. Woodley *et al.* (1991) have shown that fibronectin and types I and IV collagen induce locomotion and laminin inhibits it. Within a day or two, the cells behind the migrating front start to proliferate under the influence of TGFα and EGF (Barrandon & Green, 1987) and terminal differentiation is inhibited by the continued presence of fibronectin (Adams & Watt, 1989). It has been reported that epithelialisation is slowed in the elderly (Baker & Blair, 1968; Orentreich & Selmanowicz, 1969). Keratinocytes from old donors have a reduced response to most proliferative stimuli (Rattan & Derventzi, 1991) and increased sensitivity to inhibitors of proliferation (Peacocke *et al.*, 1989).

Angiogenesis

A variety of stimuli (e.g. TNF, extracellular matrix components) induce the migration of endothelial cells from injured vessels. Within about 24 hours, cells start to proliferate and FGF, EGF and TNF are known proliferative stimuli. Endothelial cells grow as solid tubes and secrete a basal lamina. These tubes join others and eventually form a lumen. Little is known about the effects of aging on angiogenesis.

Repair and remodelling

During this phase, collagen is produced in abundance, is remodelled and the new vessels regress to leave a mature scar. Fibronectin is removed within a few weeks and hyaluronate is largely replaced by heparan sulphate in the basement membrane and by chondroitin sulphate in the interstitium. Type III collagen is gradually replaced by type I. The regulation of collagen turnover in skin is complex and will not be discussed further. The rate of collagen synthesis in old skin is lower than in young skin and the rate of degradation is higher (Mays, 1991). When fibroblasts are cultured on plastic or on a collagen gel, EGF inhibits collagen synthesis. When these cells are cultured in a three-dimensional collagen lattice, EGF no longer inhibits collagen synthesis of fibroblasts from young donors but continues to do so for cells from old donors (Colige *et al.*, 1990).

Conclusion

Most reviews of wound healing mention age as one of the factors affecting it but very little evidence is ever presented. Likewise, many clinicians share this view even though many of their elderly patients are undernourished, uraemic, septic, jaundiced or suffering from cancer or have other systemic or local disorders that might affect wound healing, irrespective of age.

We have attempted to give an overview of our present understanding of the cellular and molecular events that occur during cutaneous wound healing. Age-related changes have been reported in many components of this process and these could conceivably be associated with impaired wound healing. The findings are often contradictory, however, and it is not known if compensatory strategies might be employed to overcome the effects of these changes. This is a very real possibility as a very prominent characteristic of cytokines, the major regulatory molecules, is their overlapping activities.

The reported studies that address the overall process of wound healing are few and littered with methodological imperfections. The best that we can say is that there probably is an age-related delay in wound healing but that this effect is not marked. A firmer conclusion must await the results of the detailed, comprehensive studies that are now underway. Probably of much greater importance for clinical practice are the numerous extrinsic factors and conditions that have a much more marked effect on wound healing.

References

Adams, J. C. & Watt, F. M. (1989). Fibronectin has been shown to inhibit terminal differentiation of human keratinocytes. *Nature*, **27**, 307–09.

Albini, A. (1988). Decline of fibroblast chemotaxis with the age of donor and cell passage number. *Coll Relat Res*, **8**, 23–37.

Baker, H. & Blair, C. P. (1968). Cell replacement in the human stratum corneum in old age. *Br J Dermatol*, **80**, 367–72.

Barbul, A. (1988). Role of the T cell dependent immune system in wound healing. *Prog Clin Biol Res*, **266**, 161–75.

Barrandon, Y. & Green, H. (1987). Cell migration is essential for sustained growth of keratinocyte colonies: the role of TGFα and EGF. *Cell*, **50**, 1131–7.

Braverman, I. M. (1989). Elastic fiber and microvascular abnormalities in aging skin. *Clin Geriatr Med*, **5**, 69–90.

Carrel, A. & DuNuoy, P. (1921). Cicatrization of wounds. *J Exp Med*, **34**, 339–48.

Clark, R. A. F. (1988). Cutaneous wound repair: an overview. In *The Molecular and Cellular Biology of Wound Repair*, ed. R. A. F. Clark & P. M. Henson, pp. 5–9. New York: Plenum Press.

Clark, R. A. F. (1991). Cutaneous wound repair: a review with emphasis on integrin receptor expression. In *Wound Healing*, ed. H. Janssen, R. Rooman & J. I. S. Robertson, pp. 7–17. Petersfield: Wrightson Biomedical Publishing.

Cohen, B. J., Danon, D. & Roth, G. S. (1987). Wound repair in mice is influenced by age and antimacrophage serum. *J Gerontol*, **42**, 295–301.

Colige, A., Nusgens, B. & Lapiere, C. M. (1990). Response to epidermal growth factor of skin fibroblasts from donors of varying age is modulated by the extracellular matrix. *J Cell Physiol*, **145**, 450–7.

Danon, D., Kowatch, M. A. & Roth, G. S. (1989). Promotion of wound repair in old mice by local injection of macrophages. *Proc Natl Acad Sci USA*, **86**, 2018–20.

Doberauber, W. (1963). Einfluß des Lebensalters auf die Heilung kunstlicher haut Defekte. *Klin Med* (*Wien*), **18**, 199–204.

Goodson, W. H. & Hunt, T. K. (1979). Wound healing and ageing. *J Invest Dermatol*, **73**, 88–91.

Gospodarowicz, D., Bialecki, H. & Thakral, T. K. (1979). The angiogenic activity of the fibroblast and epidermal growth factors. *Exp Eye Res*, **28**, 501–14.

Gospodarowicz, D., Ferrara, N., Schweigerer, L. & Neufeld, G. (1987). Structural characterization and biological functions of fibroblast growth factor. *Endocrine Rev*, **8**, 95–114.

Grigorova-Borsos, A. M., Bara, L., Aberer, E., Grochulski, A., Andre, J., Mozere, G., Peyroux, J. & Sternberg, M. (1988). Aging and diabetes increase the aggregating potency of rat skin collagen towards normal platelets. *Thromb Haemost*, **60**, 75–8.

Gross, J., Farinelli, W., Sadow, P., Anderson, R. & Burns, R. (1995). On the mechanism of skin wound 'contraction': a granulation tissue 'knockout' with a normal phenotype. *Proc Natl Acad Sci USA*, **92**, 5982–6.

Grove, G. L. (1986). Physiologic changes in older skin. *Dermatol Clin*, **4**, 425–32.

Halasz, N. A. (1968). Dehiscence of laparotomy wounds. *Am J Surg*, **116**, 210–14.

Howes, E. L. & Harvey, S. C. (1932). The age factor in the velocity of the growth of fibroblasts in the healing wound. *J Exp Med*, **55**, 577–84.

Kligman, A. M. (1979). Perspectives and problems in cutaneous gerontology. *J Invest Dermatol*, **73**, 39–46.

Kulozik, M., Heckmann, M., Mauch, C., Scharffetter, K. & Krieg, Th. (1991). Cytokine regulation of collagen metabolism during wound healing in vitro and in vivo. In *Wound Healing*, ed. H. Janssen, R. Rooman & J. I. S. Robertson, pp. 33–9. Petersfield: Wrightson Biomedical Publishing.

Kurban, R. S. & Bhavan, J. (1990). Histologic changes in skin associated with aging. *J Dermatol Surg Oncol*, **16**, 908–14.

Makinodan, T., Hahn, T. J., McDougall, S., Yamaguchi, D. T., Fang, M. & Iida-Klein, A. (1991). Cellular immunosenescence: an overview. *Exp Gerontol*, **26**, 281–88.

Mays, P. K. (1991). Age-related changes in collagen synthesis and degradation in rat tissues. *J Biochem*, **276** (part 2), 307–13.

Muggleton-Harris, A. L., Reisert, P. S. & Burghoff, R. L. (1982). *In vitro* characterisation of the response to a stimulus (wounding) with regard to aging in human skin fibroblasts. *Mech Ageing Dev*, **19**, 37–43.

Orentreich, N. & Selmanowicz, V. J. (1969). Levels of biological functions with aging. *Trans Acad Sci*, **31**, B992–B1012.

Peacocke, M., Yaar, M. & Gilchrest, B. A. (1989). Interferon and the epidermis: implications for cellular senescence. *Exp Gerontol*, **24**, 415–21.

Pienta, K. J. & Coffey, D. S. (1990). Characterisation of the subtypes of cell motility in aging human skin fibroblasts. *Mech Ageing Dev*, **56**, 99–105.

Pierce, G. F., Mustoe, T. A., Lingelbach, C., Musakowski, T., Griffin, G. L., Senior, R. M. & Deuel, T. F. (1989). Platelet-derived growth factor and transforming growth factor-beta enhance tissue repair activities by unique mechanisms. *J Cell Biol*, **109**, 429–40.

Rattan, S. I. S. & Derventzi, A. (1991). Altered cellular responsiveness during ageing. *BioEssays*, **13**, 601–6.

Regan, M. C. & Barbul, A. (1991). Regulation of wound healing by the T cell-dependent immune system. In *Wound Healing*, ed. H. Janssen, R. Rooman & J. I. S. Robertson, pp. 21–31. Petersfield: Wrightson Biomedical Publishing.

Ross, R., Raines, E. W. & Bowen-Pope, D. F. (1986). The biology of platelet-derived growth factor. *Cell*, **45**, 155–69.

Smith, L. (1989). Histopathologic characteristics and ultrastructure of aging skin. *Cutis*, **43**, 414–24.

Tamm, I., Kikuchi, T., Wang, E. & Pfeffer, L. M. (1984). Growth rate of control and beta interferon-treated human fibroblast populations over the course of their in vitro lifespan. *Cancer Res*, **44**, 2291–6.

Tonneson, M. G. (1989). Neutrophil-endothelial cell interactions: mechanisms of neutrophil adherence to vascular endothelium. *J Invest Dermatol*, **93**, 535–85.

White, H. & Cook, J. (1977). Abdominal wound dehiscence. *Ann R Coll Surg Eng*, **59**, 337–41.

Winter, G. D. (1962). Formation of the scab and the rate of epithelialization of superficial wounds in the skin of the young domestic pig. *Nature*, **193**, 293–4.

Woodley, D. T., Sarret, Y. & O'Keefe, E. J. (1991). Human keratinocyte locomotion on extracellular matrix. In *Wound Healing*, ed. H. Janssen, R. Rooman & J. I. S. Robertson, pp. 91–7. Petersfield: Wrightson Biomedical Publishing.

11

Decubitus ulceration: prevention

M. R. BLISS

Aetiology

To prevent decubitus ulcers, or pressure sores as they should more accurately be described, we need to understand their aetiology. They are not caused by nursing neglect but by peripheral circulatory failure, part of the multiorgan failure that occurs in acute illness or trauma. They principally affect patients with neurological or vascular disease and the elderly, but may occur in any very ill person.

Neurological disease

Loss or impairment of sensation prevents patients from feeling ischaemic pain in the pressure areas, and hence the normal stimulus to move which allows restoration of the blood supply and prevents tissue death. This is more important than motor paralysis. Patients with purely motor diseases (e.g. motor neurone disease, polio, muscular dystrophy) do not usually develop sores before the terminal phase (when they become acutely ill), (Raney, 1989) because normal pressure pain causes them to move themselves, or be moved, in order to obtain relief. A healthy adult makes about 16 major and 100 minor bodily movements in one night (Johnson *et al.*, 1930). Elderly patients make fewer movements than young (Bar *et al.*, 1983) and patients with neurological disease fewer still (Nicholson *et al.*, 1988), but 2–3 hourly repositioning has been shown to prevent tissue necrosis in spinal injury patients (Lowthian, 1985).

The highest incidence of pressure sores (up to 80%), and most severe sores, occur in patients with spinal cord injury (Richardson & Meyer, 1981) who not only have sensory loss and motor paralysis, but also loss of vasomotor tone (spinal shock) for up to 3 months following injury (Bogie *et al.*, 1992). It is uncertain to what extent spinal shock affects responses to pressure (Bliss, 1993) and important degenerative changes may occur later; patients with low spinal lesions and flaccid paralysis with permanent impairment of spinal reflexes have a higher incidence of pressure sores than quadrip-

154

legic patients with intact reflexes (Constantian & Jackson, 1980). Patients with chronic spinal lesions and other 'elderly immobile and insensitive subjects' at particular risk of pressure sores have been shown to have deteriorating transcutaneous gas tensions following repeated tissue loading, in contrast to the adaptive responses shown by similar patients who do not develop them (Bader, 1990), possibly depending on the degree of neuronal damage (Schubert & Fagrell, 1989). Abnormal responses to ischaemia in patients with spinal injury may help to explain why patients with other neurological diseases, e.g. multiple sclerosis, cerebrovascular disease, Parkinson's and Alzheimer's diseases, are more liable to develop pressure injury during relatively minor illness than patients who are neurologically intact. In the elderly, pressure necrosis is often associated with acute confusion, hypotension, impaired temperature regulation, incontinence and faecal stasis indicating widespread failure of brainstem and thalamic function (Blass & Plum, 1983) probably due to decreased neurotransmitter activity (Blass & Plum, 1983; Davis & Sever, 1988) and other neurodegenerative changes (Griffith & Randall, 1989). As with cognitive and other disturbances (Vasallo & Allen, 1996), susceptibility to pressure sores improves or disappears with improvement in the patient's health.

Peripheral vascular disease

Arterial insufficiency, e.g. due to atheroma, arteriolar disease or vasculitis, increases susceptability of tissues to pressure. Heel sores are common in elderly patients (Jordan, 1976) and four times commoner in smokers than non-smokers (Barton & Barton, 1981), mainly due to peripheral vascular disease. Patients undergoing surgery for atheromatous disease are also more likely to develop pressure necrosis on the operating table (sometimes mistaken for diathermy burns) (Vermillian, 1990) than other surgical patients. Virtually all diabetic foot sores are pressure sores associated with neuro-arteriopathy and abnormal tissue responses to trauma (Rayman *et al.*, 1995). Pressure sores are common in patients with rheumatoid arthritis (Salaman & Harding, 1995) in whom they are often slow to heal. However, in a survey of elderly patients in USA nursing homes, Brandeis *et al.* (1995) did not find peripheral vascular disease to be significantly associated with sores, probably because patients with vascular disease were more likely to have died before needing nursing home care.

Age

Around 70% of all pressure sores occur in patients aged over 70 years (Bond, 1993), but this is probably mainly due to the increased prevalence of neurological and vascular disease with age, and not to age itself. Alert old people with normal sensation, including those with reduced mobility, e.g. due to osteoarthritis, are at little greater risk than the young. Schubert & Fagrell (1989) did not find any difference in skin blood flow responses to pressure in subjects aged less than 35 and more than 65 years. Poor nutrition is frequently present in patients with pressure sores (Perkash & Brown, 1982), but has not been demonstrated to be important in their development (Finucane, 1995). A low plasma albumin, the only known prognostic haematological factor (Cullum & Clark, 1992), is probably mainly important as an indication of illness (Fleck & Smith, 1991). Incontinence, which is highly correlated with the development of sores (Norton *et al.*, 1975; Piloian, 1992; Ferrell *et al.*, 1993), is also usually associated with neurological disease or acute illness. Lone urinary incontinence is less significant than double incontinence, and catheterised and non-catheterised patients are equally susceptible (Piloian, 1992). This suggests that the sores are due to the patient's poor physical condition. Illness and injury are critical factors in the development of peripheral circulatory failure in patients of all ages, and the elderly are more likely to suffer from severe and terminal illness than the young. Up to 50% of elderly patients with pressure sores die within 4 months, including over 90% of those with deep sores of the trunk (Bliss & Silver, 1988).

Susceptibility to the effects of pressure in elderly patients is exacerbated by fatigue (often caused by excessive chairnursing) (Gebhardt & Bliss, 1994); and drugs, e.g. sedatives (diminishing the appreciation of pressure pain and causing hypotension and parkinsonism), beta adrenoceptor blocking agents (causing peripheral vasoconstriction), and anti-inflammatory drugs (impaired healing) (Barton & Barton, 1981).

Extrinsic sources of pressure are also more likely to affect elderly than young patients, e.g. falls resulting in a 'long lie', long waiting times in Accident and Emergency departments (Versluysen, 1986), hard hospital beds (Jeneid, 1976); waterproof sheets and incontinence pads which cause high temperatures and humidity with maceration of the skin and increased friction in the pressure areas (Flam, 1990); 'side to side' turning (Bliss *et al.*, 1966); sliding down in beds and chairs (Scales, 1982); chairnursing (Lowthian, 1975; Barbanel *et al.*, 1977; Gebhardt & Bliss, 1994), restraints (Brandeis *et al.*, 1995), bandages (Ruckley, 1988), and pressure due to deformed feet and unsuitable footwear (Bliss & Schofield, 1996).

Acute illness

Very ill unconscious or heavily sedated patients cannot feel or respond to pressure pain; however, many other factors also affect the peripheral circulation in acute illness. Tissue flaccidity (Bennet & Lee, 1985) which determines the extent of capillary distortion and occlusion in the weight bearing areas is increased by low blood pressure (Leung, 1989), dehydration, muscle paralysis (Reger *et al.*, 1990) and shock

(Guttman, 1976). Low cardiac output (Massey, 1987), and regional blood flow (Bennett, 1991), impaired respiration, tissue oxygen uptake (Shoemaker *et al.*, 1988) and mediator failure (Altura, 1986) reduce tissue oxygenation. Endothelial damage (Altura, 1986; Bhagat *et al.*, 1996) and increased coagulability of the blood occur in shock syndromes associated with sepsis (Editorial, 1991) and acute trauma (Clowes, 1987). Experimental animals with septicaemia have been shown to have enhanced susceptibility to pressure sores (Groth, 1942; Barton, 1970). In very ill patients muscle necrosis has been found to occur in even non-pressurised muscle (Helliwell *et al.*, 1989). Free radicals resulting from partial ischaemia (Knight *et al.*, 1991) and ischaemia perfusion injuries (Sinclair *et al.*, 1990) may further disrupt the cycle of capillary damage, thrombosis, thrombolysis and repair which occurs in response to pressure injury (Barton & Barton, 1981).

Pain

Pain is associated with increased susceptibility to pressure sores (Barrett, 1988). Severe pain discourages movement and raises tissue demand for oxygen due to increased skeletal muscle activity (Anderson, 1987). Pain, e.g. due to a surgical wound or fracture, is often exacerbated by the presence of pressure sores themselves. The physiological importance of pain control is well recognised in intensive care units (Rithvi, 1995), but management in general hospital wards is still far from satisfactory. Many elderly patients suffer appalling pain with only paracetamol or short-acting opiates for relief because of traditional teaching that opiates are unnecessary or dangerous. In practice, morphine in appropriate doses reduces rather than increases the risk of pressure sores by improving rest, appetite and mobility. It is often safer and more effective than sedation for the treatment of acute confusional states in the elderly.

Sore types

Pressure sores are commonly classified in four grades of severity (Maklebust, 1995), but there are two main pathological types depending on whether the source of pressure causing the original injury was primarily external or internal (Bliss, 1992). External or superficial sores are caused by objects pressing or pulling on the skin and principally affect the epidermis and dermis. Deep or interstitial sores are caused by pressure due to internal bony prominences and affect primarily the periosteal tissues. Superficial sores do not progress to become deep, but sick patients with superficial sores are at risk of developing interstitial sores if the pressure is inadequately relieved. Prosthetic devices such as catheters may also cause internal sores (Lowthian, 1985).

Prevalence

Similar prevalences of pressure sores have been found in equally ill patients of both sexes (Gosnell *et al.*, 1992) and in the community and in hospital (Barbenel *et al.*, 1977). From 5–30% of all sores are present on admission (O'Dea, 1993; Richardson, 1993; Healey, 1996) and a further 70–80% occur in the first 1–2 weeks of stay (Norton *et al.*, 1975; Versluysen, 1986) when patients are most ill. Overall, around 10% of patients in general hospitals in Britain have a skin break in the pressure areas (O'Dea, 1993), and a further 20% require pressure relief to prevent sores (Clark & Cullum, 1992). Up to 66% of elderly orthopaedic patients have been shown to suffer from pressures sores (Norton *et al.*, 1975; Versluysen, 1986). About 70% of sores occur over the sacrum and buttocks and 13–18% over the heels (Jordon, 1976; O'Dea, 1993; Healey, 1996). 90% of sores are superficial and 8–20% deep (O'Dea, 1993).

Identification of susceptible patients

One of the chief difficulties in preventing pressure sores is how to recognise susceptible patients so that pressure relief can be instituted before tissue death has occurred. Many pressure sore prediction scores have been devised but they are time consuming and have been poorly validated (Barrett, 1988). It is also difficult to know when to apply them and reliance on their use may fail to detect subsequent deterioration in a patient's condition (Healey, 1966). All are in effect measures of illness in different types of susceptible patients. A more useful approach is to identify high risk patient groups who are likely to need pressure relief during any acute illness. These are shown in Table 11.1. Only neurological patients with advanced disease and elderly patients with neurological or vascular disease are normally at risk, but this depends on the degree of illness. Hence all patients with neurological disease and all patients aged over 70 years should be considered as being potentially in need of pressure relief during illness. Acute confusion, apathy, poor appetite, dehydration, reduced mobility, new incontinence or faecal stasis are important presenting features of illness in patients with neurological disease and in the elderly and indicate the need for immediate pressure relief.

Examination of the pressure areas

The pressure areas (sacrum, greater trochanters, ischia, heels, dorsal spine) must be inspected daily. This may be difficult in incontinent or paralysed patients, or in those with severe pain, but is essential, not only to document existing lesions but because pressure sores themselves are a vital sign of illness. They virtually never occur in a

Table 11.1. *Categories of patients at risk of pressure sores*

Spinal cord injury
Neurological disease
Peripheral vascular disease
Aged over 70 years
Very ill or dying

healthy person. An area of non-blanching or persistent erythema (lasting for more than 30 minutes) is evidence of capillary thrombosis, the first stage of a pressure sore (Barton, 1983), and the need for immediate pressure relief. A rectal examination should also be carried out as faecal stasis commonly coexists with pressure sores. The patient's ability to lift his pelvis off the mattress in turning over should be noted. It is also important to realise that any patient with a new deep pressure sore is suffering from severe trauma in addition to his original illness. Destruction in the deep tissues is usually greater than in the skin and may be manifest locally only by redness or oedema. Pain and the presence of necrotic tissue activate stress hormones and complement and clotting cascades and cause inflammation, a leucocytosis and pyrexia (Clowes, 1987) without necessarily infection.

Management

Treat illness

The cause of the illness must be identified and treated, with acute or palliative care depending on the patient's underlying disease. As pressure sores in the elderly are often associated with terminal illness, resuscitative treatment will not always be appropriate (Darkovich, 1996). Good nursing is, however, essential. Dehydration should be prevented as far as possible with scrupulous mouth hygiene and frequent drinks or parenteral fluids. A nutritious diet is important if the patient can tolerate it, but artificial feeding is rarely indicated. Pain should be treated effectively, with 4 hourly morphine or a pump if required. Stimulant laxatives with a faecal softener, e.g. co-danthramer, and regular enemas will usually be needed.

Pressure relief

Pressure relief needs to be provided early (within 1–2 hours), in the community as well as in hospital. If pressure sores can be prevented in patients at home or in nursing homes, admission may be avoided.

The patient should be nursed mainly or wholly in bed with a bedcradle (or tray or pillow) to relieve the weight of the bed clothes from the heels. The bed should be clean and dry. Incontinent patients must be changed frequently (Jeter & Lutz, 1996) or catheterised. Barrier creams have not been shown to be effective in preventing pressure sores (Lowthian 1977).

If 2 hourly repositioning is to be the principal method of pressure relief, it needs to be carried out carefully. Patients should spend more time on their backs than on the hips (Lowthian, 1985). Simply turning from one side to the other is likely to cause sores over the greater trochanters (Knox *et al.*, 1994). 'Tilting' may be safer (Gunnewicht, 1996) but both turning and tilting are disliked by elderly patients. The skin must be inspected frequently – an area of unblanching erythema is a warning sign of excessive pressure and a need to change the regimen. A row of pillows placed on the mattress with gaps under bony prominences (Bliss & Silver, 1988), or a slit foam mattress (Hofman *et al.*, 1994), may help to relieve pressure. Effective 2 hourly turning, however, may be impossible in elderly patients who need to be nursed sitting up, or who are restless, confused or in pain; or for patients in the community or in wards with low staff/patient ratios. Pressure relieving supports which reduce or obviate the need for repositioning are therefore very useful. Apart from turning beds used for patients with spinal cord injury (Gunnewicht, 1996), and unsuitable for the elderly, there are two main types: constant low pressure and alternating pressure.

Constant low pressure supports

Low pressure (LP) supports aim to prevent ischaemia by distributing the body weight as widely as possible so as to prevent pressure, and hence tissue distortion, over bony prominences. The archetype of the LP support is the flotation water bed dating from the early nineteenth century (Medical Gazette, 1832). Water beds probably prevent sores (Andersen *et al.*, 1982), but the floating action makes nursing very difficult and they are unsuitable for many patients, e.g. very heavy patients, or those with unstable fractures or who require resuscitation. They have now been largely replaced by air flotation beds, e.g. low air loss (Inman *et al.*, 1993) and air fluidised bead beds (Munro *et al.*, 1989). These have a similar action, but with the advantage that flotation can be temporarily suspended to provide a firm surface when necessary. Water beds (Andersen *et al.*, 1982) and air flotation beds (Inman *et al.*, 1993) are bulky and unsuitable for emergency use. Air flotation beds are also very expensive (Inman *et al.*, 1993). Low air loss mattress replacements/overlays are more practical and cheaper (Gebhardt *et al.*, 1996), but their effectiveness has yet to be evaluated.

Non-flotation, 'soft' LP mattresses and overlays are less expensive and more practical than flotation beds. Although they may show low pressures between the support surface and the patient (Swain, 1993), and relatively well-preserved oxygen tensions at the sacrum in healthy volunteers (Colin *et al.*, 1996), they have been found to have limited clinical benefit. A bead pillow support system was shown in a randomised trial to prevent sores in elderly orthopaedic patients (Goldstone *et al.*, 1982), but was subsequently abandoned, probably because of practical difficulties. In randomised controlled trials in orthopaedic (Hofman, 1994) and long stay elderly patients (Bliss 1995), slit foam mattresses showed some reduction in the incidence of sores compared with a normal hospital mattress and shallow water (Bliss, 1995) and fibrefill overlays (Conine, 1990; Bliss, 1995), respectively. Stapleton (1986) found similar incidences of sores in orthopaedic patients on foam and fibre overlays, 41% and 35%, respectively. Only one trial of a static air overlay for preventing sores (in non-acutely ill elderly nursing home residents) has been attempted which highlighted the difficulty of maintaining correct inflation pressure in these mattresses (Lazzara & Buschmann, 1991). No difference in effectiveness was found between it and a gel overlay (which was also noted to be heavy). In summary, no non-flotation LP support has yet been shown to be able to prevent sores without additional repositioning.

Alternating pressure

Alternating pressure (AP) mattresses do not aim to provide constant low pressure, but alternation of high and low pressures on the weight bearing areas similar to that which occurs in the normal person with changes of position in response to pressure pain. The standard type consists of an air mattress with horizontal cells connected in two alternating series to a motor which causes them to inflate and deflate reciprocally underneath the patient over a 5–10 minute cycle, thus constantly changing the supporting points of pressure on the body. The diameter and pressure of the cells must be sufficient to lift the patient off the underlying mattress or bed so as to allow restoration of the blood supply in the intervening areas. Shallow mattresses with cells less than 5 cm in diameter ('small cell' AP mattresses) have been shown to be relatively ineffective at preventing sores (Bliss *et al.*, 1966; Allman *et al.*, 1987) compared with medium depth mattresses around 10 cm diameter ('large cell' AP mattresses) (Bliss *et al.*, 1966). The latter have been shown to prevent tissue necrosis in intensive care patients (Gebhardt *et al.*, 1996) and in acute (Gebhardt *et al.*, 1994) and long stay (Bliss, 1995) elderly patients with infrequent or no repositioning. In a randomised trial in a district general hospital including general medical, elderly, orthopaedic and intensive care patients, AP supports showed an overall reduction in incidence of sores in patients with Norton pressure sore prediction scores (Norton *et al.*, 1975) of less than 13, to 13% compared with 34% on similarly priced LP supports (AP £3.13 and LP £5.22 per patient per day) (Gebhardt *et al.*, 1994). AP mattresses have the disadvantage compared with static LP supports of having an electrical pump which is liable to malfunction, but AP overlays are generally easier to carry and to install on the mattress of a patient's bed by one person than most LP supports.

Deeper AP overlays and mattress replacements with double layered (Exton Smith *et al.*, 1982) or rectangular cells (Devine, 1995) (diameter around 15 cm) and with electronically adjustable inflation pressures according to the weight and position of the patient are available, but are more expensive and less portable than simple large-cell overlays. They are helpful for very heavy or bony patients. In the UK they are mainly used for healing sores (Devine, 1995) for which they appear to be as effective as flotation beds.

Some patients, particularly alert, younger patients and those with severe pain, e.g. due to rheumatoid arthritis or cancer, find AP mattresses uncomfortable (Conine *et al.*, 1990) and a few refuse to tolerate them. Up to 60% of patients, however, are unaware of their presence. A blanket placed over the mattress lessens the impact of the pressure changes and also improves humidity and may help to prevent superficial sores. The original Pegasus Airwave mattress (Exton Smith *et al.*, 1982) had a full length nursing fleece which did not impair its performance and which may have contributed to its better results compared with the Large Cell Ripplebed. Pillows, and thick or multiple incontinence pads, must not, however, be placed between the body and an AP support. Heel bootees are also contraindicated and restrict movement. Otherwise patients may be nursed on AP mattresses as on ordinary beds. Backrests are normally placed over the support, but some types can be profiled over a backrest to protect the back and shoulders. Patients may be turned on AP supports, including on their hips if necessary. A pillow should be used to prevent pressure between the knees.

Removing pressure relieving supports

Many patients who complain of the discomfort of AP mattresses will recover sufficiently from their acute illness to be no longer in need of them. Like most other life support equipment, e.g. intravenous infusions and ventilators, pressure relieving mattresses are normally only necessary for 1 or 2 weeks. Once patients are well enough to spend most of the day out of bed in ordinary armchairs without developing pressure marks on the skin, the special mattresses should be removed. AP mattresses hinder rehabilitation by making it difficult for patients to move or to get on and off their beds unaided. Their general condition and pressure areas should continue to be examined daily and if either show signs of deterioration the support should be replaced for a further period. A few patients with advanced neurological disease or chronically ill or dying patients may need them indefinitely.

Servicing and training

Pressure relieving mattresses and overlays must be robust and regularly serviced. They must have a warning device to indicate malfunction and staff need to be properly trained in their use. Lack of servicing, poor training and the use of small-celled and semi-disposable mattresses which constantly broke down were probably the main reasons for the poor performance of AP supports in the past (Bliss, 1979; Lowthian, 1985; Clark & Cullum, 1992). A soft mattress which allows the patient to bottom through it cannot prevent pressure necrosis and merely provides a false sense of security (Lowthian, 1975).

Chairs

Pressure relieving supports are much less effective in the sitting position in chairs (Chow & Odell, 1978) than in the lying position in bed. For this reason, and because patients at risk of pressure sores are ill and unfit to spend long periods sitting up, they should be nursed mainly in bed. Spinal injury patients are nursed in bed (Rogers, 1986) until spinal shock has resolved or existing sores have healed, and they have been taught suitable strategies for protecting themselves from pressure in their wheelchairs. It is important to remember, however, that elderly patients, including elderly spinal injury patients (Zarb, 1987), do not have the strength to do 'lift ups' in their chairs to relieve pressure on the ischial tuberosities. Cushions for relieving pressure in healthy people in wheelchairs are also unsuitable for nursing elderly patients in armchairs. Most old people are more comfortable, and can move more freely, in well-designed chairs of the correct height for their leg length without a cushion on the seat. Back cushions should be used to support the lumbar spine. Pillows may also be placed vertically on either side to relieve pressure over prominent dorsal vertebrae, or under the forearms to prevent sores on the elbows. Cushions should always be placed on either side of, never directly under, the vulnerable area. Fleecy pads may be helpful. Patients should not be sat out of bed for more than 2 hours per session until they are well enough to maintain their sitting balance and preferably to relieve their own pressure areas. Physiotherapy and walking exercises should be given as appropriate.

Anticoagulation

Spinal injury patients who have sustained a major trauma are at high risk of venous thrombosis and are therefore normally anticoagulated during the first 3 months while they are in bed (Silver & Noori, 1991). It has been suggested that anticoagulation may also help to prevent pressure sores by reducing capillary thrombosis (Frankel, 1991). However, except for patients with femoral neck fracture or other trauma (Drugs and Therapeutics Bulletin 1992), routine low dose heparin is probably unnecessary for old people in bed. The velocity of blood flow in the veins is greatly increased in the horizontal compared with the sitting position (Ashby *et al.*, 1995).

Accident and Emergency

Elderly patients have been shown to wait for up to 12 hours in the Accident and Emergency department, on hard trolleys without fluids, food or pain relief (Versluysen, 1986). Presure sore prevention policies (Royal College of Physicians, 1989) have tried to ensure that they are admitted within 1 hour, but this is not always practicable (Legge, 1995). An immediate pressure-relieving strategy is therefore important. Depending on their condition and the likelihood of surgery in the next few hours, fluid (e.g. tea) (Debra *et al.*, 1995) and food should be given and pain treated. AP supports are less suitable for use on trolleys than on beds and a LP overlay, e.g. slit foam, is probably sufficient. Patients with femoral neck fracture or stroke should have pillows placed under the calves to ensure that the heels are free from pressure. Most patients will be adequately protected for a few hours by these means.

Operating theatre

Patients probably suffer more from pressure necrosis sustained during the pre- and postoperative periods than on the operating table itself. Long periods spent lying on their backs, sedated, without fluid or food, waiting to go to theatre (Versluysen, 1986), and subsequent delay in returning to the ward, can result in tissue death in the pressure areas which may only become apparent next day. Vulnerable patients should be nursed on AP supports and if possible sent to theatre on their beds. Most AP mattresses have devices to maintain inflation during transit; they can then be reconnected to a power source in the recovery room ready to receive the patient at the end of the operation. Some patients, e.g. those undergoing prolonged cardiovascular operations, may also require protection on the operating table such as soft foam overlays (Lowthian, 1989). Anaesthetics, muscle relaxants, hypotensives and sympathomimetic drugs increase the risk of peripheral circulatory failure. It has been suggested that monitoring techniques used in cardiac surgery should be employed for all patients with heart disease undergoing non-cardiac operations, including those being given regional anaesthesia (Anderson, 1987). This is primarily to prevent perioperative cardiac complications but could also help to reduce the incidence of peripheral tissue infarction.

The future

Over the past few years the incidence of sores, particularly of deep sores, in some British hospitals appears to be reducing (Bond & Challands, 1996; Healey, 1996; McSweeney, 1996). This is probably partly the result of increased awareness due to the Government's 1994/95 NHS Priorities and Planning Guidance encouraging Health Authorities to set annual targets for a 5% reduction of sores (McSweeney, 1996), and partly due to the earlier use of AP supports (Healey, 1996). AP mattresses are more effective at preventing deep than superficial sores, the latter being exacerbated by humidity and friction (Jeter & Lutz, 1996). The incidence of superficial sores is therefore less likely to respond to pressure relieving supports alone without additional repositioning. This may account for the disappointing finding of Clark & Cullum (1992) that increasing the supply of pressure relieving equipment was associated with an increased prevalence of sores. Over-dependence on ineffective equipment, including small-celled and faulty AP mattresses, and a greater interest in reporting sores (Healey, 1996), have also contributed.

Clark & Cullum stressed the importance of measuring the incidence of sores developed following admission rather than prevalence which includes sores present on admission. Richardson (1993) showed an increase of 35% in the number of patients admitted with sores between 1990 and 1991. Shorter hospital stays and increased community care for very disabled and sick patients is likely to result in a greater proportion of sores occurring outside hospital. Barbenel *et al.* (1977) found that the prevalence was similar in equally ill patients in hospital and in the community; however, general practitioners and community nurses are less likely to be aware of patients at risk, and pressure relieving aids such as AP mattresses are not always readily available for patients at home or in nursing homes (Parham, 1995). The Department of Health advises that technical equipment which would normally be used for patients in hospital should be freely available for patients in nursing homes (Department of Health, 1995a), but there is little mention of pressure relieving supports in its 1994 Video and Booklet for patients and carers: 'Don't get sore – get moving' (Department of Health, 1995b).

Greater emphasis on resuscitative medical treatment for very old people (Sinclair & Woodhouse, 1996) is resulting in the survival of more and more patients with recurrent acute illness at high risk of developing pressure sores. Prevalence rates may not therefore fall significantly despite improved preventive techniques. Furthermore, however cost-effective pressure relieving aids may be in the short term, they are likely to contribute to increased overall cost. Like artificial feeding and other life support therapies, AP mattresses may permit earlier discharge from hospital, but increase the need for long-term nursing care. Death from pressure sores is lingering and distressing and few would argue that we should not make every effort to prevent them. But, we do need to think why we seek to prolong the lives of some very sick old people and perhaps to develop alternative strategies of palliative care, similar to those used by hospices, with emphasis on comfort and dignity rather than survival. Finally, it is important to recognise that some dying patients may occasionally develop widespread peripheral tissue necrosis in the final few days of life despite meticulous pressure care (Hanson *et al.*, 1991). These sores remain cold without a normal hyperaemic response or natural debridement (Barton, 1983). Antibiotics and surgery are inappropriate and ineffective.

References

Allman, R. M., Walker, J. M., Hart, M. K., Lapsade, C. A., Noel, L. B. & Smith, C. R. (1987). Air fluidised or conventional therapy for pressure sores. *Ann Intern Med*, **107**, 641–8.

Altura, B. M. (1986). Endothelial and reticuloendothelial cell function: roles in injury and low flow states. In *The Scientific Basis for the Care of the Critically Ill*, ed. R. A. Little & K. N. Frayne, pp. 259–74. Manchester: Manchester University Press.

Andersen, K. E., Jensen, O., Kvorning, S. A. & Bach, E. (1982). Decubitus prophylaxis – a prospective trial of the efficacy of an alternating pressure air mattress, and a water mattress. *Acta Dermatol (Stockholm)*, **63**, 227–30.

Anderson, W. G. (1987). Anaesthesia for patients with cardiac disease. Postoperative care. *Br J Hosp Med*, **37**, 411–18.

Ashby, E. C., Ashford, N. S. & Campbell, M. J. (1995). Posture, blood velocity in the common femoral vein and prophylaxis of venous thromboembolism. *Lancet*, **345**, 419–21.

Bader, D. L. (1990). The recovery characteristics of soft tissues following repeated tissue loading. *J Rehab Res Devel*, **27**, 141–50.

Bar, C. A., Lloyd, S., Pathy, M. S. & Chawler, J. C. (1983). A system to monitor gross positional changes in recumbent patients. *Care Sci Practice*, **2**, 4–7.

Barbenel, J. C., Jordan, M. M., Nicol, S. M. & Clark, M. O. (1977). Incidence of pressure sores in the Greater Glasgow Health Board Area, *Lancet*, **ii**, 548–50.

Barrett, E. (1988). A review of risk assessment methods. *Care Sci Practice*, **6**, 49–52.

Barton, A. A. (1970). *The pathogenesis and inhibition of pressure sores.* MD Thesis, University of London.

Barton, A. A. (1983). Pressure sores. In *Pressures Sores*, ed. J. C. Barbenel, C. D. Forbes & G. D. O. Lowe, pp. 53–7. London: MacMillan Press.

Barton, A. & Barton, M. (1981). *The Management and Preventions of Pressures Sores.* London: Faber and Faber.

Bennett, E. D. (1991). Regional blood flow. **46** (*Critical Care*, **91**, Suppl.) 25 (abstract).

Bennett, L. & Lee, B. Y. (1985). Pressure versus shear in pressure sore causation. In *Chronic Ulcers of the Skin*, ed. B. Y. Lee, pp. 39–56. New York: McGraw Hill.

Bhagat, K., Collier, J. & Vallance, P. (1996). Brief exposure to endotoxin produces prolonged endothelial dysfunction in humans. *Clin Sci*, **90** (Suppl. 4), 22.

Blass, J. P. & Plum, F. (1983). Metabolic encephalopathy in older adults. In *The Neurology of Ageing*, ed. R. Katzman & R. Terry, pp. 189–220. Philadelphia: Davis.

Bliss, M. R. (1979). The use of Ripplebeds in hospitals. *Hosp Health Services Rev*, **74**, 190–3.

Bliss, M. R. (1992). Acute pressure area care: Sir James Paget's legacy. *Lancet*, **339**, 113–221.

Bliss, M. R. (1993). Aetiology of pressure sores. *Rev Clin Gerontol*, **3**, 379–97.

Bliss, M. R. (1995). Preventing pressure sores in elderly patients. A comparison of seven mattress overlays. *Age Ageing*, **24**, 297–302.

Bliss, M. R., McLaren, R. & Exton Smith, A. N. (1966). Mattresses for preventing pressure sores in geriatric patients. *Monthly Bull Min Health*, **25**, 238–68.

Bliss, M. & Schofield, M. (1996). Leg ulcers caused by pressure and oedema. *J Tissue Viab*, **6**, 17–19.

Bliss, M. R. & Silver, J. R. (1988). Pressure sores. In *Skin Disorders in the Elderly*, ed. B. E. Monk, R. A. C. Brown Graham & I. Sarkany, pp. 97–117. Oxford: Blackwell Scientific Publications.

Bogie, K. M., Nuseibeh, I. & Bader, D. L. (1992). Transcutaneous gas tensions in the sacrum during the acute phase of spinal cord injury. Proceedings of the Institute of Mechanical Engineers. Part H. *J Eng Med*, **206**, 1–6.

Bond, M. (1993). North Derbyshire Health Authority pressure sore surveys. *J Tissue Viabil*, **3**, 114–22.

Bond, M. & Challands, A. (1996). An update on the North Derbyshire pressure sore prevalence surveys. *J Tissue Viab*, **6**, 24.

Brandeis, G. H., Berlowitz, D. R., Hossain, M. & Morris, J. N. (1995). Pressure ulcers: the minimum data set and the resident assessment protocol. *Adv Wound Care*, **8**, 18–25.

Chow, W. W. & Odell, E. I. (1978). Deformations and stresses in soft body tissues in a sitting person. *J Biomechan Eng*, **100**, 79–87.

Clark, M. & Cullum, N. (1992). Matching patient need for pressure sore prevention with the supply of pressure redistributing mattresses. *J Adv Nursing*, **17**, 310–16.

Clowes, G. (1987). The metabolic response to trauma. *Med Int*, **2**, 1561–6.

Colin, D., Loyant, R., Abraham, P. & Saumet, J. L. (1996). Changes in sacral transcutaneous oxygen tension in the evaluation of different mattresses in the prevention of pressure sores. *Adv Wound Care*, **9**, 25–8.

Conine, T. A., Daechsel, D. & Laus, M. S. (1990). The role of alternating air and silicone overlays in preventing decubitus ulcers. *Int J Rehab Res*, **13**, 57–65.

Constantian, M. B. & Jackson, H. S. (1980). Factors affecting pressure ulcer development. In *Pressure ulcers. Principles and Techniques of Management*, ed. M. B. Constantian, pp. 143–8. Boston: Little Brown.

Cullum, N. & Clark, M. (1992). Intrinsic factors associated with pressure sores in elderly people. *J Adv Nursing*, **17**, 427–31.

Darkovich, S. I. (1996). When is no treatment the right treatment? *Adv Wound Care*, **9**, 6–7.

Davis, I. B. & Sever, P. S. (1988). Adrenoceptor function. In *Autonomic Failure*, ed. R. Bannister, pp. 348–66. Oxford: Oxford University Press.

Debra, K., Haigh, R., Sherwin, R., Murphy, J. & Kerr, D. (1995). The effect of acute and chronic caffeine use on the cerebrovascular, cardiovascular and hormonal responses to orthostasis in healthy volunteers. *Clin Sci*, **89**, 475–80.

Department of Health. (1995a). NHS responsibilities for meeting continuing health care needs. London.

Department of Health. (1995b). Don't get sore – get moving. London: Crown Business Communications, CFL Vision, PO Box 35, Wetherby, Yorkshire, LS23 7EX.

Devine, B. (1995). Alternating pressure air mattresses in the management of established pressure sores. *J Tissue Viab*, **5**, 94–8.

Drugs and Therapeutics Bulletin. (1992). Preventing and treating deep vein thrombosis. **30**, 9–12.

Editorial. (1991). Endotoxin bound and gagged. *Lancet*, **337**, 588–90.

Exton Smith, A. N., Overstall, P. W., Wedgewood, J. & Wallace, G. (1982). Use of the 'Airwave system' to prevent pressure sores in hospital. *Lancet*, **i**, 1288–90.

Ferrell, B. A., Osterweil, D. & Christensen, P. A. (1993). Randomised trial of low air loss beds for the treatment of pressure ulcers. *JAMA*, **269**, 494–7.

Finucane, T. E. (1995). Malnutrition, tube feeding and pressure sores: data are incomplete. *J Am Geriatr Soc*, **43**, 447–51.

Flam, E. (1990). Skin maintainance in the bedridden patient. *Osteotomy/ Wound Man*, May/June, 48–54.

Fleck, A. & Smith, G. (1991). An assessment of malnutrition in elderly patients. *Lancet*, **337**, 793.

Frankel, H. L. (1991). The spinal injury patient. London: Queen Mary and Westfield College: Tissue Viability Society Autumn Conference.

Gebhardt, K. S. & Bliss, M. R. (1994). Preventing pressure sores in orthopaedic patients – is prolonged chair nursing detrimental? *J Tissue Viabil*, **4**, 51–4.

Gebhardt, K. S., Bliss, M. R. & Winwright, P. L. (1994). A randomised controlled trial to compare the efficacy and cost of alternating pressure and constant low pressure supports for preventing pressure sores in hospital. *Age Aging*, **23** (Suppl. 2), 9.

Gebhardt, K. S., Bliss, M. R., Winwright, P. L. & Thomas, J. M. (1996). Pressure relieving supports in an ICU. *J Wound Care*, **5**, 116–21.

Goldstone, L. A., Norris, M., O'Reilly, M. & White, J. A. (1982). Clinical trial of a bead bed system for the prevention of pressure sores in elderly orthopaedic patients. *J Adv Nursing*, **7**, 545–8.

Gosnell, D. J., Johannsen, J. & Ayres, M. (1992). Pressure ulcer incidence and severity in a community hospital. *Decubitus*, **5**, 56–62.

Griffith, J. & Randall, M. (1989). Nitric oxide comes of age. *Lancet*, **2**, 875–6.

Groth, K. E. (1942). Klinische Beobachtungen und experimentelle Studien uber die Entstehung des Dekubitus. *Acta Chir Scand*, **87** (Suppl 76).

Gunnewicht, B. R. (1996). Management of pressure sores in a spinal injuries unit. *J Wound Care*, **5**, 36–9.

Guttman, L. (1976). The prevention and treatment of pressure sores. In *Bedsore Biomechanics*, ed. R. M. Kenedi, J. M. Cowden & J. T. Scales, pp. 153–9. London: MacMillan Press.

Hanson, D., Langemo, D. K., Olson, B., Hunter, S., Sauvage, T. R., Burd, C. & Cathcart-Silberberg, T. (1991). The prevalence and incidence of pressure ulcers in the hospice setting: analysis of two methadologies. *Am J Hosp Palliative Care*, **5**, 18–22.

Healey, F. (1996). Using incidence data to improve risk assessment. *J Tissue Viabil*, **6**, 3–9.

Helliwell, T. R., Griffiths, R. D., Coakley, J. H., McLelland, P., Williams, P. S., Campbell, I. T. & Bone, J. M. (1989). Necrosis of muscle in critically ill patients. *Br J Hosp Med*, **42**, 140.

Hofman, A., Geelkerken, R. H., Wilk, J., Hamming, J. J., Hermans, J. & Breslau, P. J. (1994). Pressure sores and pressure decreasing mattresses: controlled clinical trial. *Lancet*, **343**, 568–71.

Inman, K. J., Sibbald, W. J. & Rutledge, F. S. (1993). Clinical utility and cost effectiveness of an air suspension bed in the prevention of pressure ulcers. *JAMA*, **269**, 494–7.

Jeneid, P. (1976). Static and dynamic support surfaces – pressure differences on the body. In

Bedsore Biomechanics, ed. R. M. Kenedi, J. M. Cowden & J. T. Scales, pp. 287–99. London: MacMillan Press.

Jeter, K. F. & Lutz, J. B. (1996). Skin care in the frail elderly dependent, incontinent patient. *Adv Wound Care*, **9**, 29–34.

Johnson, H. M., Swan, T. H. & Weigard, G. E. (1930). In what position do healthy people sleep? *J Am Med Assoc*, **94**, 2058–62.

Jordan, M. M. (1976). *Report on pressure sores in the elderly*. Further information from the survey of the patient community of the Greater Glasgow Health Board Area.

Knight, K. R., Angel, M. F., Lepore, D. A., Abbey, P. A., Arnold, L. I., Gray, K. A., Mellow, C. G. & O'Brien, B. McC. (1991). Secondary ischaemia in rabbit skin flaps; the roles played by thromboxane and free radicals. *Clin. Sci*, **80**, 235–40.

Knox, D. M., Anderson, T. M. & Anderson, P. S. (1994). Effects of different turn intervals on skin of healthy older adults. *Adv Wound Care*, **7**, 48–56.

Lazzara, D. J. & Buschmann, M. T. B. (1991). Prevention of pressure sores in elderly nursing home residents: are special supports the answer? *Decubitus*, **4**, 42–6.

Legge, A. (1995). Poor hip fracture care points to bigger problems for the elderly. *Care Elderly*, **7**, 20–1.

Leung, K. H. (1989). Interface pressure: can blood pressure be the equation? *Decubitus*, **2**, 8.

Lowthian, P. (1977). A review of pressure sore prophylaxis. *Nursing Mirror Suppl*, March 17th, VII–XV.

Lowthian, P. (1985). Preventing pressure sores. *Nursing Mirror*, **160**, 18–20.

Lowthian, P. (1989). Pressure sore prevention. *Nursing*, **3**, 17–23.

Lowthian, P. T. (1975). Pressure sores. Practical prophylaxis. *Modern Geriatr*, **5**, 25–30.

McSweeney, P. (1996). Improving pressure care in North Essex – report of a study and progress. *J Tissue Viabil*, **6**, 11–14.

Maklebust, J. A. (1995). Pressure ulcer stageing systems. *Adv Wound Care*, **8**. (4) (National Pressure Ulcer Advisory Panel Proceedings): 28/11–28/14.

Massey, S. A. & Burton, G. W. (1987). Anaesthesia for patients with cardiac disease. Preoperative management. *Br J Hosp Med*, **37**, 386–96.

Medical Gazette (1832). *Dr Arnott's hydrostatic bed for invalids*. **10**, 712–14.

Munro, B. H., Brown, L. & Heitman, B. B. (1989). Pressure ulcers: one bed or another. *Geriatr Nursing*, **10**, 190–2.

Nicholson, P. W., Leeman, A. L., O'Neill, C. J. A., Dobbs, S. M., Deshmukh, A. A. & Denman, M. J. (1988). Pressure sores: effect of Parkinson's disease and cognitive function on spontaneous movement in bed. *Age Ageing*, **17**, 111–15.

Norton, D., McLaren, R. & Exton Smith, A. N. (1975). *An Investigation of Geriatric Nursing Problems in Hospital*. Edinburgh: Churchill Livingstone.

O'Dea, K. (1993). Prevalence of pressure damage in hospital patients in the UK. *J Wound Care*, **2**, 221–5.

Parham, J. (1995). *Tissue Viabil*, **5**, 74.

Perkash, A. & Brown, M. (1982). Anaemia in patients with traumatic spinal cord injury. *Paraplegia*, **20**, 235–6.

Piloian, B. B. (1992). Defining characteristics of the nursing diagnosis 'high risk for impaired skin integrity'. *Decubitus*, **5**, 32–47.

Raney, J. P. (1989). A comparison of the prevalence of pressure sores in hospitalised ALS and MS patients. *Decubitus*, **2**, 48–9.

Rayman, G., Malik, R. A., Sharma, A. K. & Day, J. L. (1995). Microvascular response to tissue injury and capillary ultrastructure in the foot skin of Type 1 diabetic patients. *Clin Sci*, **89**, 467–74.

Reger, S. I., McGovern, T. F. & Chung, K. C. (1990). Biomechanics of tissue distortion and stiffness by magnetic resonance imaging. In *Pressure Sores. Clinical Practice and Scientific Approach*, ed. D. L. Bader, pp. 177–190. Basingstoke: MacMillan Press.

Richardson, B. (1993). Hospital versus community acquired pressure sores: should prevalence rates be separated. *J Tissue Viabil*, **3**, 13–15.

Richardson, B. R. & Meyer, P. R. (1981). Prevalence and incidence of pressure sores in acute spinal injuries. *Paraplegia*, **19**, 235–47.

Rithvi, R. (1995). *Pain Medicine: a Comprehensive Review*. St. Louis: Mosby.

Rogers, M. A. (1986). *Living with Paraplegia*. London: Faber and Faber, pp. 46–63.

Royal College of Physicians. (1989). Fractured neck of femur: prevention and management. Summary and recommendations of a report. *J R Coll Phys* (Lond), **23**, 8–12.

Ruckley, C. V. (1988). *A Colour Atlas of Surgical Management of Venous Disease*. London: Wolfe Medical Publications.

Salaman, R. A. & Harding, K. G. (1995). The aetiology and healing rates of chronic leg ulcers. *J Wound Care*, **7**, 320–3.

Scales, J. T. (1982). Pressure sore prevention. *Care Science Practice*, **2**, 9–17.

Schubert, V. & Fagrell, B. (1989). Local skin pressure and its effects on the microcirculation as evaluated by Laser Doppler Fluxmetry. *Clin Physiol*, **9**, 535–45.

Shoemaker, W. C., Apel, P. L. & Kram, H. B. (1988). Tissue oxygen debt as a determinant of lethal and non lethal post operative organ failure. *Critical Care Med*, **16**, 1117–20.

Silver, J. R. & Noori, Z. (1991). Pulmonary embolism following anticoagulation therapy. *Int Disabil Studies*, **13**, 16–19.

Sinclair, A. J., Barnett, A. H. & Lunec, J. (1990). Free radicals and antioxidant systems in health and disease. *Br J Hosp Med*, **43**, 334–44.

Sinclair, A. J. & Woodhouse, K. W. (1996). *Acute Medical Illness on Old Age*. London: Chapman and Hall Medical.

Stapleton, M. (1986). Preventing pressure sores: an evaluation of three products. *Geriatr Nursing*, **6**, 23–5.

Swain, I. (1993). PSI *Evaluation: Foam Mattresses*. London: HMSO.

Vasallo, M. & Allen, S. C. (1996). Autonomic impairment in elderly patients with pneumonia. *Age Aging*, **25** (Suppl 1), 28.

Vermillian, C. (1990). Operating room acquired ulcers. *Decubitus*, **3**, 26–9.

Versluysen, M. (1986). How elderly patients with femoral neck fracture develop pressure sores in hospital. *Br Med J*, **292**, 1311–13.

Zarb, G. (1987). Ageing and paraplegia. *Spinal Injuries Association Newsletter*, **43**, 11–12.

12

Cardiovascular control

J. DUGGAN

Introduction

One of the major determinants of outcome following injury in the elderly is the response of the aging cardiovascular system to injury. The cardiovascular response to injury depends on the heart rate, blood pressure, cardiac output, peripheral resistance and baroreceptor responses in the elderly. Aging and disease in the elderly influence these cardiovascular parameters and may alter the cardiovascular response to injury in the aging. In this chapter, the effect of age on these parameters is outlined and the implications for responses to injury in the aging are discussed. Throughout the chapter, an attempt is made to distinguish between the effects of normal aging and the effects of age-associated cardiovascular disease on cardiovascular control mechanisms, as both could influence responses to injury.

The chapter is divided into three sections: Cardiovascular response to injury, Age and the cardiovascular system, and Cardiovascular response to injury in the elderly.

Cardiovascular response to injury

The cardiovascular response to injury depends on the type, severity and duration of the injury. It is now known, for example, that even a moderate injury, such as a hip fracture, is associated with a blood loss of up to 2 litres in humans (i.e. 40% of blood volume). The reflex response of the cardiovascular system is crucial in determining outcome following injury. There are three important reflexes involved in the cardiovascular response to injury – arterial baroreceptors, arterial chemoreceptors and cardiac c-fibre afferents. There is some information regarding the effect of age on baroreceptor function (see later) however, little is known about aging and chemoreceptor or cardiac c-fibre function.

Baroreceptors respond to changes in blood pressure, pulse pressure and heart rate.

This is especially important in the response to haemorrhage, where after a loss of up to 10% of the blood volume, mean blood pressure remains constant, but the baroreceptors are activated by a reduction in pulse pressure (Kirkman & Little, 1988).

An injury which results in a fall in arterial blood pressure activates the baroreceptor reflex which causes a reflex increase in sympathetic activity to the heart and peripheral blood vessels. An increase in cardiac output and total peripheral resistance thereby occurs, and blood pressure returns towards the original, pre-injury level.

The arterial chemoreceptors respond to changes in oxygen tension, carbon dioxide levels and arterial blood pH. Stimulation, for example by haemorrhage, results in increased respiration (Heymans & Neil, 1958) and bradycardia and vasoconstriction (Daly, 1983). The primary cardiovascular effects are modified by the increased respiration which inhibits both the increased vagal and sympathetic activity (Spyer, 1984).

Stimulation of cardiac c-fibre afferents leads to hypotension, bradycardia, and a fall in skeletal muscle and renal vascular resistance. These receptors are activated under physiological conditions such as exercise (Thorén, 1977) and pathological conditions such as acute severe haemorrhage where they are stimulated by a tearing and squeezing of the myocardium due to vigorous contractions of the left ventricle around an almost empty chamber (Öberg & Thorén, 1972b).

The role of these reflexes in the cardiovascular response to injury has been investigated; the influence of age, if any, is not known. Furthermore, the cardiovascular response to injury has been studied in a systematic way with studies of response to haemorrhage alone, tissue injury and haemorrhage plus injury combined.

Haemorrhage alone

Acute haemorrhage leads to activation of the baroreceptor reflex producing a progressive increase in heart rate and vascular resistance (Secher & Bie, 1985) which is so efficient in young, healthy people that mean arterial pressure is maintained near pre-haemorrhage levels despite blood losses of up to 10–15% of blood volume. In this situation, the baroreceptor reflex undergoes an increase in sensitivity (Little *et al.*, 1984). A severe haemorrhage (more than 20% of blood volume) leads to bradycardia and a profound drop in blood pressure which may cause syncope (Barcroft *et al.*, 1944; Secher *et al.*, 1984; Secher & Bie, 1985; Sander-Jensen *et al.*, 1986) due to cardiac c-fibre afferent activation (Öberg & Thorén, 1972a).

The arterial chemoreceptors may prevent further falls in blood pressure and cause the increase in respiration observed following severe haemorrhage (D'Silva *et al.*, 1966). The enhanced respiratory activity may attenuate the bradycardia following severe haemorrhage as increased respiration reduces the reflex bradycardia produced by stimulation of cardiac c-fibre afferents (Daly *et al.*, 1988).

Tissue injury

Tissue injury, in contrast, produces an increase in arterial blood pressure and a tachycardia. These cardiovascular responses occur because of a simultaneous reduction in sensitivity and rightward resetting of the baroreflex (Anderson *et al.*, 1988).

Haemorrhage plus injury

In this situation, the cardiovascular responses to haemorrhage are dramatically attenuated. The tachycardia observed following haemorrhage resulting in the loss of 11% of blood volume is attenuated 30 minutes after the production of bilateral hindlimb ischaemia in the rat (Little *et al.*, 1989), possibly due to attenuation of the baroreflex following injury. When injury is associated with severe haemorrhage the cardiovascular response is greatly modified because the profound bradycardia is prevented (Little *et al.*, 1989). There appears to be relative protection against the fall in blood pressure produced by severe haemorrhage in injured animals because equivalent haemorrhages produce smaller decrements in blood pressure in injured than control animals (Little *et al.*, 1989). The long-term survival of the injured animal, however, is not improved, suggesting that the better blood pressure homeostasis is achieved at the expense of tissue blood flow resulting in exacerbation of the injury (Kirkman & Little, 1988).

In summary, cardiovascular reflexes are crucial in the response to haemorrhage and injury. The cardiovascular response to haemorrhage alone involves baroreceptor-initiated tachycardia and increased vascular resistance. Of crucial importance in this response is the protection of brain and myocardial blood flow. To this end the activation of sympathetic supply to different vascular beds is not uniform. Some vascular beds, therefore, experience more intense vasoconstriction than others (Kirchheim, 1976). In this way, the baroreflex maintains blood flow to tissues critically dependent on oxygen delivery (e.g. brain and myocardium) at the expense of flow to other organs (e.g. skeletal muscle and gut) where oxygen delivery in the short term is less essential. The effect of age on these responses has not been investigated.

Baroreceptor reflex activity is augmented by an increase in sensitivity and possibly by chemoreceptor reflex activation. As the haemorrhage continues towards 20% of blood volume a different response occurs i.e. bradycardia plus hypotension due to activation of the vagal cardiac c-fibre afferents which may protect the heart by reducing cardiac work when coronary blood flow is inadequate. Tissue injury alone is associated with a contrasting response to that of haemorrhage alone, i.e. an increase in blood pressure and heart rate and reduced baroreflex sensitivity. When haemorrhage and injury occur together, the cardiovascular response to injury blunts that to haemorrhage and dramatically attenuates the 'depressor' response to a large haemorrhage. As a result, blood pressure is better maintained following a combined injury than with haemorrhage alone, but this may occur at the expense of intense vasoconstriction in other vascular beds which may exacerbate the injury and not improve survival. The influence of age on these responses has not been studied.

Age and the cardiovascular system

Aging and cardiovascular disease

Coronary artery atherosclerosis begins in young adults and increases progressively with age (Tejada *et al.*, 1968). Furthermore, the prevalence of vessel narrowing and stenosis increases with age with a more than 50% prevalence of occlusion of at least one of the three major coronary arteries by age 55–64 years (Elveback & Lie, 1984). Coronary artery disease is present in an occult form in many people during life; however, although they may be asymptomatic, the coronary stenosis may affect myocardial function (Lakatta, 1988). This becomes important when one attempts to assess the impact of age on cardiovascular function; it is imperative to exclude those with occult coronary artery disease to assess the impact of age alone. In more recent studies of aging and cardiovascular function, in particular the Baltimore Longitudinal Study of Aging (BLSA), exercise stress testing combined with thallium imaging has been used to screen for the presence of occult coronary disease prior to inclusion in the investigation (Gerstenblith *et al.*, 1980; Rodeheffer *et al.*, 1984). The findings of these studies of aging and cardiovascular function differ from the findings of previous investigations (Brandfonbrenner *et al.*, 1955; Julius *et al.*, 1967), which suggests that the earlier studies included patients with occult coronary disease and were not necessarily studies of aging itself. This is an important distinction to make, not only for academic reasons, but because assumptions about the ability of the cardiovascular system of an elderly patient to respond to the stress of injury, for example, should not be made on the basis of studies which were flawed. On the other hand, it is true to say that the elderly who are injured will include people who are free of occult coronary artery disease, those with occult coronary disease and those with overt cardiovascular disease. Therefore, the cardiovascular response to injury in the elderly will often depend on factors in addition to age.

Aging, blood pressure and arterial stiffness

Blood pressure increases with age in Western societies (Kannel, 1980). The exact mechanisms underlying this increase are not clear but the increased stiffness of blood vessels which occurs with aging certainly contributes. The increased stiffness appears to be due to alterations within the vascular media, in particular, an increase in collagen and a change in the structure of elastin (Wolinsky, 1972). An increase in intracellular calcium could also contribute to increased stiffness (Fleckenstein *et al.*, 1983). Using the platelet as a model for the vascular smooth muscle cell in humans, we have recently found an increase in platelet intracellular free calcium with age in healthy human subjects (Duggan *et al.*, 1991). Whatever the underlying mechanism, the increased stiffness increases the resistance to blood flow from the heart, thus, for a given volume of blood ejected, the pressure is higher than in normal arteries (Lakatta, 1984). Arterial pulse wave velocity gives an index of the degree of arterial stiffening or distensibility and has been shown to increase with age. There is doubt, however, as to whether increased arterial stiffness is a feature of normal aging or due to associated cardiovascular disease. Epidemiological studies suggest that changing from a low to high sodium diet accelerates the tendency for vascular stiffness and blood pressure to increase with age (Avolio *et al.*, 1985). It is also clear that even those studies which have excluded subjects with occult coronary disease have found a significantly higher resting systolic blood pressure in elderly subjects (Rodeheffer *et al.*, 1984).

In addition to an increase in the amplitude of the aortic pressure with age, the peak occurs later (Lakatta, 1984). The late peak of aortic systolic pressure may be due to early reflected pulse waves, due to the augmented pulse wave velocity associated with increased arterial stiffening (O'Rourke, 1986).

Cardiac output at rest

The increase in systolic blood pressure augments the workload on the heart and leads to age-related changes in cardiac function (Lakatta, 1987). Stroke work (i.e. stroke volume times blood pressure) increases with age (Brandfonbrenner *et al.*, 1955; Rodeheffer *et al.*, 1984) and this leads to a modest increase in left ventricular (LV) wall thickness (Sjögren, 1971; Gerstenblith *et al.*, 1977; Gardin *et al.*, 1979) and estimated LV mass (Gardin *et al.*, 1979). Furthermore, there is a correlation between blood pressure and the degree of LV wall thickness (Lakatta, 1987). Resting heart rate does not change with age (Rodeheffer *et al.*, 1984; Lakatta, 1990) but there is an age-related delay in the onset of ventricular filling which is detected by kinetocardiographic techniques as a prolongation of the interval between closure of the aortic valve and opening of the mitral valve, i.e. an increase in the isovolumic relaxation time (Harrison *et al.*, 1964). Resting early diastolic filling rate, observed as a reduction in the E-F slope of the M-mode echocardiogram (Gerstenblith *et al.*, 1977), during gated blood pool scans (Gerstenblith *et al.*, 1983) and from Doppler echocardiograms (Swinne *et al.*, 1989), declines with age, with almost a 50% decrement between age 20 and 80 years. The decline in early diastolic filling does not, however, lead to a reduction in end-diastolic volume (Rodeheffer *et al.*, 1984), which implies that atrial contraction must make a relatively greater contribution to ventricular filling in the elderly. This has been confirmed in a Doppler echocardiography study of healthy men and women (Swinne *et al.*, 1989). Furthermore, despite the above changes with age in the timing of ventricular filling, cardiac output at rest does not change with age in healthy adults who are screened to exclude occult coronary disease (Rodeheffer *et al.*, 1984). This is in contrast to the findings of previous studies, where volunteers were not so rigorously screened, and a decline in resting cardiac output was reported, almost certainly due to inclusion of some subjects with occult coronary diseases (Brandfonbrenner *et al.*, 1955; Julius *et al.*, 1967). Other indices of pump function, such as ejection fraction and velocity of ejection, do not change with age in a screened population. Therefore, the modest cardiac hypertrophy, described earlier, which was found in a subset of the same screened population, represents an adaptive mechanism to normalise the increased ventricular stress due to increased blood pressure in the elderly. In this way, normal ventricular ejection is possible despite the increased afterload (Lakatta, 1987).

In summary, therefore, in subjects who are free of overt or occult coronary disease, there is an age-related increase in systolic blood pressure and arterial stiffening but no change in cardiac output or pump function. Normal ejection fraction, stroke volume, end-diastolic volume and end-systolic volume are attained by adaptations, which include a moderate increase in LV thickness, prolonged contraction, atrial enlargement and increased atrial contribution to LV filling. Prolonged contraction maintains the load-bearing capacity of the aging heart for a longer period during systole which seems to be an important adaptation in the presence of increased arterial stiffening.

In terms of the response to injury in the elderly, therefore, as far as resting cardiac function goes, there is no reason why the elderly should not be able to respond in a similar fashion to young subjects. This is true for elderly subjects who are free of overt or occult cardiac disease. In contrast, those elderly subjects who have occult coronary disease will have the disadvantage of impaired resting cardiac output (Brandfonbrenner *et al.*, 1955; Julius *et al.*, 1967) and if they are injured this could compromise their ability to respond.

Age and baroreflex function

The crucial role played by the baroreceptor reflex has been outlined earlier. Any change in baroreceptor sensitivity with age could have important implications in terms of the ability of the elderly to respond to injury. Gribben and colleagues (1971) were the first group to demonstrate that baroreflex sensitivity changed with age. They calculated baroreflex sensitivity by relating the increase in pulse interval in milliseconds to the transient rise in systolic blood pressure induced by injecting the alpha-agonist phenylephrine. They found a linear relation between pulse interval and systolic blood pressure and the slope of the line gave a measure of baroreflex sensitivity. The steeper the slope, implying a greater increase in pulse interval per mmHg rise in blood pressure, the more sensitive the reflex. These investigators documented a significant and progressive decline in baroreflex sensitivity with age in both normotensives and hypertensives (Gribben *et al.*, 1971). There are, however, methodological problems with this study. First, it was not a study of 'normal aging' as no screening of subjects was carried out. Second, in the analysis borderline hypertensives were included with the normotensive group. Finally, only five of the normotensives were over 50 years of age. In a more recent study (Shimada *et al.*, 1985), baroreflex sensitivity was assessed in 54 normal subjects aged 14–77 years who were screened by history, physical examination, electrocardiogram (ECG), chest radiography and fasting blood glucose to exclude the presence of disease. Baroreflex sensitivity was measured as a change in the R-R interval per unit change in systolic blood pressure during phase 4 of the Valsalva manoeuvre. There was an age-related decline in baroreflex sensitivity which occurred independently of the associated increase in systolic blood pressure and noradrenaline. We have recently documented, in an investigation of responses to angiotensin II infusion in healthy young and elderly subjects, that heart rate fell significantly in the young but not in the elderly following the increase in blood pressure due to ANG II (Duggan *et al.*, 1993). These findings are compatible with reduced baroreceptor sensitivity in the elderly, although ANG II also exerts effects on the sympathetic nervous system (Peach, 1977) and on the myocardium (Freer *et al.*, 1976; Knape & Zweiten, 1988) and possible differences in response at these sites with age cannot be excluded (Duggan *et al.*, 1993).

It would appear, therefore, that baroreceptor sensitivity declines with age. This could have important implications in terms of response to injury in the elderly with an impaired ability to mount a tachycardia in response to a fall in blood pressure following haemorrhage.

Cardiac output response to stress

There is little or no information in the literature concerning the effect of age on the cardiovascular response to the stress of injury. In contrast, the effect of age on the cardiovascular response to the stress of exercise has been widely studied (Becklake *et al.*, 1965; Julius *et al.*, 1967; Gerstenblith *et al.*, 1976; Port *et al.*, 1980; Rodeheffer *et al.*, 1984; Fleg *et al.*, 1988). Data from older studies (Port *et al.*, 1980) suggest that the cardiac output response to exercise is significantly reduced in the elderly. When subjects with occult coronary artery disease are excluded, however, no significant age-related change in exercise cardiac output is observed (Rodeheffer *et al.*, 1984).

There is a change, however, in the way in which cardiac output is augmented in response to exercise. Elderly subjects do not increase their heart rate to the same extent as the young but instead increase their end-diastolic volume and stroke volume to a greater extent than the young. The elderly, therefore, during exercise utilise the Frank–Starling mechanism to augment cardiac output and thereby respond to the stress of exercise. Despite their ability to augment stroke volume during exercise, there is a smaller increment in ejection fraction in the elderly because the reduction in end-systolic volume is less in elderly than young subjects. Those elderly subjects who are free of disease, however, are capable of increasing their ejection fraction above the resting level. This contrasts with elderly subjects in previous studies in whom occult coronary disease was not excluded and who were unable to increase their ejection fraction above the resting level and therefore exhibited a dramatic age-related decline in exercise-induced increment in ejection fraction.

Similarities have been shown between the cardiovascular response to exercise in the elderly (reduced heart rate response, greater end-diastolic, end-systolic and stroke volumes) and exercise in younger subjects in the presence of beta-adrenergic blockade (Lakatta, 1990). The elderly increase their plasma adrenaline and noradrenaline levels to a greater extent than the young during exercise (Fleg *et al.*, 1985). It is postulated that the age-related alterations in the cardiovascular response to the stress of exercise are due to reduced beta-adrenergic cardiovascular responsiveness with age (Lakatta, 1990).

Injury often leads to intravascular volume depletion, either directly due to haemorrhage or indirectly because of poor intake, fever, excessive diuretics, pharmacological vasodilation, decreased plasma oncotic pressure or increased microvascular permeability. Because of the greater reliance on the Frank–Starling mechanism in the elderly, it might be expected that intravascular volume depletion would be more harmful in the elderly. Following tilting from supine to 60° both elderly and young subjects respond with a similar increase in heart rate and blood pressure (Shannon *et al.*, 1986). Following preload reduction with diuretics, however, the elderly sustain a symptomatic fall in blood pressure. This occurs because the elderly are unable to mount a tachycardia in response to tilt whereas young subjects produce a dramatic increase in heart rate (Shannon *et al.*, 1986).

In summary, with regard to responses to injury, it would appear that a healthy elderly person who is free of coronary artery disease should be able to mount a cardiac output response similar to that of a young person albeit by a different mechanism. Those elderly patients who do have occult coronary disease are less likely to augment their cardiac output to the level of a younger person in response to injury and are unlikely to be capable of increasing their ejection fraction above the resting level.

Aerobic capacity and response to stress

The maximum oxygen consumption rate ($\dot{V}O_2$ max) achieved during stress, for example the stress of exercise, is an accepted standard of level of fitness. $\dot{V}O_2$ is also one of the cardiorespiratory variables measured in intensive care following injury. to interpret $\dot{V}O_2$ max in elderly injured subjects it is first necessary to examine the influence of 'normal' aging on $\dot{V}O_2$. There is some evidence to suggest that there is an age-related decline in work capacity and $\dot{V}O_2$ max (Lakatta, 1990). There is a major debate, however, as to whether central (cardiopulmonary) or peripheral (arteriovenous oxygen extraction) mechanisms are the major cause of this deterioration.

As discussed earlier, information from the Baltimore Longitudinal Study on Aging suggests that maximal cardiac output shows only a minor (nonsignificant) decline with age (Rodeheffer *et al.*, 1984). Although $\dot{V}O_2$ max was not measured directly in that study, there was a decline in maximal exercise time with age. Assuming that $\dot{V}O_2$ max also declined, it would appear that peripheral rather than central factors are the major cause of the decline in $\dot{V}O_2$ max with age. Skeletal muscle mass is one important peripheral factor which determines $\dot{V}O_2$ max. Skeletal muscle mass declines with age and if $\dot{V}O_2$ max is normalised for muscle mass instead of body weight, the decline in $\dot{V}O_2$ max attributable to age falls from 60% to 4% in men and from 50% to 8% in women (Fleg *et al.*, 1988). Physical conditioning is also an important determinant of $\dot{V}O_2$ max, i.e. athletes improve their ability to extract oxygen from tissues. Elderly healthy sedentary men when compared with age-matched athletes have a significantly reduced $\dot{V}O_2$ max. Two-thirds of this large difference in $\dot{V}O_2$ max is due to increased arteriovenous oxygen difference, i.e. an increased ability of athletes to extract oxygen (Fleg *et al.*, 1988).

In summary, therefore, $\dot{V}O_2$ max data in injured elderly patients should be interpreted with caution. Aging in normal subjects is probably associated with a decline in $\dot{V}O_2$ max and this is primarily due to peripheral factors such as a decline in muscle mass and reduced physical conditioning associated with a sedentary lifestyle rather than due to changes in central or cardiopulmonary factors.

Regional blood flow

Age and cerebral blood flow

It is widely believed that cerebral blood flow declines with age in normal individuals. This would have important implications in terms of response to injury in the elderly as severe hypotension, for example following haemorrhage, might be expected to cause cerebral ischaemia more easily in the elderly than the young because of reduced cerebral blood flow.

There appears to be little doubt that cerebral blood flow (CBF) undergoes a rapid decline during puberty until the age of 20 years (Kety, 1956); this, however, is a 'maturational' change rather than a true aging change. It has been suggested in many reports that CBF declines with advancing age after age 20 years also (Kety, 1956; Melamed *et al.*, 1980; Pantano *et al.*, 1984; Shirahata *et al.*, 1985). Dastur (1985), however, found no real change in cerebral blood flow and metabolism with normal aging except a small fall in the brain's utilisation of glucose. Different criteria employed in selecting elderly normal subjects and less accurate experimental methodology may account for the findings of earlier studies. In a recent study (Waldemar *et al.*, 1991), the contributions of age, sex and atrophy to variations in global CBF were investigated using multiple regression analysis. There was a significant negative correlation of global CBF with cortical atrophy but not with ventricular size, sex or age. Although global cerebral blood flow did not change with age, there were age-related changes in regional CBF (Waldemar *et al.*, 1991). In particular, frontal cortex CBF decreased significantly with age. The clinical significance of these findings has not yet been established but these areas of the brain may be at greater risk of ischaemia following injury in the elderly.

Aging and autoregulation of cerebral blood flow

CBF is autoregulated very well between arterial blood pressures of 60 and 140 mmHg. Consequently, arterial pressure can fall acutely (e.g. following haemorrhage) as low as 60 mmHg or increase as high as 140 mmHg (e.g. following injury), and CBF will not change significantly (Guyton, 1991). The autoregulatory range shifts to higher pressure levels (180–200 mmHg) in patients with hypertension. As blood pressure increases with age, one might expect a similar, although perhaps less pronounced, shift in the autoregulatory range in the elderly although there are no studies to support this. If arterial pressure falls below 60 mmHg, cerebral blood flow is severely compromised. If arterial pressure rises above the upper limit of autoregulation, blood flow increases rapidly and may lead to severe overstretching of the cerebral blood vessels and possibly cerebral oedema. The effect of age, if any, on autoregulation of cerebral blood flow remains to be established.

Age and gastrointestinal blood flow

Stimulation of the sympathetic supply to the gastrointestinal tract causes profound arteriolar vasoconstriction and severely diminished blood flow. After a few minutes, however, the flow returns to normal by means of an 'autoregulatory escape' mechanism. This occurs because local metabolic vasodilator mechanisms elicited by ischaemia override the sympathetic vasoconstriction and thus redilate the arterioles with resultant return of blood flow to the gastrointestinal tract, glands and muscle (Guyton, 1991).

When increased blood flow is needed elsewhere, e.g. during exercise by skeletal muscle and heart or during injury/haemorrhage by brain and heart, sympathetic vasoconstriction in the gastrointestinal tract allows shutting off of the tract and other splanchnic blood flow for as long as an hour. Sympathetic stimulation also causes intense constriction of the intestinal and mesenteric veins. In addition, there is no 'escape' of this vasoconstriction and it decreases the volume of these veins making large amounts of blood available for other parts of the circulation, as much as 200–300 ml in haemorrhagic shock (Guyton, 1991). The effect of age, if any, on this response is not known.

Age and liver blood flow

Approximately 1100 ml of blood flows from the portal vein to the liver sinusoids each minute and 350 ml into the sinusoids via the hepatic artery giving an average liver blood flow of approx 1450 ml/min which amounts to 29% of the cardiac output (Guyton, 1991). Recent evidence suggests that liver blood flow declines with age in healthy individuals (Wynne *et al.*, 1989). With regard to injury in the elderly, there is information to suggest that following femur fracture, there is no further decline in liver blood flow; however, nothing further is known about injuries of greater severity in the elderly (M. Horan, personal communication).

Age and renal blood flow

Renal blood flow remains in the normal range despite large changes in arterial pressure because of autoregulation of renal blood flow. Thus, the normal renal blood flow of 1200 ml/min is maintained despite falls in arterial pressure to 75 mmHg or increases as high as 160 mmHg. The most important mechanism autoregulating renal blood flow is the so-called 'afferent arteriolar vasodilator mechanism' (Guyton, 1991). Thus, if renal blood flow falls to a certain level, it causes a decline in glomerular filtration rate (GFR). The decline in GFR causes a feedback effect at the juxtaglomerular complex to dilate the afferent arteriole, thus increasing blood flow to the glomerulus and returning renal blood flow and GFR to normal.

Both the afferent and efferent arterioles are innervated by the sympathetic nervous system. Slight to moderate sympathetic stimulation has minimal effects on renal blood flow and GFR, probably because renal autoregulatory mechanisms override the sympathetic stimuli. In contrast, pronounced, acute sympathetic stimulation (e.g. following haemorrhage) constricts renal arterioles to such an extent that renal blood flow declines temporarily to 10–30% of normal and urine output may fall to zero. If this powerful sympathetic stimulation continues, however, renal blood flow, GFR and urine output recover within 30 minutes despite continued stimulation. Renal blood flow is well maintained until approximately the fourth decade of life and then declines by about 10% per decade (Hollenberg *et al.*, 1974). The effect of age on renal autoregulation has not been studied.

Cardiovascular response to injury in the elderly

Few, if any, studies have been designed to look specifically at the effect of age on the cardiovascular response to injury. This applies to both human and animal work and any available information comes from surgical studies of outcome following the injury of surgery. Shoemaker & Kram (1990) have recently published data on outcome following surgery in the elderly. This appears to be a retrospective analysis of data from a previously published study (Bland *et al.*, 1985) which was not specifically designed to look at the effect of age on responses to surgery. Nevertheless, it does provide some information on the topic.

These investigators conducted invasive haemodynamic monitoring on 220 critically ill surgical patients judged by clinical evaluation to have a high risk of surgical complication or death and excluded those with markedly abnormal preoperative haemodynamic values (Bland *et al.*, 1985). In the re-analysis (Shoemaker & Kram, 1990) divided patients into 'elderly' (more than 65 years) and 'non-elderly' (less than 65 years, hereafter referred to as 'younger'), and into survivors and non-survivors. With regard to survivors, before operation, the haemodynamic and oxygen transport patterns of the elderly and younger patients were similar. Before operation and at their lowest point, the cardiac index (CI), oxygen consumption ($\dot{V}O_2$) and oxygen delivery (DO_2) were slightly lower and mean pulmonary artery pressure (MPAP) and right cardiac work index (RCWI) slightly higher than in younger patients.

The intraoperative and postoperative responses to surgical injury were similar in elderly and younger patients although the responses were blunted in the elderly, which the authors felt reflected some limitation of pulmonary and cardiac reserve function and relatively lower inherent metabolic needs (Shoemaker & Kram, 1990). The elderly, for example, increased their CI by 20% compared with a 40% increase in the younger patients. Elderly patients increased their $\dot{V}O_2$ by approximately 55% with half being due to the increased CI and DO_2 and half due to increased O_2 extraction. Elderly patients produced early and sustained increases in MAP and systemic vascular resistance index (SVRI) which did not occur in younger patients.

With regard to non-survivors, elderly and younger patients responded in a broadly similar fashion. Preoperative cardiac function was predominantly within the normal range. Cardiac reserve was reduced, however, as evidenced by the elevated filling pressures (CVP and pulmonary artery wedge pressure (WP)) necessary to maintain resting cardiac function. Left ventricular stroke work index (LVSWI) in particular was very low while left cardiac work index (LCWI) was within normal limits primarily because of an elevated resting heart rate. MPAP, Qsp/Qt and $P(A-a)O_2$ were higher before operation in elderly compared with younger patients which the authors interpreted as being due to prior illnesses, other stresses or the ageing process itself (Shoemaker & Kram, 1990).

In summary, in this group of patients, postoperative stress responses in elderly and younger patients were similar because both responded to the injury of surgery with an increased cardiac function. There was a major difference, however, between the age groups in terms of the magnitude of response. Shoemaker & Kram (1990) felt that the pattern of limited augmentation of cardiac function in response to surgery in the elderly survivors and non-survivors was similar to that of younger non-survivors. In particular, LVSWI was particularly abnormal in the elderly as it remained low both before and after operation, being only transiently within the normal range.

Although this study (Bland *et al.*, 1985; Shoemaker & Kram, 1990) was not designed specifically to examine the response to injury in the elderly, it does provide some information. In terms of their cardiovascular response the elderly performed less well than younger patients. The question remains as to whether the impaired performance was due to age itself or, as seems more likely, due to the increased prevalence of disease (cardiovascular and other) both symptomatic and asymptomatic, in the elderly subjects.

Tacchino *et al.* (1986) have studied the relation between age and development of postinjury myocardial depression (MD) in previously healthy but multiply injured trauma victims. They found that those aged 13–30 years had an incidence of myocardial depression of 21% while those aged 65 or over had a 32% incidence, which was associated with reductions in cardiac ejection fraction, ventricular function, cardiac index and oxygen consumption. Mortality rose to 60% when myocardial depression appeared (Siegel, 1988). This study provides important information on cardiovascular responses to trauma in the elderly and suggests that myocardial depression is commoner in the elderly, although it is likely that these findings are due to the greater prevalence of cardiovascular disease in the elderly than to age itself.

Siegel (1988) has recently reviewed the factors influencing oxygen consumption in injured elderly patients. Oxygen consumption ($\dot{V}O_2/M^2$) is primarily dependent on total body flow (cardiac index) (Siegel *et al.*, 1987). In all forms of shock and in hypermetabolic states an increase in CI results in an increase in oxygen consumption until a critical level of flow is reached at which delivery meets demand. The ability of the elderly to augment $\dot{V}O_2$ in this fashion has been questioned (Siegel, 1988), primarily because of the false assumption that CI declines with age, which as discussed earlier is not true of 'normal' aging but may be true in elderly patients with overt or asymptomatic coronary artery disease. When the effect of age on oxygen consumption in 165 trauma patients was examined it was found that $\dot{V}O_2/M^2$ declined significantly from 173 ml/min per M^2 in the young (13–30 years) to 129 ml/min per M^2 in the elderly (age

65 years or more) (Siegel *et al.*, 1987). This decline in $\dot{V}O_2$ was primarily due to a significantly lower ejection fraction in elderly compared with young. The lower ejection fraction in these elderly patients is more likely to reflect age-related disease than age itself.

The quality of ejection of blood from the heart is determined by intrinsic myocardial contractility and by the impedance to blood flow (peripheral resistance). The influence of age on peripheral resistance has been examined in the same trauma patients (Siegel *et al.*, 1987). CI was presented as a function of the total peripheral resistance. Those older post-trauma patients who had myocardial depression were found to have a reduced total peripheral resistance for a given level of flow, although the reduced cardiac afterload and myocardial oxygen consumption were associated with a poor outcome.

The influence of age on the relation between left ventricular end diastolic volume (LVEDV) and cardiac output using Starling–Sarnoff ventricular function curves has been examined in the same group of 165 post-trauma patients (Tacchino *et al.*, 1986; Siegel *et al.*, 1987). Patients of all ages who did not have myocardial depression tended to have an augmented cardiac output for any given LVEDV, i.e. their ventricular function curve was shifted to the left, with a higher cardiac output per unit LVEDV. Those patients with myocardial depression had curves which were shifted to the right, i.e. lower cardiac output per unit LVEDV. When the authors examined age as a contributory factor in myocardial depression they found that the elderly post-trauma patients with reduced ejection fraction were found to operate at the lower end of the LVEDV range. This was interpreted as being due to their greater tendency to develop overt cardiac failure and/or pulmonary oedema as LVEDV and left atrial pressure increased acutely with rapid volume infusion. Younger patients, in contrast, with comparable or more severe reductions in ejection fraction were able to maintain a near-normal cardiac output by being able to tolerate a higher LVEDV (Siegel *et al.*, 1987). The authors interpreted the findings as being due to age- or disease-related chronic myocardial fibrosis leading to a less compliant ventricle; thus, a smaller rise in LVEDV produces a greater increase in ventricular end-diastolic pressure than normal, potentiating pulmonary transcapillary transudation. The younger patients, therefore, were operating at a higher point on the Starling–Sarnoff curve, and were able to compensate for poor contractile function, due to a negative inotropic effect, by being able to handle a greater ventricular fibre length preload. These findings are, however, at variance with the finding (described earlier) in health-status-defined normal volunteers, of the greater use of the Frank–Starling mechanism in the elderly to augment cardiac output during the stress of exercise. The findings described by Siegel *et al.* (1987), therefore, may be due to the increased prevalence of cardiovascular disease in elderly patients rather than to age itself. Nevertheless, they provide important information on cardiovascular responses to injury in elderly patients.

It is worth emphasising that operative mortality (i.e. response to surgery in the elderly) has been related to the number of systems involved with degenerative cardiovascular disease, increasing from 25% with four or fewer cardiovascular abnormalities to 67% in patients with five or more (Powers, 1968). It is important, therefore, to put any effect of age itself in perspective with the impact of various disease states on the cardiovascular response to injury in the elderly (Siegel, 1988).

Conclusion

Much is known about the cardiovascular response to injury. In addition, there is an accumulating, detailed literature on the effect of age on the cardiovascular system. In contrast, there is a dearth of information regarding the effect of age on the cardiovascular response to injury. Research in this area, both animal studies and studies in humans, is urgently required. In particular, investigations must strive to separate the effects of age from those of age-associated disease. With information from carefully conducted studies, we will be in a better position to assess and manage elderly victims of injury. Doctors who look after injured elderly patients will also be better informed in their decisions regarding accepting or denying invasive monitoring or treatment of elderly patients on the basis of age alone.

References

Anderson, I. D., Little, R. A. & Heath, D. F. (1988). Human baroreflex suppression after injury. *Circ Shock*, **24**, 193.

Avolio, A. P., Fa-Quan, D., We-Qiang, L., Yao-Fei, L., Zhen-Dong, H., Lian-Fen, X. & O'Rourke, M. F. (1985). Effects of aging on arterial distensibility in populations with high and low prevalence of hypertension: comparison between urban and rural communities in China. *Circulation*, **71**, 202–10.

Barcroft, H., Edholm, O. G., McMichael, J. & Sharpey-Schafer, E. P. (1944). Posthaemorrhagic fainting. Study by cardiac output and forearm flow. *Lancet*, **1**, 489–91.

Becklake, M. R., Frank, H. & Dagenais, G. R. (1965). Influence of age and sex on exercise cardiac output. *J Appl Physiol*, **20**, 938–47.

Bland, R. D., Shoemaker, W. C., Abraham, E. & Cobo, J. C. (1985). Hemodynamic and oxygen transport patterns in surviving and nonsurviving postoperative patients. *Crit Care Med*, **13**, 85–90.

Brandfonbrenner, M., Landowne, M. & Shock, N. W. (1955). Changes in cardiac output with age. *Circulation*, **12**, 447–566.

Daly, M de B. (1983). Peripheral arterial chemoreceptors and the cardiovascular system. In *Physiology of the Peripheral Arterial Chemoreceptors*, ed. H. Acker & R. G. O'Regan, pp. 325–93. Amsterdam: Elsevier Science Publishers.

Daly, M de B., Kirkman, E. & Wood, L. M. (1988). Cardiovascular responses to stimulation of cardiac receptors in the cat and their modification by changes in respiration. *J Physiol*, **407**, 349–62.

Dastur, D. K. (1985). Cerebral blood flow and metabolism in normal human aging, pathological aging, and senile dementia. *J Cereb Blood Flow Metab*, **5**, 1–9.

D'Silva, J. L., Gill, D. & Mendel, D. (1966). The effects of acute haemorrhage on respiration in the cat. *J Physiol*, **187**, 369–77.

Duggan, J., Kilfeather, S., O'Brien, E. & O'Malley, K. (1991). Platelet intracellular free calcium concentration in ageing and hypertension. *J Hypertens*, **9**, 845–50.

Duggan, J., Nussberger, J., Kilfeather, S. & O'Malley, K. (1993). Ageing and hormonal and pressor responsiveness to angiotensin II infusion with simultaneous measurement of exogenous and endogenous angiotension II. *Am J Hypertens*, **6**, 641–7.

Elveback, L. & Lie, J. T. (1984). Combined high incidence of coronary artery disease at autopsy in Olmstead County, Minnesota, 1950–1979. *Circulation*, **70**, 345–9.

Fleckenstein, A., Frey, M. & Leder, O. (1983). Prevention by calcium antagonists of arterial calcinosis. In *New Calcium Antagonists: Recent Developments and Prospects*, ed. A. Fleckenstein, pp. 15–31. New York: G. Fischer, Stuttgart.

Fleg, J. L., Schulman, S. & Gerstenblith, G. (1988). Central versus peripheral adaptations in highly trained seniors. *Physiologist*, **31**, A158.

Fleg, J. L., Tzankoff, S. P. & Lakatta, E. G. (1985). Age-related augmentation of plasma catecholamines during exercise in healthy males. *J Appl Physiol*, **59**, 1033–9.

Freer, R. J., Pappano, A. J., Peach, M. J., Bing, K. T., McLean, M. J., Vogel, B. & Sperelakis, N. (1976). Mechanism for the positive inotropic effect of angiotensin II on isolated cardiac muscle. *Circ Res*, **39**, 178–83.

Gardin, J. M., Henry, W. L. & Savage, D. D. (1979). Echocardiographic measurements in normal subjects: evaluation of an adult population without clinically apparent heart disease. *J Clin Ultrasound*, **7**, 439–47.

Gerstenblith, G., Fleg, J. L. & Becker, L. C. (1983). Maximum left ventricular filling rate in healthy individuals measured by gated blood pool scans: effect of age. *Circulation*, **68** (Part II), 101–11.

Gerstenblith, G., Fleg, J. L., Vantosh, A., Becker, L., Kallmann, C., Andres, R., Weisfeldt, M. & Lakatta, E. G. (1980). Stress testing redefines the prevalence of coronary artery disease in epidemiological studies. *Circulation*, **62**, 111–308.

Gerstenblith, G., Fredericksen, J., Yin, F. C. P., Fortunin, N. J., Lakatta, E. G. & Weisfeldt, M. L. (1977). Echocardiographic assessment of a normal aging population. *Circulation*, **56**, 273–8.

Gerstenblith, G., Lakatta, E. G. & Weisfeldt, M. L. (1976). Age changes in myocardial function and exercise response. *Prog Cardiovasc Res*, **19**, 1–21.

Gribben, B., Pickering, T. G., Sleight, P. & Peto, R. (1971). Effect of age and high blood pressure on baroreflex sensitivity in man. *Circ Res*, **29**, 424–31.

Guyton, A. C. (1991). *Testbook of Medical Physiology*, 8th edn. Philadelphia: W. B. Saunders.

Harrison, T. R., Dixon, K., Russell, R. O., Bidwai, P. S. & Coleman, H. N. (1964). The relation of age to the duration of contraction, ejection and relaxation of the normal human heart. *Am Heart J*, **67**, 189–99.

Heymans, C. & Neil, E. (1958). *Reflexogenic Areas of the Cardiovascular System*. London: Churchill.

Hollenberg, N. K., Adams, D. F., Solomon, H. S., Rashid, R., Abrams, H. L. & Merrill, J. P. (1974). Senescence and the renal vasculature in normal man. *Circ Res*, **34**, 309–16.

Julius, S., Antoon, A., Whitlock, L. S. & Conway, J. (1967). Influence of age on the haemodynamic response to exercise. *Circulation*, **36**, 222–30.

Kannel, W. B. (1980). Host and environmental determinants of hypertension. Perspective from the Framingham study. In *Epidemiology of Arterial Blood Pressure*, ed. H. Kestleloot & J. Joossens, pp. 265–95. The Hague: Martinus Nijhoff.

Kety, S. (1956). Human cerebral blood flow and oxygen consumption as related to aging. *J Chron Dis*, **3**, 478–86.

Kirchheim, H. (1976). Systemic arterial baroreceptor reflexes. *Physiol Rev*, **56**, 100–76.

Kirkman, E. & Little, R. A. (1988). The pathophysiology of trauma and shock. In *Clinical Anaesthesiology: Fluid Resuscitation*, ed. R. Little.

Knape, J. T. & Zweiten, P. A. (1988). Positive chronotropic activity of angiotensin II in the pithed normotensive rat is primarily due to activation of cardiac beta-1 adrenoreceptors. *Naunyn Schmeidebergs Arch Pharmacol*, **338**, 185–90.

Lakatta, E. G. (1984). Cardiovascular reserve and aging. In *Blood Pressure Regulation and Ageing*, ed. M. J. Horan, G. M. Steinberg, J. B. Dunbar & E. C. Hadley. New York: Biomedical Information.

Lakatta, E. G. (1987). Do hypertension and ageing have a similar effect on the myocardium? *Circulation*, **75** (Suppl. 1), 169–77.

Lakatta, E. G. (1988). Cardiovascular system. In *Human Ageing Research: Concepts and Techniques, Ageing*, vol. 34, ed. B. Kent & R. Butler.

Lakatta, E. G. (1990). Changes in cardiovascular function with aging. *Eur Heart J*, **11** (Suppl. C), 22–9.

Little, R. A., Marshall, H. W. & Kirkman, E. (1989). Attenuation of the acute cardiovascular response to haemorrhage by tissue injury in the conscious rat. *Q J Exp Physiol*, **74**, 825–33.

Little, R. A., Randall, P. E., Redfern, W. S., Stoner, H. B. & Marshall, H. W. (1984). Components of injury (haemorrhage and tissue ischaemia) affecting cardiovascular reflexes in man and rat. *Q J Exp Physiol*, **69**, 753–62.

Melamed, E., Lavy, S., Bentin, S., Cooper, G. & Rinot, Y. (1980). Reduction in regional cerebral blood flow during normal aging in man. *Stroke*, **11**, 31–5.

Öberg, B. & Thorén, P. (1972a). Studies on left ventricular receptors signalling in non-medullated vagal afferents. *Acta Physiol Scand*, **85**, 145–63.

Öberg, B. & Thorén, P. (1972b). Increased activity in left ventricular receptors during haemorrhage or occlusion of the caval veins in the cat. A possible cause of the vasovagal reaction. *Acta Physiol Scand*, **85**, 164–73.

O'Rourke, M. F. (1986). *Arterial Function in Health and Disease*, p. 275. New York: Churchill Livingstone.

Pantano, P., Baron, J.-C., Lebrun-Grandie, P., Duquesnoy, N., Bousser, M.-G. & Comar, D. (1984). Regional cerebral blood flow and oxygen consumption in human aging. *Stroke*, **15**, 635–41.

Peach, M. J. (1977). Renin–angiotensin system: biochemistry and mechanisms of action. *Physiol Rev*, **57**, 313–70.

Port, E., Cobb, F. R., Coleman, R. E. & Jones, R. H. (1980). Effect of age on the response of the left ventricular ejection fraction to exercise. *New Engl J Med*, **303**, 1133–7.

Powers, J. H. (1968). Coexisting debilitating and degenerative diseases: preoperative investigation and management of elderly patients. In *Surgery of the Aged and Debilitated Patient*, ed. J. H. Powers. Philadelphia: W. B. Saunders.

Rodeheffer, R., Gerstenblith, G., Becker, L. C., Fleg, J. L., Weisfeldt, M. L. & Lakatta, E. G. (1984). Exercise cardiac output is maintained with advancing age in healthy human subjects:

cardiac dilatation and increased stroke volume compensate for a diminished heart rate. *Circulation*, **69**, 203–13.

Sander-Jensen, K., Secher, N. H., Bie, P., Warberg, J. & Schwartz, T. W. (1986). Vagal slowing of the heart during haemorrhage: observations from 20 consecutive hypotensive patients. *Br Med J*, **292**, 364–6.

Secher, N. H. & Bie, P. (1985). Bradycardia during reversible haemorrhagic shock: a forgotten observation? *Clin Physiol*, **5**, 315–23.

Secher, N. H., Sander-Jensen, K., Werner, C., Warberg, J. & Bie, P. (1984). Bradycardia during severe but reversible hypovolaemic shock in man. *Circ Shock*, **14**, 267–74.

Shannon, R. P., Wei, J. Y. & Rosa, R. M. (1986). The effect of age and sodium depletion on cardiovascular response to orthostasis. *Hypertension*, **8**, 438–43.

Shimada, K., Kitazumi, T., Sadakane, N., Ogura, H. & Ozawa, T. (1985). Age-related changes of baroreflex function, plasma norepinephrine and blood pressure. *Hypertension*, **7**, 113–17.

Shirahata, N., Henriksen, L., Vorstrup, S., Holm, S., Lauritzen, M., Paulson, P. B. & Lassen, N. A. (1985). Regional cerebral blood flow assessed by ^{133}Xe inhalation and emission tomography: normal values. *J Comput Assist Tomogr*, **9**, 861–6.

Shoemaker, W. C. & Kram, H. B. (1990). Perioperative monitoring and management of normal, stressed and elderly high risk patients. In *Geriatric Surgery: Comprehensive Care of the Elderly Patient*, ed. M. R. Katlic, pp. 311–27. Baltimore-Munich: Urban & Schwarzenberg.

Siegel, J. H. (1988). The heart and its functions in the aged. In *Surgical Care of the Elderly*, ed. J. J. Meakins & J. C. McClaren, pp. 88–120. Chicago: Year Book Medical Publishers Inc.

Siegel, J. H., Linberg, S. E. & Wiles, C. E. (1987). Hemodynamic evaluation and cardiovascular therapy of low flow shock states. In *Trauma: Emergency Surgery and Critical Care*, pp. 201–84. New York: Churchill-Livingstone.

Sjögren, A. L. (1971). Left ventricular wall thickness determined by ultrasound in 100 subjects without heart disease. *Chest*, **60**, 341–6.

Spyer, K. M. (1984). Central control of the cardiovascular system. *Recent Adv Physiol*, **10**, 163–200.

Swinne, C. J., Fleg, J. L., Lima, J. A. C., Lima, S. D. & Shapiro, E. P. (1989). Age-related changes in left ventricular performance during isometric exercise. *J Am Coll Cardiol*, **13**, 56A.

Tacchino, R. M., Siegel, J. H., Chiarly, C. *et al.* (1986). Incidence and therapy of myocardial depression in critically ill post-trauma patients. *Circ Shock*, **18**, 360.

Tejada, C., Strong, J. P., Montenegro, M. R., Restropo, C. & Solberg, L. A. (1968). Distribution of coronary and aortic atherosclerosis by geographic location, race and sex. *Lab Invest*, **18**, 49–66.

Thorén, P. (1977). Characteristics of left ventricular receptors with non-medullated vagal afferents in the cat. *Circ Res*, **40**, 415–21.

Waldemar, G., Hasselbach, S. G., Anderesen, A. R., Delecluse, F., Petersen, P., Johnsen, A. & Paulson, O. B. (1991). ^{99m}Tc-d,1–HMPAO and SPECT of the brain in normal aging. *J Cer Blood Flow Metab*, **11**, 508–21.

Wolinsky, H. (1972). Long-term effects of hypertension on the rat aortic wall and their relation to concurrent aging changes. Morphological and chemical studies. *Circ Res*, **30**, 301–9.

Wynne, H. A., Cope, L. H., Mutch, E., Rawlins, M. D., Woodhouse, K. W. & James, O. F. W. (1989). The effect of age upon liver volume and apparent liver blood flow in healthy man. *Hepatology*, **9**, 297–301.

13

Aging in muscle

W. J. K. CUMMING

Introduction

In muscle, which can be considered as the end organ of the anterior horn cell, the commonest change seen with advancing age, in the absence of any signs of associated disease, is atrophy in terms both of the size of the individual fibre and the overall muscle bulk (Jennekens *et al.*, 1971; Grimby *et al.*, 1982; Lexel *et al.*, 1983a,b, 1986; Munsat, 1984; Cumming, 1992; Jennekens, 1992).

Normal muscle

The anterior horn cell, its associated axon and the muscle fibres that it innervates are collectively known as the motor unit. This motor unit is not static throughout life, as changes occur both as a consequence of disease and as a consequence of aging (Larsson, 1992). Muscle fibres are of two major types: type I or 'slow twitch' fibres and type II or 'fast twitch' fibres. The proportion of these fibre types differs according to the specialisation of the individual muscle although the proportion of type I and type II fibres of any given muscle are relatively constant between individuals. The metabolism of type I (slow twitch) and type II (fast twitch) fibres differs considerably. Slow twitch fibres (which are fatigue resistant) have a high myoglobin content and depend on oxidative energy for metabolism. Type II fibres can be divided into two groups: fast fibres which are fatigue resistant (type IIa), show a high myoglobin content and have a combination of oxidative and glycolytic metabolism, and fast rapidly fatiguable fibres (type IIb) which have low myoglobin content and show glycolytic energy metabolism (Slater & Harris, 1988; Landon, 1992).

These varying metabolic pathways form the basis of the different histochemical stains that are used to differentiate muscle fibres in fresh frozen biopsy samples.

It has become increasingly recognised in this last decade that 'normal' has to be specified for age, in that the normal appearances of a muscle at age 20 years are

189

very different from the comparable appearances from a normal individual of age 80 years.

This has led to confusion in the literature relating to some disease states. For example, it had previously been considered that there were changes seen in muscle biopsy in motor neuron disease (MND) which were indicators of the rapidity of progression of that disease. When such changes were reviewed in the light of the 'normal' for age (Kristmundsdottir *et al.*, 1990), it was clear that the apparent pathological changes were not specific for MND, but reflected the age of the individuals. This indicates, as stated above, that there is considerable apparent abnormality of muscle pathology with age.

Clearly, the complexity of the anterior horn cell, the axon, the neuromuscular junction and the enzymatic function in muscle implies that there could be more than one pathway involved in the changes seen in aging muscle.

Muscle response to varied demand

Muscle fibres exhibit a remarkable ability to change their characteristics in response to altered functional demands. It is recognised that once the fibres have differentiated the total number of fibres appears constant. Therefore any changes that occur subsequently have to occur in terms of size and functional property. It is well recognised that exercise stimulates the growth of skeletal muscle and depending on the type of exercise employed, then the changes produced include hypertrophy of muscle fibres, increase in mitochondrial protein concentration, increased percentage of type IIa fibres and decreased percentage of IIb fibres (Grimby *et al.*, 1982; Vandervoort *et al.*, 1986; Klitgaard *et al.*, 1990; Frontera *et al.*, 1991; Sipilae & Suominen, 1991; Aniansson *et al.*, 1992; Phillips *et al.*, 1992, 1993). These changes are usually seen more obviously in females than males (Phillips *et al.*, 1993). Similar changes are seen in aging animal muscle (Phillips *et al.*, 1991; Brown *et al.*, 1992). Allied to this is an increased resistance to fatigue. With any type of exercise that induces a higher rate of mechanical work, the greater is the deviation from the muscles' resting chemical composition in terms of proportions of high energy phosphate, lactate and glycogen concentrations (Barnard *et al.*, 1992; Bittles, 1992; Byrne & Dennett, 1992).

In contrast, atrophy of muscle can be produced by a diverse range of agents, the commonest being malnutrition, disuse and denervation (Jennekens, 1992).

In malnutrition, muscle changes are mainly those of a general reduction of fibre diameter with increased variation of fibre size, but with little evidence of intrinsic muscle fibre pathology. Disuse atrophy also involves reduction in the size but not the number of type II fibres, whereas denervation atrophy characteristically is first seen as small groups of atrophic fibres. In addition, there are structural changes in the muscle fibre (e.g. target, targetoid, ringbinden).

In attempting therefore to address the problem of aging in muscle, one of the greatest problems is to differentiate between external factors such as exercise (or lack of it), malnutrition and changes that are associated with aging alone.

Aging in muscle

The most obvious finding in aging muscle is the loss of muscle volume. This is seen not only in humans but also in animal material (Ansved & Larsson, 1990; Arabadjis *et al.*, 1990; Ansved & Edstrom, 1991; Clark & White, 1991; Peinemann *et al.*, 1991; Baumgartner *et al.*, 1992; Coggan *et al.*, 1992; Einsiedel & Luff, 1992a,b). Volume loss in the muscle appears to start at the age of 25 years and by the age of 50 years some 10% of muscle volume has been lost. The rate of loss of muscle volume increases with advancing age so that by the age of 80 years almost half the muscle will appear to be wasted. The loss of muscle volume is not reflected across the fibre types, unfortunately, in that type I fibres appear to remain well preserved with advancing age, whereas type II fibres (particularly type IIa fibres) appear to be reduced both in number and in size.

The involutional or physiological processes that underlie the loss of muscle mass appear to involve the anterior horn cell and also to a lesser extent the axon. There is a marked increase in lipofuscin (as much as 75–95% of cell volume) by the seventh decade at the expense of other intracellular substances. With progressive age, anterior horn cells may appear shrunken and hypochromatic, whereas the remaining cells appear swollen and distorted by lipofuscin and there is in addition diffuse gliosis of the anterior horn cell (Tomlinson & Irving, 1977). Thus, the changes occurring in the anterior horn cell and the axon lead to progressive fractionation of the motor unit.

Clinically, atrophy of muscle in the elderly, in the absence of any underlying disease, is most marked in the lower extremities and is more severe distally. This loss of muscle strength has been recognised for many years and has more recently been the subject of more detailed investigation (Vandervoort *et al.*, 1986). In studies looking at ankle flexion and extension, hand grip and elbow flexion, the percentage decline in strength with age varied between 17 and 59%. The results were consistent between the muscles tested, indicating that the pattern of strength lost was similar for the different groups irrespective of whether they were proximally or distally located in the upper or the lower limbs. In addition, although there are some views to the contrary (Phillips *et al.*, 1993), there appears to be little difference between males and females (Grimby *et al.*, 1982; Vandervoort *et al.*, 1986; Sipilae & Suominen, 1991).

These studies have shown that by the age of 70 years there is about a 20% decrease in maximum voluntary contraction compared with younger age groups and that with advancing age the fall off in maximum and voluntary contraction can reach 50%.

There are two possible explanations for the lower strength levels seen in the elderly which could be due either to factors interfering with volitional activation of muscles or factors contributing to reduced excitable muscle mass.

It is possible that apparent depression of motor unit activation could be due to lack of motivation or to an additional contribution from painful joints or the presence of a motor neuron lesion. In elderly individuals with no evidence of underlying disease process (Campbell *et al.*, 1973; McComas, 1991), high levels of muscle excitation could be produced in isometric tests of ankle dorsiflexion and plantar flexion. These results indicate that older, as well as younger subjects, retained the ability to activate the muscles under test conditions. It would appear therefore that age itself does not render the individual unable to use their muscles optimally in generating force (Phillips *et al.*, 1992).

Therefore, if the elderly individual can fully activate their muscles, yet the strength of those muscles is decreased, the excitable muscle mass must be reduced. This area has been addressed in detail in Lexel and his colleagues (Lexell *et al.*, 1983a,b, 1986, 1992; Lexell & Downham, 1991, 1992; Lexell & Taylor, 1991; Sjoestroem *et al.*, 1992) who have employed the technique of looking at whole cross sections of the vastus lateralis muscle in the age ranges of younger (19–37 years) and older (70 + years) subjects. In the very elderly they have shown a fall out of fibres of about 25% and have shown that type II fibres are preferentially affected in terms of smaller size.

Consistent with the loss of type II fibres is the finding that the compound muscle axon potential, generated by maximum excitation of the motor nerve and recorded by surface electromyograph (EMG), is diminished in the elderly to approximately the same degree as the loss of strength (Campbell *et al.*, 1973). This has been interpreted as providing anatomical and physiological support for the theory that aging in muscle has caused a reduction in the number of functioning motor neurons.

The type II fibre atrophy observed in aging is much less likely to be associated with compensatory type I fibre hypertrophy (40% in the elderly, 85 + % in young individuals) (Lexell & Taylor, 1991) and it would therefore appear that other factors, other than just abnormalities of the motor neuron due to perturbation of the anterior horn cell, are operating in this situation.

It has been shown (Grimby *et al.*, 1982) that type II fibre atrophy can be reversed by physical activity in muscle training even up to the age of 80 years (Greig *et al.*, 1993). Lexell & Taylor (1991) have therefore suggested that there is an interplay between neurogenic factors affecting the motor unit and also a change in the physical activity pattern of the elderly, which contribute to the type II fibre atrophy. Functional demands over a long period of time differ and therefore muscle fibres develop different properties. As the movement of the aged individual is in general more restricted, the functional demands of the fibre population with respect to force, thrust and duration is also changed or decreased, resulting in more homogeneous dispersion of fibre properties (Lexell *et al.*, 1983b; Lexell & Downham, 1991, 1992).

There are now several studies which show that mitochondrial abnormalities occur in skeletal muscle fibres in both the aged rat and human (Mueller-Hoecker, 1990; Schonk *et al.*, 1990; Katayama *et al.*, 1991; Miquel, 1991; Cooper *et al.*, 1992; Edstroem *et al.*, 1992; Mueller-Hoecker *et al.*, 1993). These mitochondrial abnormalities are of a respiratory chain type and are mostly associated with mitochondrial DNA deletions. Indeed, abnormalities of the mitochondrial genome, for example deletion on site 4374 which normally leads to the development of the MELAS syndrome (multiple stroke-like episodes with a mitochondrial myopathy), can be shown to be present as a normal finding in aged muscle (Zhang *et al.*, 1992). Indeed up to 50% of the muscle fibres of the elderly population have been shown to contain abnormalities of mitochondrial DNA. These abnormalities in the mitochondrial genome are not regularly associated with major evidence of mitochondrial dysfunction as judged by histochemical stains for mitochondrial function or by studies of mitochondrial respiratory chain function (Byrne & Dennett, 1992; Cooper *et al.*, 1992).

In the mitochondrial myopathies, where clear ultrastructural changes within the mitochondria are seen, it has been suggested that the abnormal mitochondria in some way contribute to the muscle weakness that the patient experiences. The same is also true in myotonic dystrophy where there is an increasing amount of abnormal mitochondrial DNA with advancing muscle weakness. Clearly in myotonic dystrophy, the gene abnormality (Sahashi *et al.*, 1992) in the nuclear genome (Ptacek *et al.*, 1993) and the findings of mutant mitochondrial DNA in limb muscle remain to be explained.

Although there is persuasive evidence to suggest that increased abnormalities of peroxidation can lead to increasingly damaged mitochondrial DNA (Hruszkewycz, 1992) this may well occur in the anterior horn cell and could be a contributing factor to anterior horn cell loss in association with aging (Wallace, 1992). It is more difficult, however, to understand the mechanism whereby increased mitochondrial genomic deletions in muscle fibres would lead to abnormalities within the muscle fibre in terms of its loss of size and volume and consequent loss of strength. The exact relation therefore between mitochondrial DNA deletions and skeletal muscle of aging remains to be elucidated.

It would appear therefore that at the present time the most likely prominent mechanism in the loss of muscle fibre bulk with age relates to anterior horn cell changes leading to denervation with ineffective reinnervation within the muscle.

References

Aniansson, A., Grimby, G. & Hedberg, M. (1992). Compensatory muscle fiber hypertrophy in elderly men. *J Appl Physiol*, **73**, 812–16.
Ansved, T. & Edstrom, L. (1991). Effects of age on fibre structure, ultrastructure and expression of desmin and spectrin in fast- and slow-twitch rat muscles. *J Anat*, **174**, 61–79.

Ansved, T. & Larsson, L. (1990). Effects of denervation on enzyme-histochemical and morphometrical properties of the rat soleus muscle in relation to age. *Acta Physiol Scand*, **139**, 297–304.

Arabadjis, P. G., Heffner, R. R., Jr & Pendergast, D. R. (1990). Morphologic and functional alterations in aging rat muscle. *J Neuropath Exp Neurol*, **49**, 600–9.

Barnard, R. J., Lawani, L. O., Martin, D. A., Youngren, J. F., Singh, R. & Scheck, S. H. (1992). Effects of maturation and aging on the skeletal muscle glucose transport system. *Am J Physiol*, **262**, E619–E626.

Baumgartner, R. N., Rhyne, R. L., Troup, C., Wayne, S. & Garry, P. J. (1992). Appendicular skeletal muscle areas assessed by magnetic resonance imaging in older persons. *J Gerontol*, **47**, M67–M72.

Bittles, A. H. (1992). Evidence for and against the causal involvement of mitochondrial DNA mutation in mammalian ageing. *Mutat Res DNAging Genet Instability Aging*, **275**, 217–25.

Brown, M., Ross, T. P. & Holloszy, J. O. (1992). Effects of ageing and exercise on soleus and extensor digitorum longus muscles of female rats. *Mechn Ageing Dev*, **63**, 69–77.

Byrne, E. & Dennett, X. (1992). Respiratory chain failure in adult muscle fibres: relationship with ageing and possible implications for the neuronal pool. *Mutat Res DNAging Genet Instability Aging*, **275**, 125–31.

Campbell, M. J., McComas, A. J. & Petito, F. (1973). Physiological changes in ageing muscles. *J Neurol Neurosurg Psychiatry*, **36**, 174–82.

Clark, K. I. & White, T. P. (1991). Neuromuscular adaptations to cross-reinnervation in 12– and 29-mo-old Fischer 344 rats. *Am J Physiol*, **260**, C96–C103.

Coggan, A. R., Spina, R. J., King, D. S., Rogers, M. A., Brown, M., Nemeth, P. M. & Holloszy, J. O. (1992). Histochemical and enzymatic comparison of the gastrocnemius muscle of young and elderly men and women. *J Gerontol*, **47**, B71–B76.

Cooper, J. M., Mann, V. M. & Schapira, A. H. V. (1992). Analyses of mitochondrial respiratory chain function and mitochondrial DNA deletion in human skeletal muscle: effect of ageing. *J Neurol Sci*, **113**, 91–8.

Cumming, W. J. K. (1992). Aging and neuromuscular disease. In *Textbook of Geriatric Medicine and Gerontology*, 4 edn, ed. J. C. Brocklehurst, R. C. Tallis & H. M. Fillit, pp. 834–42. Edinburgh: Churchill Livingstone.

Edstroem, L., Larsson, H. & Larsson, L. (1992). Neurogenic effects on the palatopharyngeal muscle in patients with obstructive sleep apnoea: a muscle biopsy study. *J Neurol Neurosurg Psychiatry*, **55**, 916–20.

Einsiedel, L. J. & Luff, A. R. (1992a). Alterations in the contractile properties of motor units within the ageing rat medial gastrocnemius. *J Neruol Sci*, **112**, 170–7.

Einsiedel, L. J. & Luff, A. R. (1992b). Effect of partial denervation on motor units in the ageing rat medial gastrocnemius. *J Neurol Sci*, **112**, 178–84.

Frontera, W. R., Hughes, V. A., Lutz, K. J. & Evans, W. J. (1991). A cross-sectional study of muscle strength and mass in 45–to 78–yr-old men and women. *J Appl Physiol*, **71**, 644–50.

Greig, C. A., Botella, J. & Young, A. (1993). The quadriceps strength of healthy elderly people remeasured after eight years. *Muscle & Nerve*, **16**, 6–10.

Grimby, G., Danneskiold-Samse, B., Hvid, K. & Saltin, B. (1982). Morphology and enzyme capacity in arm and leg muscles in 78–81 year old men and women. *Acta Physiol Scand*, **115**, 125–34.

Hruszkewycz, A. M. (1992). Lipid peroxidation and mtDNA degeneration. A hypothesis. *Mutat Res DNAging Genet Instability Aging*, **275**, 243–8.

Jennekens, F. G. I. (1992). Disuse, cachexia and aging. In *Skeletal Muscle Pathology*, 2nd edn, ed. F. L. Mastaglia & J. N. Walton, pp. 753–67. Edinburgh: Churchill Livingstone.

Jennekens, F. G. I., Tomlinson, B. E. & Walton, J. N. (1971). Histochemical aspects of five limb muscles in old age: an autopsy study. *J Neurol Sci*, **14**, 259–76.

Katayama, M., Tanaka, M., Yamamoto, H., Ohbayashi, T., Nimura, Y. & Ozawa, T. (1991). Deleted mitochondrial DNA in the skeletal muscle of aged individuals. *Biochem Int*, **25**, 47–56.

Klitgaard, H., Mantoni, M., Schiaffino, S., Ausoni, S., Gorza, L., Laurent-Winter, C. Schnohr, P. & Saltin, B. (1990). Function, morphology and protein expression of ageing skeletal muscle: a cross-sectional study of elderly men with different training backgrounds. *Acta Physiol Scand*, **140**, 41–54.

Kristmundsdottir, F., Mahon, M., Froes, M. M. Q. & Cumming, W. J. K. (1990). Histomorphometric and histopathological study of the human cricopharyngeus muscle: in health and in motor neuron disease. *Neuropathol Appl Neurobiol*, **16**, 461–75.

Landon, D. N. (1992). Skeletal muscle: normal morphology, development and innervation. In *Skeletal Muscle Pathology*, 2nd edn, ed. F. L. Mastaglia & Lord Walton of Detchant, pp. 1–94. Edinburgh: Churchill Livingstone.

Larsson, L. (1992). Is the motor unit uniform? *Acta Physiol Scand*, **144**, 143–54.

Lexell, J. & Downham, D. Y. (1991). The occurrence of fibre-type grouping in healthy human muscle: a quantitative study of cross-sections of whole vastus lateralis from men between 15 and 83 years. *Acta Neuropathol (Berl)*, **81**, 377–81.

Lexell, J. & Downham, D. (1992). What is the effect of ageing on type 2 muscle fibres? *J Neurol Sci*, **107**, 250–1.

Lexell, J., Downham, D. & Sjöström, M. (1986). Distribution of different fibre types in human skeletal muscles: fibre type arrangements in m. vastus lateralis from three groups of healthy men between 15 and 82 years. *J Neurol Sci*, **72**, 211–22.

Lexell, J., Henriksson-Larsén, K. & Sjöström, M. (1983a). Distribution of different fibre types in human skeletal muscle: 2. A study of cross sections of whole m. vastus lateralis. *Acta Physiol Scand*, **117**, 115–22.

Lexell, J., Henriksson-Larsén, K., Winblad, B. & Sjöström, M. (1983b). Distribution of different fibre types in human skeletal muscles: effects of aging studied in whole muscle cross section. *Muscle Nerve*, **6**, 588–95.

Lexell, J., Sjoestroem, M., Nordlund, A.-S. & Taylor, C. C. (1992). Growth and development of human muscle: a quantitative morphological study of whole vastus lateralis from childhood to adult age. *Muscle Nerve*, **15**, 404–9.

Lexell, J. & Taylor, C. C. (1991). Variability in muscle fibre areas in whole human quadriceps muscle: effects of increasing age. *J Anat*, **174**, 239–49.

McComas, A. J. (1991). Invited review: motor unit estimation: methods, results and present status. *Muscle Nerve*, **14**, 585–97.

Miquel, J. (1991). An integrated theory of aging as the result of mitochondrial DNA mutation in differentiated cells. *Arch Gerontol Geriatr*, **12**, 99–117.

Mueller-Hoecker, J. (1990). Cytochrome c oxidase deficient fibres in the limb muscle and diaphragm of man without muscular disease: an age-related alteration. *J Neurol Sci*, **100**, 14–21.

Mueller-Hoecker, J., Seibel, P., Schneiderbanger, K. & Kadenbach, B. (1993). Different *in situ* hybridization patterns of mitochondrial DNA in cytochrome c oxidase-deficient extraocular muscle fibres in the elderly. *Virchows Arch A Pathol Anat Histopathol*, **422**, 7–15.

Munsat, T. L. (1984). Aging of the neuromuscular system. In *Clinical Neurology of Aging*, ed. M. L. Albert, pp. 404–24. New York: Oxford University Press.

Peinemann, F., Wagner, M., Franke, U., Kulle, M. & Reiss, J. (1991). Prenatal deletion detection in a sporadic case of Duchenne muscular dystrophy without genotype information from the affected individual *Eur J Pediatr*, **150**, 256–8.

Phillips, S. K., Bruce, S. A. & Woledge, R. C. (1991). In mice, the muscle weakness due to age is absent during stretching. *J Physiol (Lond)*, **437**, 63–70.

Phillips, S. K., Bruce, S. A., Newton, D. & Woledge, R. C. (1992). The weakness of old age is not due to failure of muscle activation. *J Gerontol*, **47**, M45–M49.

Phillips, S. K., Rook, K. M., Siddle, N. C., Bruce, S. A. & Woledge, R. C. (1993). Muscle weakness in women occurs at an earlier age than in men, but strength is preserved by hormone replacement therapy. *Clin Sci*, **84**, 95–8.

Ptacek, L. J., Johnson, K. J. & Griggs, R. C. (1993). Mechanisms of disease: genetics and physiology of the myotonic muscle disorders. *New Engl J Med*, **328**, 482–9.

Sahashi,K., Tanaka, M., Tashiro, M., Ohno, K., Ibi, T., Takahashi, A. & Ozawa, T. (1992). Increased mitochondrial DNA deletions in the skeletal muscle of myotonic dystrophy. *Gerontology*, **38**, 18–29.

Schonk, D., Van, D. P., Riegmann, P., Trapman, J., Holm, C., Willcocks, T. C., Sillekens, P., Van, V. W., Wimmer, E., Geurts, van K. A., Ropers, H.-H. & Wieringa, B. (1990). Assignment of seven genes to distinct intervals on the midportion of human chromosome 19q surrounding the myotonic dystrophy gene region. *Cytogenet Cell Genet*, **54**, 15–19.

Sipilae, S. & Suominen, H. (1991). Ultrasound imaging of the quadriceps muscle in elderly athletes and untrained men. *Muscle Nerve*, **14**, 527–33.

Sjoestroem, M., Lexell, J. & Downham, D. Y. (1992). Differences in fiber number and fiber type proportion within fascicles: a quantitative morphological study of whole vastus lateralis muscle from childhood to old age. *Anat Rec*, **234**, 183–9.

Slater, C. R. & Harris, J. B. (1988). The anatomy and physiology of the motor unit. In *Disorders of Voluntary Muscle*, 5th edn, ed. J. N. Walton, pp. 1–26. Edinburgh: Churchill Livingstone.

Tomlinson, B. E. & Irving, D. (1977). The number of limb motor neurones in the human lumbosacral cord throughout life. *J Neurol Sci*, **34**, 213–19.

Vandervoort, A. A., Hayes, K. C. & Belanger, A. Y. (1986). Strength and endurance of skeletal muscle in the elderly. *Physiotherapy Can*, **38**, 167–73.

Wallace, D. C. (1992). Mitochondrial genetics: a paradigm for aging and degenerative diseases. *Science*, **256**, 628–32.

Zhang, C., Baumer, A., Maxwell, R. J., Linnane, A. W. & Nagley, P. (1992). Multiple mitochondrial DNA deletions in an elderly human individual. *FEBS Lett*, **297**, 34–8.

14

Metabolic responses

R. A. LITTLE

Introduction

The metabolic changes were among the first of the responses to injury to be subjected to scientific study (for reviews see Cuthbertson, 1980a,b). In an attempt to minimise the influence of constitutional factors, such as the presence of intercurrent disease, these studies were often limited to previously healthy young people. Unfortunately, as discussed elsewhere in this volume, accidental injuries and surgery are not uncommon in the elderly who seem to be more vulnerable than the young to their adverse consequences. A recent review highlighted the dearth of information on the biological responses to injury in the aged (Horan *et al.*, 1988). In the present review a number of the features of the metabolic response to injury (for a fuller discussion see Barton *et al.*, 1990) and how they might be expected to be different in the elderly are briefly discussed. The responses are considered in relation to time after injury. Traditionally the early and late phases of the responses have been termed 'ebb' and 'flow' (Cuthbertson, 1942). Although there is now some debate about the changes implicit in these terms they are still useful and will be used here.

Metabolic rate and body temperature

'Ebb' phase

The concept of the 'ebb' phase as a period of reduced energy metabolism arises from experimental studies which showed that after injury oxygen consumption and body temperature, at ambient temperatures below the thermoneutral range, were reduced. This impairment of heat production could not be reversed by reinfusion of blood or the administration of 100% inspired oxygen which are effective after simple haemorrhage. Thus although the fall in heat production after haemorrhage can be ascribed to a failure of oxygen delivery this is not the case after tissue injury. In such cases

197

nociceptive afferent impulses triggered at the site of injury activate noradrenergic neurons in the hind brain from whence axons ascend in the ventral noradrenergic bundle liberating noradrenaline in the region of the dorsomedial nucleus of the hypothalamus. The result is an inhibition of both thermoregulatory heat production and heat loss mechanisms. Thus lower temperatures have to be applied to the skin or the hypothalamus to induce shivering in skeletal muscle and higher temperatures have to be applied to the hypothalamus to initiate an increase in heat loss (Stoner, 1972). The inhibition of thermoregulatory heat production by injury in the rat, which involves both skeletal muscle and brown adipose tissue (Stoner, 1971, 1974), can eventually be overcome by lowering ambient temperature sufficiently or by the injection of exogenous noradrenaline. This supports the suggestion that the reduction in heat production in the 'ebb' phase of the response to injury in experimental animals is due to a change in central control rather than to an impairment of peripheral effector mechanisms.

The evidence for a similar pattern of change after injury in humans is not so good. Body temperature is reduced acutely after injury and the reduction is directly related to its severity (Little & Stoner, 1981). It is, however, difficult to conclude that these changes are central in origin because plasma lactate concentrations are elevated after the most serious injuries and an impairment of oxygen transport cannot be excluded. There is some evidence for a change in thermoregulatory control at this time: patients do not shiver despite having body temperatures below the normal threshold for its onset and also the appreciation of thermal comfort is modified (Little *et al.*, 1986). Measurements of metabolic rate at this time after injury have not provided convincing evidence for a controlled reduction in metabolic rate measured by, for example indirect calorimetry (Little & Stoner, 1981).

Oxygen consumption calculated by a modification of the Fick equation is often higher than predicted in severely injured patients both before and after resuscitation (Cournand *et al.*, 1943; Edwards *et al.*, 1988). A possible limitation of this approach, especially after treatment, is that any manoeuvre which increases cardiac output might also be expected to 'increase' oxygen consumption the calculation of which includes cardiac output. The consensus is that there is no evidence for a reduction in body temperature and metabolic rate acutely after injury in humans that cannot be attributed to a failure of oxygen transport or necrobiosis. This may not be too surprising if it is remembered that many of the measurements have been made at ambient temperatures close to or within the thermoneutral range, which may of course be extended after injury.

It is also important to realise that the continuous thermoregulatory variable in humans is heat loss and not heat production as in the rat. Thus although changes in heat production (oxygen consumption) have been studied in the rat clinical studies would, perhaps, be better focused on the mechanisms of heat loss at this time. Indeed a detailed study of heat balance has shown an inhibition of heat loss and an upward resetting of thermoregulation to achieve an increase in heat content within the first 12 hours after burning injury in children (Childs *et al.*, 1989).

'Flow' phase

The characteristic features of the 'flow' phase are increases in metabolic rate, body temperature and urinary nitrogen excretion and reductions in body weight and, most importantly, lean body mass.

The increase in metabolic rate has been claimed to be directly related to the severity of injury with the largest increases occurring after burns exceeding 40–50% of body surface area (Wilmore, 1977). This relation is not, however, always very obvious because the hypermetabolic response to injury is often superimposed on a background of reduced food intake and loss of muscle mass, both of which will reduce metabolic rate. The situation can be further complicated by treatment, for example after head injury the use of neuromuscular blockade and steroids – the latter exacerbating the catabolic loss of lean body mass (Greenblatt *et al.*, 1989).

Metabolic rate may also be limited by the supply of oxygen to the tissues. It has been suggested that in the severely injured patient oxygen delivery should be increased to supranormal levels by the use of inotropic agents and artificial ventilation with high inspired oxygen concentrations to ensure that oxygen consumption is not limited by its supply (Edwards, 1990). If agents such as dopamine or dobutamine are used it is important to realise that they, of themselves, increase oxygen consumption even in normal subjects (Regan *et al.*, 1990). When oxygen delivery is inadequate and oxygen consumption cannot be maintained by increasing oxygen extraction then a vicious cycle of anaerobic metabolism, depletion of energy stores and increasing tissue damage will occur: the 'necrobiotic' phase of the response to injury (Stoner, 1961).

If it is accepted that metabolic rate is increased in the flow phase it is important to understand its pathogenesis. Burns (Chapter 20) in which there are large increases in evaporative water loss have been most comprehensively studied. The energy cost of the latent heat of evaporation has to be met by an increase in metabolic rate and although the water loss can be reduced by the use of impermeable dressing (Lamke *et al.*, 1977) there is no agreement on the effect this has on metabolic rate (Davies, 1982). There is also little agreement on the effects of off-setting the increase in evaporative heat loss by reducing dry heat losses by increasing ambient temperature. In some hands this abolishes the hypermetabolism (Arturson, 1978), while Wilmore and his colleagues have been able to demonstrate only a small reduction (Aulick *et al.*, 1979). Indeed Wilmore has concluded that the dissociation between the evaporative water loss and hypermetabolism and the persistence of an elevated metabolic rate at a raised environmental temperature are evidence for an upward resetting in hypothalamic thermoregulatory control. He makes the case that the latent heat of evaporation of water from the surface of a burn is a convenient route for the dissipation of the excess energy produced by the increase in metabolic rate (Wilmore, 1977).

This upward resetting of thermoregulation after thermal injury leads to an increase in sympathetic nervous activity and it is the increase in catecholamine release which mediates the increase in energy production. There is a positive relation between urinary catecholamine excretion and metabolic rate which can be reduced by combined adrenergic blockade (Wilmore et al., 1974). Although plasma catecholamine concentrations remain increased during the flow phase response to burns and to severe head injury (Hadfield et al., 1992) they have returned to normal after severe musculoskeletal injuries (Frayn et al., 1984).

One way in which increased sympathetic activity may stimulate metabolic rate is by the enhanced exchange between non-esterified fatty acids (NEFAs) and triacylglycerol both within adipose tissue and via plasma NEFAs, which can be blocked by propranolol (Wolfe et al., 1987). In addition there is a concomitant increase in exchange between glucose and glycolytic products and it has been calculated that at least 15% of the 'flow' phase increase in metabolic rate can be accounted for by this substrate cycling (Wolfe et al., 1987).

The wound, which can be considered as an extra organ, contributes to the glucose-cycling (Wilmore, 1986). Lactate, produced by anaerobic glycolysis in the wound, is transported to the liver where it is converted to glucose (via the Cori cycle) which is then returned to fuel the wound. The wound will also contribute to the increase in metabolic rate in a number of other ways. It has a hyperaemic circulation, which is not under neural control, and will require an increase in cardiac output incurring extra energy expenditure by the heart. The inflammatory cells localised in the wound are themselves metabolically very active and will release a number of cytokines which have been implicated in the generation of fever via a prostaglandin-mediated upward resetting of hypothalamic set point (Rothwell, 1989).

Response in the elderly

Aging has always been associated with a reduction in resting metabolic expenditure, a change attributed to a loss of lean body mass (Durnin, 1959; Rudman, 1985). Recently it has been shown that predictive formulae (for example the Harris and Benedict equations) markedly underestimate metabolic rate in the elderly and that the reduction in metabolic rate with age is not as great as previously supposed (Owen, 1988). This author emphasised that although skeletal muscle may represent as much as 35–40% of total body weight it is responsible for only 20% of resting energy expenditure whereas brain and liver which together represent less than 5% of body weight throughout life are responsible for 40% of total energy expenditure. The better maintenance of metabolic rate with increasing age may be the result of improvements in the lifestyle of the elderly such that the negative influences of restricted calorie intake and inactivity on energy expenditure are now less marked.

Although the influence of a reduction in skeletal muscle mass on resting energy expenditure may be small its effects on shivering thermogenesis, which is reduced in the elderly on exposure to cold (Krag & Kountz, 1950), may be of greater significance. This reduction in skeletal muscle mass may be associated with the lower increases in metabolic demands (oxygen consumption) associated with postoperative shivering in the elderly compared with younger patients (Frank *et al.*, 1995). Other aspects of thermoregulation are also impaired in the elderly; for example they have a reduced ability to discriminate differences in environmental temperature and to select thermal comfort (Collins *et al.*, 1981). The control of heat loss is also impaired (Collins *et al.*, 1977) and the reduction in heat production due to an impairment of shivering may be exacerbated by pre-existing protein malnutrition. Elderly undernourished patients, compared with normally nourished aged controls, have a reduced increase in metabolic rate on cold exposure and this is associated with a fall, rather than the expected rise, in plasma catecholamine concentrations (Fellows *et al.*, 1985). Aged animals have been shown to have reduced pyrogenic and thermogenic responses to, for example, endotoxin (Chapter 8) and also a reduced thermogenic response to a nutrient load (Thorne & Wahren, 1990). In the latter clinical study, a reduced response in the elderly was tentatively ascribed to a reduced oxidative capacity in skeletal muscle. Thus it seems likely that the effects of the inhibition of thermoregulation elicited acutely by injury would be exaggerated in the elderly who have a pre-existing impairment of thermoregulation, but little data are available to test this hypothesis. One study of the responses of elderly men to elective surgery suggests that they experience greater disturbances in thermal balance and pulmonary gas exchange than their younger counterparts (Renck, 1969). It has been suggested that the impairment in lower body thermoregulatory activity induced by epidural anaesthesia may be more marked in the elderly (Frank *et al.*, 1994).

The ability to mount a prolonged flow phase increase in metabolic rate may also be reduced in the elderly, although the magnitude of the hypermetabolic responses on days 2 or 3 after severe injury are similar in elderly and young patients (Jeevanandam *et al.*, 1990a). Such an increase in metabolic rate is dependent on concomitant increases in cardiac output and oxygen transport; however, the myocardium of the elderly becomes infiltrated with collagen and they are less able to maintain an increase in cardiac output (Weisfeldt *et al.*, 1971; Rothbaum *et al.*, 1974). Also pulmonary function is limited in the elderly by a reduction in compliance of the rib cage, loss of muscle from the diaphragm and an impairment of gas exchange in the lungs, reflected in a reduction in arterial oxygen tension (Klocke, 1977; Mahler *et al.*, 1986; Blom *et al.*, 1988). A failure to achieve the sustained increase in tissue oxygen delivery needed to fuel the hypermetabolic flow phase may be one of the reasons why the elderly are so vulnerable to the effects of injury.

Fat metabolism

The increased activity of the sympathetic nervous system acutely after injury leads to the mobilisation of energy substrates as part of the fight or flight response.

Plasma concentrations of NEFAs and glycerol are raised acutely after injury reflecting this mobilisation of triacylglycerol stores in adipose tissue. The relation with severity is complex, for example plasma NEFA concentrations are lower after severe than after moderate injuries. This may be related to either metabolic (e.g. stimulation of re-esterification within adipose tissue by the raised lactate levels associated with severe injuries) or circulatory (e.g. poor perfusion of fat depots) factors.

This pattern of fuel mobilisation does not seem to be modified by the site of injury but the age and sex of the patient may influence the changes seen. For example, for a given severity of injury there is a suggestion that the plasma concentrations of lipid metabolites (NEFA, glycerol and ketone bodies) are higher in elderly patients. This may be explained by the preponderance in this age group of females who exhibit greater lipolysis than men after surgical trauma (for a review see Horan *et al.*, 1988). These findings must, however, be interpreted in the light of the finding of increased 'resting' triacylglycerol and NEFA concentrations in the elderly (Greenfield *et al.*, 1980).

Studies in aged rodents have shown a reduced lipolytic response to injury which was attributed to a reduced responsiveness to catecholamines (Hrůza & Jelínková, 1963; Hrůza *et al.*, 1965). This is consistent with *in vitro* studies showing a reduction with age in β-adrenergic receptors in adipose tissue (Roth, 1979) although *in vivo* studies have failed to show a difference between old and younger people in the increase in NEFA caused by noradrenaline infusion (Eisdorfer *et al.*, 1965).

During the flow phase plasma NEFA concentrations fall as the sympathetic drive to lipolysis wanes although after major injuries such as severe burns they may remain high (Batstone *et al.*, 1976; Frayn *et al.*, 1984). Fatty acid oxidation is, however, greater than expected from the plasma NEFA concentration (Birkhahn *et al.*, 1981; Frayn *et al.*, 1984). Turnover which is normally directly proportional to concentration is also disproportionately increased (Nordenström *et al.*, 1983) although there is no clear relation between NEFA turnover and oxidation. The turnover of endogenous and of infused triacylglycerol is also enhanced in the hypermetabolic state (Wilmore *et al.*, 1973; Nordenström *et al.*, 1983; Wolfe *et al.*, 1985). Injury causes similar changes in the relation between the turnover and plasma concentration of glycerol. Thus in patients with burns glycerol turnover is increased in relation to its concentration and also to the turnover of NEFAs implying increased re-esterification within adipose tissue (Wolfe *et al.*, 1987). In the fasted uninjured subject fat oxidation is suppressed by insulin released by the intravenous administration of large amounts of glucose, a response that is preserved in the aged (Davidson, 1979). In hypermetabolic patients this suppression is incomplete and fat oxidation continues (for a review see Barton *et al.*, 1990). The contributions of fat oxidation and NEFA/triacylglycerol cycling to total energy expenditure in the hypermetabolic flow phase have recently been shown to be less in the elderly than in younger injured patients (Jeevanandam *et al.*, 1990a).

Carbohydrate metabolism

In addition to the effects on lipolysis the increased activity of the sympathetic nervous system acutely after injury also stimulates glycogenolysis. The main stimulus for the breakdown of glycogen in both skeletal muscle and liver is adrenaline although glucagon and vasopressin may also have a role in the liver. This glycogenolysis leads to hyperglycaemia either directly due to liberation of glucose from the liver or indirectly, via the Cori cycle, from lactate released from skeletal muscle. The hyperglycaemia, which is directly related to the severity of injury (Stoner *et al.*, 1979), is potentiated after severe injuries by the reduction of glucose utilisation in skeletal muscle following the inhibition of insulin secretion by raised adrenaline levels and by the development of intracellular insulin resistance. The mechanism of this early insulin resistance is unclear although both glucocorticoids and cytokines may be involved.

A similar acute hyperglycaemic response to accidental injury and elective surgery is found in the elderly, in fact after minor injuries the response is exaggerated (Horan *et al.*, 1988; Desai *et al.*, 1989).

The changes in carbohydrate metabolism in the 'ebb' phase can be interpreted as defensive. In addition to providing a fuel for fight or flight the hyperglycaemia may also play a role in the compensation of post-traumatic fluid loss both through the mobilisation of water associated with glycogen and through its osmotic effects. The decrease in glucose clearance associated with insulin resistance can also be considered protective in that it prevents the wasteful use of the mobilised glucose, which is an essential fuel for the brain and the wound, at a time when a supply of nutrients may be limited.

Hyperglycaemia and inappropriately high plasma insulin concentrations are features of the flow phase although an exception to this pattern may be seen after very severe injuries, such as burns, where the prolonged rise in plasma catecholamine concentrations maintains adrenergic suppression of insulin secretion. There is also an exaggerated pancreatic insulin response to glucose which may be related to the increased plasma concentration of arginine, an insulin secretagogue (Fajans et al., 1967; Frayn et al., 1984). The concomitant elevations of plasma glucose and plasma insulin concentration are the hallmarks of insulin resistance which involves both liver and muscle. Also hepatic glucose production is not inhibited as expected by hyper-glycaemia and hyperinsulinaemia during the flow phase.

There is an increase in glucose turnover at this time although because of the prevailing insulin resistance the peripheral utilisation of glucose is less than expected from the raised glucose and insulin concentrations (for a review see Barton et al., 1990). This impairment of glucose disposal has been demonstrated using glucose/insulin clamp techniques after thermal and non-thermal injuries and also in septic surgical patients (Black et al., 1982; Brooks et al., 1984; White et al., 1987; Henderson et al., 1991). As expected part of insulin resistance is found in uninjured skeletal muscle. The relation between glucose uptake and plasma insulin concentration shows a marked reduction in both the maximum response and sensitivity to insulin (Henderson et al., 1991) suggesting changes in both receptor binding of insulin and intracellular path-ways (Kahn, 1978).

Aging itself causes marked changes in carbohydrate metabolism but little is known of the interaction with the response to injury (Watters et al., 1994). An impairment of peripheral glucose uptake is associated with aging (Davidson, 1979; Fink, et al., 1983; Watters et al., 1994). This does not seem to be due to the loss of muscle mass and although immobility and an impairment of insulin secretion may play a part the major factor seems to be a reduction in peripheral tissue sensitivity to insulin (Jackson et al., 1982; Pagano et al., 1984; Fukagawa et al., 1988; Watters et al., 1994). This decrease in sensitivity does not involve loss of insulin receptors but may be a result of a decrease in membrane glucose transporters (Fink et al., 1986). Notwithstanding this aging-related reduction in whole body glucose disposal a further reduction has been reported 2–5 days after accidental injury (Injury Severity Score; (ISS) 17–30) in the elderly (Watters et al., 1994). One other study of elderly patients following accidental injury has suggested that post-traumatic insulin resistance may last for longer in the aged than in younger patients (Frayn et al., 1983). This may be a result of the persistent elevation of plasma cortisol concentrations which is a feature of the response to injury in the elderly (see Chapter 16).

An important role has been suggested for cortisol and the other counterregulatory hormones (e.g. glucagon, adrenaline, and growth hormone) in the pathogenesis of insulin resistance. The plasma concentrations of all these hormones are elevated at some time during the response to injury (Barton, 1987). Infusions of glucagon, adren-aline and cortisol over a 3 day period mimic some of the features of the flow phase: peripheral insulin resistance and increases in metabolic rate and urinary nitrogen excretion (Gelfand *et al.*, 1984; Bessey *et al.*, 1984). The plasma concentrations of these hormones needed to elicit this pattern of response are closer to those found in the acute 'ebb' phase rather than in the 'flow' phase when the endogenous levels of these hormones are falling, except after the most severe injuries, to or close to normal (Frayn, 1986). The suggestion is that other humoral factors may have a role and the cytokines are likely candidates. They are able to reproduce by central and peripheral mechanisms many of the acute and flow phase responses to injury such as acute phase protein synthesis (Gauldie *et al.*, 1987), central resetting of metabolic activity (Dinarello, 1984), muscle protein catabolism (Clowes *et al.*, 1983) and glucose homoeostasis (Del Rey & Besedovsky, 1987; Tredget *et al.*, 1988). Although it is perhaps an oversimplification to assume that any single cytokine is predominant they may, by acting collectively in a coordinated way, both locally and systemically, be very important.

Protein metabolism

Although the major changes in protein metabolism following injury are associated with the 'flow' phase the acute phase plasma protein response (Fleck, 1988) is initiated during the 'ebb' phase. A number of plasma proteins increase in concentration (e.g. C-reactive protein (CRP) and fibrinogen) although there is always a lag of approximately 6 hours before changes are seen. The cytokine interleukin 6 (IL-6) released from activated macrophages, etc. after injury may be responsible for inducing the hepatic synthesis of such acute phase proteins (Gauldie *et al.*, 1987). After surgery it has been shown that the rise in IL-6 precedes that of CRP and a weak but significant positive correlation has been demonstrated between their serum levels (Cruickshank *et al.*, 1990). Such a delay or lag is not seen for the proteins that show an acute phase decrease in concentration after injury. The rapid fall in, for example, albumin concentration cannot be attributed to a reduction in its rate of synthesis but is due to changes in its distribution between intra- and extravascular compartments secondary to an increase in microvascular permeability (Fleck *et al.*, 1985; Fleck, 1988). No data are available for the acute phase response to injury in elderly patients although the CRP response to the stress of an infection is preserved (Kenny *et al.*, 1984).

The increased urinary output of nitrogen and the muscle wasting observed by Cuthbertson (1930) during the 'flow' phase led to the suggestion that an increased rate of amino acid oxidation was largely responsible for fuelling the hypermetabolism at this time. It now seems that the contribution of protein oxidation is not as great as previously assumed, representing no more than 20% of whole body expenditure in the severely catabolic patient (Duke *et al.*, 1970). An exception may be after head injuries where, even in the absence of steroid treatment, the contribution of protein oxidation is as high as 30% (Hadfield & Little, 1992).

Whole body protein turnover is increased after injury with the balance between synthesis and breakdown being modified by the severity of injury and the influence of nutritional intake on synthesis (Clague *et al.*, 1983). Thus increasing severities of injury cause increasing rates of both synthesis and breakdown while undernutrition reduces synthesis. After the most severe injuries, however, the increase in breakdown predominates and cannot be countered by even the most aggressive nutritional support (Streat *et al.*, 1987).

The most obvious site of the net increase in protein breakdown is skeletal muscle although it is likely that, just as in starvation, muscle in the diaphragm, the wall of the gut and the heart is also affected. The breakdown of myofibrillar protein is reflected by the increase in urinary excretion of 3–methylhistidine which is directly related to the amount of damaged muscle rather than to ISS (Threlfall *et al.*, 1981). However the use of 3–methylhistidine as a specific marker of skeletal muscle breakdown is complicated by its liberation from other organs such as the gut (Rennie & Millward, 1983). The increase in urinary creatine after injury is, however, directly related to ISS although much of the creatine comes from muscle distant from the site of injury emphasising the general nature of the catabolic flow phase (Threlfall *et al.*, 1984).

Once again little is known of the effects of aging on these responses although Stableforth (1986) concluded from a study of nitrogen balance in elderly female patients with fractures of the femoral neck that age *per se* did not affect the response. This finding is supported by a recent study of protein and energy balance, again following femoral neck fracture, which also suggested that the anabolic response (assessed from whole body leucine kinetics) to parenteral feeding was unaltered in the injured elderly (Nelson *et al.*, 1995). It has been suggested that the decrease in protein turnover associated with aging will reduce the net nitrogen loss after injury (Clague *et al.*, 1983); however, the response to injury will be complicated by the concomitant immobility which increases protein breakdown and turnover in the elderly (Lehmann *et al.*, 1989). The elevated plasma cortisol levels associated with immobility (but see Chapter 16) may be partly responsible for the higher rates of protein turnover noted in this study. Urinary nitrogen excretion represents the balance between the rates of protein breakdown and synthesis in different organs. The relative contributions of such organs changes with age, for example, skeletal muscle which accounts for approximately 30% of whole body protein turnover in young men contributes only 20% in elderly men. Visceral organs, on the other hand, make a greater contribution as age increases (Winterer *et al.*, 1976; Young, 1990).

As alluded to above, the increase in proteolysis provides amino acids as precursors for hepatic gluconeogenesis. Although the plasma levels of a number of amino acids, such as alanine, fall at this time, their hepatic extraction is increased because of increases in hepatic blood flow (for a review see Barton *et al.*, 1990). The increase in hepatic gluconeogenesis, at a time when plasma concentrations of glucose and insulin are increased, is one of the facets of insulin resistance discussed in Chapter 16. One amino acid of particular interest is glutamine, the intracellular concentration of which falls from its normally high levels after injury. The glutamine released from muscle is an important fuel for the lymphocytes and macrophages activated by injury. Also it has been implicated in the maintenance of the gut mucosa (O'Dwyer *et al.*, 1989), the integrity of which is compromised after injury. It is possible that the reduced contribution made by skeletal muscle to overall protein metabolism may limit this homoeostatic mobilisation of amino acids from peripheral sites and thereby impair the resistance of the elderly to injury (Young, 1990). There is little evidence to substantiate this suggestion although a recent study has shown that the reduction in plasma amino acid concentrations associated with severe trauma is less pronounced in the elderly (Jeevanandam *et al.*, 1990b).

References

Arturson, M. G. S. (1978). Metabolic changes following thermal injury. *World J Surg*, **2**, 203–14.

Aulick, L. H., Hander, E. H., Wilmore, D. W., Mason, A. D. & Pruitt, B. A. (1979). The relative significance of thermal and metabolic demands on burn hypermetabolism. *J Trauma*, **19**, 559–66.

Barton, R. N. (1987). The neuroendocrinology of physical injury. In *Clinical Endocrinology and Metabolism: Neuroendocrinology of Stress*, ed. A. Grossman, pp. 355–74. London: Baillière Tindall.

Barton, R. N., Frayn, K. N. & Little, R. A. (1990). Trauma, burns and surgery. In *The Metabolic and Molecular Basis of Acquired Disease*, 1st edn, vol. 1, ed. R. D. Cohen, B. Lewis, K. G. M. M. Alberti & A. M. Denman, pp. 684–717. London: Baillière Tindall.

Batstone, G. F., Alberti, K. G. M. M., Hinks, L., Smythe, P., Laing, J. E., Ward, C. M., Ely, D. W. & Bloom, S. R. (1976). Metabolic studies in subjects following thermal injury. Intermediary metabolites, hormones and tissue oxygenation. *Burns*, **2**, 207–25.

Bessey, P. Q., Watters, J. M., Aoki, T. T. & Wilmore, D. W. (1984). Combined hormonal infusion simulates the metabolic response to injury. *Ann Surg*, **200**, 264–80.

Birkhahn, R. H., Long, C. L., Fitkin, D. L., Busnardo, A. C., Geiger, J. W. & Blakemore, W. S. (1981). A comparison of the effects of skeletal trauma and surgery on the ketones of starvation in man. *J Trauma*, **21**, 513–18.

Black, P. R., Brooks, D. C., Bessey, P. Q., Wolfe, R. R. & Wilmore, D. W. (1982). Mechanisms of insulin resistance following injury. *Ann Surg*, **196**, 420–35.

Blom, H., Mulder, M. & Verweij, W. (1988). Arterial oxygen tension and saturation in hospital patients: effect of age and activity. *Br Med J*, **297**, 720–1.

Brooks, D. C., Bessey, P. Q., Black, P. R., Aoki, T. T. & Wilmore, D. W. (1984). Post-traumatic insulin resistance in uninjured forearm tissue. *J Surg Res*, **37**, 100–7.

Childs, C., Stoner, H. B., Little, R. A. & Davenport, P. J. (1989). A comparison of some thermoregulatory responses in healthy children and in children with burn injury. *Clin Sci*, **77**, 425–9.

Clague, M. B., Keir, M. J., Wright, P. D. & Johnston, I. D. A. (1983). The effects of nutrition and trauma on whole-body protein metabolism in man. *Clin Sci*, **65**, 165–75.

Clowes, G. H. A., George, B. C., Villee, C. A. & Saravis, C. A. (1983). Muscle proteolysis induced by a circulating peptide in patients with sepsis or trauma. *New Engl J Med*, **308**, 545–52.

Collins, K. J., Dore, C., Exton-Smith, A. M., Fox, R. H. MacDonald, I. C. & Woodward, P. M. (1977). Accidental hypothermia and impaired temperature homeostasis in the elderly. *Br Med J*, **1**, 353–6.

Collins, K. J., Exton-Smith, A. M. & Dore, C. (1981). Urban hypothermia: preferred temperature and thermal perceptions in old age. *Br Med J*, **1**, 175–7.

Cournand, A., Riley, R. L., Bradley, S. E., Breed, E. S., Noble, R. P., Lauson, H. D., Gregersen, M. I. & Richards, D. W. (1943). Studies of the circulation in clinical shock. *Surgery*, **13**, 964–95.

Cruickshank, A. M., Fraser, W. D., Burns, H. J. G., VanDamme, J. & Shenkin, A. (1990). Responses to serum interleukin 6 in patients undergoing elective surgery of varying severity. *Clin Sci*, **79**, 161–5.

Cuthbertson, D. P. (1930). The disturbance of metabolism produced by bony and non-bony injury, with notes on certain abnormal conditions of bone. *Biochem J*, **24**, 1244–63.

Cuthbertson, D. P. (1942). Post-shock metabolic response. *Lancet*, **1**, 433–7.

Cuthbertson, D. P. (1980a). Alterations in metabolism following injury: part 1. *Injury*, **11**, 175–89.

Cuthbertson, D. P. (1980b). Alterations in metabolism following injury: part II. *Injury*, **11**, 286–303.

Davidson, M. B. (1979). The effect of ageing on carbohydrate metabolism: a review of the English literature and a practical approach to the diagnosis of diabetes mellitus in the elderly. *Metabolism*, **28**, 688–705.

Davies, J. W. L. (1982). *Physiological Responses to Burning Injury*. New York: Academic Press.

Del Ray, A. & Besedovsky, H. (1987). Interleukin 1 affects glucose homeostasis. *Am J Physiol*, **253**, R794–R798.

Desai, D., March, R. & Watters, J. M. (1989). Hyperglycemia after trauma increases with age. *J Trauma*, **29**, 719–23.

Dinarello, C. A. (1984). Interleukin 1. *Rev Infect Dis*, **6**, 51–95.

Duke, J. H., Jorgensen, S. B., Broell, J. R., Long, C. L. & Kinney, J. M. (1970). Contribution of protein to caloric expenditure following injury. *Surgery*, **68**, 168–74.

Durnin, J. V. G. A. (1959). The use of surface area and of body weight as standards of reference in studies on human energy expenditure. *Br J Nutr*, **13**, 68–71.

Edwards, J. D. (1990). Acute circulatory failure – shock. *Care Crit Ill*, **6**, 59–61.

Edwards, J. D., Redmond, A. D., Nightingale, P. & Wilkins, R. G. (1988). Oxygen consumption following trauma: a reappraisal in severely injured patients requiring mechanical ventilation. *Br J Surg*, **75**, 690–2.

Eisdorfer, C., Powell, A. H., Silverman, G. & Bogdonoff, M. D. (1965). The characteristics of lipid mobilization and peripheral disposition in aged individuals. *J Gerontol*, **20**, 511–14.

Fajans, S. S., Floyd, J. C., Knopf, R. F. & Conn, J. W. (1967). Effect of amino acids and proteins on insulin secretion in man. *Recent Progr Hormone Res*, **23**, 617–62.

Fellows, I. W., Macdonald, I. A., Bennett, T. A. & Allison, S. P. (1985). The effect of undernutrition on thermoregulation in the elderly. *Clin Sci*, **69**, 525–32.

Fink, R. I., Kolterman, O. G., Griffin, J. & Olefsky, J. M. (1983). Mechanisms of insulin resistance in ageing. *J Clin Invest*, **71**, 1523–35.

Fink, R. I., Wallace, P. & Olefsky, J. M. (1986). Effects of aging on glucose-mediated diposal and glucose transport. *J Clin Invest*, **76**, 149–55.

Fleck, A. (1988). Nutrition, protein metabolism and fluid balance. In *Bailliere's Clinical Anaesthesiology – Fluid Resuscitation* 2, ed. W. J. Kox & J. Gamble, pp. 625–48. London: Baillière Tindall.

Fleck, A., Colley, C. M. & Myers, M. A. (1985). Liver export proteins and trauma. *Br Med Bull*, **41**, 265–73.

Frank, S. M., Fleisher, L. A., Olson, K. F., Gorman, R. B., Higgins, M. S., Breslow, M. J., Sitzmann, J. V. & Beattie, C. (1995). Multivariate determinants of early postoperative oxygen consumption in elderly patients: Effects of shivering, body temperature, and gender. *Anesthesiology*, **83**, 241–9.

Frank, S. M., Shir, Y., Raja, S. N., Fleisher, L. A. & Beattie, C. (1994). Core hypothermia and skin-surface temperature gradients. Epidural versus general anesthesia and the effects of age. *Anesthesiology*, **80**, 502–8.

Frayn, K. N. (1986). Hormonal control of metabolism in trauma and sepsis. *Clin Endocrinol*, **24**, 577–99.

Frayn, K. N., Little, R. A., Stoner, H. B. & Galasko, C. S. B. (1984). Metabolic control in non-septic patients with musculoskeletal injuries. *Injury*, **16**, 73–9.

Frayn, K. N., Stoner, H. B., Barton, R. N., Heath, D. F. & Galasko, C. S. B. (1983). Persistence of high plasma glucose, insulin and cortisol concentrations in elderly patients with proximal femoral fractures. *Age Ageing*, **12**, 70–6.

Fukagawa, N. K., Minaker, K. L., Rowe, J. W., Matthews, D. E., Bier, D. M. & Young, V. R. (1988). Glucose and amino acid metabolism in aging men: differential effects of insulin. *Metabolism*, **37**, 371–7.

Gauldie, J., Richards, C., Harnish, D. *et al.* (1987). Interferon β_2/β-cell stimulating factor type 2 shares identity with monocyte-derived hepatocyte-stimulating factor and regulates the major acute plasma protein response in liver cells. *Proc Natl Acad Sci USA*, **84**, 7251–6.

Gelfand, R. A., Matthews, D. E., Bier, D. M. & Sherwin, R. S. (1984). Role of counterregulatory hormones in the catabolic response to stress. *J Clin Invest*, **74**, 2238–48.

Greenblatt, S. H., Long, C. L., Blakemore, W. S., Dennis, R. S., Rayport, M. & Geiger, J. W. (1989). Catabolic effect of dexamethasone in patients with major head injuries. *J Parent Ent Nutr*, **13**, 372–6.

Greenfield, M. S., Kraemer, F., Tobey, T. & Reaven, G. (1980). Effect of age on plasma triglyceride concentrations in man. *Metabolism*, **29**, 1095–9.

Hadfield, J. M. & Little, R. A. (1992). Substrate oxidation and the contribution of protein oxidation to energy expenditure after severe head injury. *Injury*, **23**, 183–6.

Hadfield, J. M., Little, R. A. & Jones, R. A. C. (1992). Measured energy expenditure and plasma substrate and hormonal changes following severe head injury. *Injury*, **23**, 177–82.

Henderson, A. A., Frayn, K. N., Galasko, C. S. B. & Little, R. A. (1991). Dose–response relationships for the effects of insulin on glucose and fat metabolism in injured patients and control subjects. *Clin Sci*, **80**, 25–32.

Horan, M. A., Barton, R. N. & Little, R. A. (1988). Ageing and the response to injury. In *Advanced Geriatric Medicine*, vol. 7, ed. J. Grimley Evans & F. I. Caird, pp. 101–35. London: Wright.

Hrůza, Z. & Jelínková, M. (1963). The metabolism of fat and proteins in trauma and adaptation to trauma in rats of different ages. *Gerontologia*, **8**, 36–45.

Hrůza, Z., Jelínková, M. & Hlaváčková, V. (1965). Metabolism following a turpentine abscess in old age. *Exp Gerontol*, **1**, 127–31.

Jackson, R. A., Blix, P. M., Matthews, J. A., Hamling, J. B., Din, B. M., Brown, D. C., Belin, J.,

Rubenstein, A. H. & Nabarro, J. D. N. (1982). Influence of ageing on glucose homeostasis. *J Clin Endocrinol Metab*, **55**, 840–8.

Jeevanandam, M., Young, D. H. & Schiller, W. R. (1990a). Energy cost of fat-fuel mobilization in geriatric trauma. *Metabolism*, **39**, 144–9.

Jeevanandam, M., Young, D. H., Ramias, L. & Schiller, W. R. (1990b). Effect of major trauma on plasma free amino acid concentrations in geriatric patients. *Am J Clin Nutri*, **51**, 1040–5.

Kahn, C. R. (1978). Insulin resistance, insulin insensitivity, and insulin unresponsiveness: a necessary distinction. *Metabolism*, **27** (Suppl 2), 1893–902.

Kenny, R. A., Hodkinson, H. M., Cox, M. L., Caspi, D. & Pepys, M. B. (1984). Acute phase protein response to infection in elderly patients. *Age Ageing*, **13**, 89–94.

Klocke, R. A. (1977). In *Handbook of the Biology of Aging*, ed. C. E. Finch & L. Hayflick, pp. 432–44. New York: Van Nostrand Reinhold.

Krag, C. L. & Kountz, W. B. (1950). Studies of body function in the aged. 1. Effect of exposure of the body to cold. *J Gerontol*, **5**, 227–35.

Lamke, L.-O., Nilsson, G. E. & Reithner, H. L. (1977). The evaporative water loss from burns and the water vapour permeability of grafts and artificial membranes used in the treatment of burns. *Burns*, **3**, 159–65.

Lehmann, A. B., Johnston, D. & James, O. F. W. (1989). The effects of old age and immobility on protein turnover in human subject with some observations on the possible role of hormones. *Age Ageing*, **18**, 148–57.

Little, R. A. & Stoner, H. B. (1981). Body temperature after accidental injury. *Br J Surg*, **68**, 221–4.

Little, R. A., Stoner, H. B., Randall, P. & Carlson, G. (1986). An effect of injury on thermoregulation in man. *Q J Exp Physiol*, **71**, 295–306.

Mahler, D. A., Rosiello, R. A. & Loke, J. (1986). The ageing lung. *Clin Geriatr Med*, **2**, 215–25.

Nelson, K. M., Richards, E. W., Long, C. L., Martin, K. R., Geiger, J. W., Brooks, S. W., Gandy, R. E. & Blackemore, W. S. (1995). Protein and energy balance following femoral neck fracture in geriatric patients. *Metabolism*, **44**, 59–66.

Nordenström, J., Carpentier, Y. A., Askanazi, J., Robin, A. P., Elwyn, D. H., Hensle, T. W. & Kinney, J. M. (1983). Free fatty acid mobilisation and oxidation during total parenteral nutrition in trauma and infection. *Ann Surg*, **198**, 725–35.

O'Dwyer, S. T., Smith, R. J., Hwang, T. L. & Wilmore, D. W. (1989). Maintenance of small bowel mucosa with glutamine-enriched parenteral nutrition. *J Parent Ent Nutr*, **13**, 579–85.

Owen, O. E. (1988). Resting metabolic requirements of men and women. *Mayo Clin Proc*, **63**, 503–10.

Pagano, G., Cassader, M., Cavallo-Perin, P., Bruno, A., Masciola, P., Ozzello, A., Dall'Ormo, A. M. & Foco, A. (1984). Insulin resistance in the aged: a quantitative evaluation of *in vivo* sensitivity and *in vitro* glucose transport. *Metabolism*, **33**, 976–81.

Regan, C. J., Duckworth, R., Fairhurst, J. A., Maycock, P. F., Frayn, K. N. & Campbell, I. T. (1990). Metabolic effects of low-dose dopamine infusion in normal volunteers. *Clin Sci*, **79**, 605–11.

Renck, H. (1969). The elderly patient after anaesthesia and surgery. *Acta Anaesthesiol Scand*, Suppl. **34**.

Rennie, M. J. & Millward, D. J. (1983). 3–Methylhistidine excretion and the urinary 3–methylhistidine/creatinine ratio are poor indicators of skeletal muscle protein breakdown. *Clin Sci*, **65**, 217–25.

Roth, G. S. (1979). Hormone receptor changes during adulthood and senescence: significance for aging research. *Fed Proc*, **38**, 1910–14.

Rothbaum, D. A., Shaw, D. J., Angell, C. S. & Shock, N. W. (1974). Age difference in the baroreceptor response of rats. *J Gerontol*, **29**, 488–92.

Rothwell, N. J. (1989). CRF is involved in the pyrogenic and thermogenic effects of interleukin 1β in the rat. *Am J Physiol*, **256**, (*Endocrinol Metab*, **19**), E111–E115.

Rudman, D. (1985). Growth hormone, body composition and ageing. *J Am Geriatr Soc*, **33**, 800–7.

Stableforth, P. G. (1986). Supplement feeds and nitrogen and caloric balance following femoral neck fracture. *Br J Surg* , **73**, 651–5.

Stoner, H. B. (1961). Critical analysis of traumatic shock models. *Fed Proc*, **20** (Suppl 9), 38–48.

Stoner, H. B. (1971). Effect of injury on shivering thermogenesis in the rat. *J Physiol*, **214**, 599–615.

Stoner, H. B. (1972). Effect of injury on the responses to thermal stimulation of the hypothalamus. *J Appl Physiol*, **33**, 665–71.

Stoner, H. B. (1974). Inhibition of thermoregulatory non-shivering thermogenesis by trauma in cold acclimated rats. *J Physiol*, **238**, 657–70.

Stoner, H. B. (1993). Responses to trauma: fifty years of ebb and flow. *Circ Shock*, **39**, 316–19.

Stoner, H. B., Frayn, K. N., Barton, R. N., Threlfall, C. J. & Little, R. A. (1979). The relationships between plasma substrates and hormones and the severity of injury in 277 recently injured patients. *Clin Sci*, **56**, 563–73.

Streat, S. J., Beddoe, A. H. & Hill, G. L. (1987). Aggressive nutritional support does not prevent protein loss despite fat gain in septic intensive care patients. *J Trauma*, **27**, 262–6.

Thorne, A. & Wahren, J. (1990). Diminished meal-induced thermogenesis in elderly man. *Clin Physiol*, **10**, 427–37.

Threlfall, C. J., Maxwell, A. R. & Stoner, H. B. (1984). Post-traumatic creatinuria. *J Trauma*, **24**, 516–23.

Threlfall, C. J., Stoner, H. B. & Galasko, C. S. B. (1981). Patterns in the excretion of muscle markers after trauma and orthopaedic surgery. *J Trauma*, **21**, 140–7.

Tredget, E. E., Yu, Y. M., Zhong, S., Burini, R., Okusawa, S., Gelfand, J. A., Dinarello, C. A., Young, V. R. & Burke, J. F. (1988). Role of interleukin and tumor necrosis factor on energy metabolism in rabbits. *Am J Physiol*, **255**, E760–E768.

Watters, J. M., Moulton, S. B., Clancey, S. M., Blakslee, J. M. & Monaghan, M. (1994). Aging exaggerates glucose intolerance following injury. *J Trauma*, **37**, 786–91.

Weisfeldt, M. L., Loeven, W. A. & Shock, N. W. (1971). Resting and active mechanical properties of trabeculae carneae from aged male rats. *Am J Physiol*, **220**, 1921–7.

White, R. H., Frayn, K. N., Little, R. A., Threlfall, C. J., Stoner, H. B. & Irving, M. H. (1987). Hormonal and metabolic responses to glucose infusion in sepsis studied by the hyperglycemic glucose-clamp technique. *J Parent Ent Nutr*, **11**, 345–53.

Wilmore, D. W. (1977). *The Metabolic Management of the Critically Ill*. New York: Plenum Press.

Wilmore, D. W. (1986). The wound as an organ. In *The Scientific Basis for the Care of the Critically Ill*, ed. R. A. Little & K. N. Frayn, pp. 45–59. Manchester: Manchester University Press.

Wilmore, D. W., Long, J. M., Mason, A. D., Skreen, R. W. & Pruitt, B. A. (1974). Catecholamines: mediator of the hypermetabolic response to thermal injury. *Ann Surg*, **180**, 653–68.

Wilmore, D. W., Moylan, J. A., Helmkamp, G. M. & Pruitt, B. A. (1973). Clinical evaluation of

10% intravenous fat emulsion for parenteral nutrition in thermally injured patients. *Ann Surg*, **178**, 503–12.

Winterer, J., Steffee, W. P., Perera, W. D. A., Uauy, R., Scrimshaw, N. S. & Young, V. R. (1976). Whole body protein turnover in aging man. *Exp Gerontol*, **11**, 79–87.

Wolfe, R. R., Herndon, D. N., Jahoor, F., Miyoshi, H. & Wolfe, M. (1987). Effect of severe burn injury on substrate cycling by glucose and fatty acids. *New Engl J Med*, **317**, 403–8.

Wolfe, R. R., Shaw, J. H. F. & Durkot, M. J. (1985). Effect of sepsis on VLDL kinetics: responses in basal state and during glucose infusion. *Am J Physiol*, **248**, E732–E740.

Young, V. R. (1990). Protein and amino acid metabolism with reference to aging and the elderly. *Prog Clin Biol Res* (*New York*), **326**, 279–300.

15

Water and electrolyte metabolism

P. A. O'NEILL

This is why we grow old, some at one age, others at another, sooner or later, because we either are from the beginning by nature excessively dry, or become so either from circumstances, or diet, or disease, or worry, or some such cause. *Galen*

Introduction

Galen in his treatise on hygiene expounded a common theory of ageing in antiquity which equated the wrinkling of the skin to a progressive dehydration. More importantly, he recognised the influence of external factors on these changes. In considering the effect of injury on water and electrolyte balance in elderly people, a reasonable starting point is to examine what is known about the changes in water and electrolyte homeostasis that occur with age, determining what additional effects the presence of disease might have. This understanding can be used as a framework to consider the response to trauma and how it might or might not be influenced by the age of the victim.

In this context the practical management of the patient can be discussed using the relevant research and also highlighting areas where further work is needed.

Water homeostasis

General

The preservation of water balance is crucial to the survival of the organism. Intake is primarily controlled by learnt behaviour and social habit with increasing thirst being perceived once intake is insufficient to meet requirements. The internal 'sensing' system responds to changes in plasma osmolality by secretion of arginine vasopressin (AVP, antidiuretic hormone). The target organ of AVP is the kidney which reacts by excreting urine of increasing concentration and a high osmolality. Changes with age in all these systems have been investigated, together with their interrelationships. It should be appreciated that, as one might expect in an important biological system, water homeostasis does not depend solely on this simple mechanism and other hormone systems also influence water balance; these will be discussed where appropriate.

Thirst

Other than the widely held belief that thirst diminishes with age (Wolf, 1958; Hodkinson, 1980), the scientific evidence relies heavily on two studies (Phillips *et al.*, 1984; Crowe *et al.*, 1987). One study (Phillips *et al.*, 1984) studied seven normal men during 24 hours of dehydration. Thirst was reduced compared to the young controls, but interpretation of the results is difficult because of the presence of a sham infusion at the end of the period. The second study (Crowe *et al.*, 1987) examined changes in thirst following an oral water load, during which time the sensation gradually rose in the young but not the elderly male group.

In contrast we have reported that in a group of elderly health status defined subjects (Ligthart *et al.*, 1984) there were no differences in thirst perception during a hypertonic saline infusion compared to a young control group (McLean *et al.*, 1991a,b).

The majority of patients who have suffered trauma have pre-existing medical problems that may affect thirst, but there have not been any well conducted studies in the elderly with specific disease states. Mukherjee *et al.* (1973) reported that only one of six elderly patients complained of thirst when deprived of fluid for 54 hours. Little detail was provided as to their antecedent clinical conditions, although one had had a previous femoral neck fracture. Miller *et al.* (1982) studied six patients with hypodipsia who had had a stroke. In spite of severe hypernatraemia no attempts were made to drink readily accessible water and it was postulated that this was due to diffuse cerebrovascular disease.

From the above, there is no consensus on what changes occur in thirst in normal or pathological aging. Furthermore, there are other factors which may influence the perception of thirst in the period following trauma, including electrolyte (particularly sodium) disturbance, neuroendocrine responses, volume changes in the vascular, extracellular and intracellular spaces, and oropharyngeal sensation, none of which has been adequately studied.

Arginine vasopressin

In contrast to most homeostatic functions, it has been reported that the osmoreceptor sensitivity is increased with advancing age. This conclusion was drawn from the work of Helderman *et al.* (1978) who studied a group of subjects with a mean age of only 59 years. These results were confirmed in a much older group by Bevilacqua *et al.* (1987), but detailed data were not presented. In our own work, using carefully screened elderly individuals, we found that the relation of plasma osmolality to arginine vasopressin was curvilinear with a reduced responsiveness with increasing age (McLean *et al.*, 1991a). These results were supported by the study of Li *et al.* (1984) into the response to dehydration, but the methodology they used was flawed. The evidence is patchy for neurohypophyseal dysfunction in disease states. Acutely ill elderly people who were dehydrated had a clear preservation of neurohypophyseal responsiveness (Kirkland *et al.*, 1984). In Alzheimer's disease (Albert *et al.*, 1989) the response was impaired following overnight dehydration.

Renal changes

It is widely accepted that glomerular filtration rate decreases with increasing age (Davies & Shock, 1950), although there is also an increasing variance in the magnitude of the change observed (Rowe *et al.*, 1976a).

Glomerular filtration rate and creatinine clearance are used as general indicators of renal function. It is of equal importance to determine how the specific mechanisms present in the glomerulotubular unit and its associated vascular supply vary with age. Sodium handling alters, with a decreased capacity to excrete a sodium load either with or without volume expansion (Yamada *et al.*, 1979; Myers *et al.*, 1982), although this view was contradicted by the study of Karlberg & Tolagen (1977). At the opposite extreme, under conditions of sodium restriction, the elderly population excreted a higher percentage of the filtered load compared with young controls (Macias Nuñez *et al.*, 1987).

Similarly for potassium, there was a significant reduction in the renal excretion of the cation in the elderly (Kirkland *et al.*, 1983), but if this was corrected according to the reduction in glomerular mass, the fraction excreted was elevated (Macias Nuñez *et al.*, 1987), indicating a greater elimination per nephron.

There is a decrease in the renal concentrating mechanism with age (Dontas *et al.*, 1972), which has been linked to the reduction in the glomerular filtration rate, causing an osmotic diuresis at the remaining glomeruli (Kleeman, 1972). This is not supported by all the available data (Rowe *et al.*, 1976a, Ledingham *et al.*, 1987). The response to a water load also alters (McLean *et al.*, 1991b) with a diminution in the maximum diluting capacity of the kidney and Crowe *et al.* (1987) also reported a delayed excretion of a water load.

Water compartmentation

In aging there are changes in total body water and also in the intracellular and extracellular compartments. Shock *et al.* (1963) demonstrated significant decreases in total body water and intracellular volume, which were confirmed by Lesser &

Markotsky (1979), although a more recent longitudinal study by Steen *et al.* (1985) reported that the decline in total body water was more closely related to a decrease in extracellular water. The consequences of these changes leave an elderly person with a reduced homeostatic capacity to cope with any stresses such as restriction of fluid input or an increase in losses.

General effects of pathology

The above short review has concentrated on the changes that are found with normal aging. As the reader is probably aware there are great difficulties in the semantics of the description 'normal'. Most elderly people are not examples of the 'successful aging' described by Rowe & Kahn (1987), but lie somewhere in the continuum from 'usual aging' through to the presence of single or multiple pathological states. In the case of the injured person, it has already been discussed (Chapter 2) that they most likely belong to the 'frail elderly' (Woodhouse *et al.*, 1988) with covert or overt pathological processes.

Sodium

Elderly people in hospital have a high incidence of sodium, potassium and water abnormalities. It has been reported that 11% of acutely ill elderly patients and 22% of those living in institutions have a plasma sodium of less than 130 mEq/l, which is a greater incidence than that found in general hospitalised populations (Kleinfeld *et al.*, 1979; Sunderam & Mankikar, 1983; Mahowald & Himmelstein, 1981). Both hyper- and hyponatraemia are associated with a high morbidity and mortality (Arieff & Guisado, 1976; Bhatnagar & Weinkove, 1988). The aetiologies of disorders of sodium balance are numerous and the reader is advised to consult a more general textbook for a full description. Following injury, particularly fractured neck of femur in an elderly population, there are no accurate data on the prevalence of electrolyte abnormalities; most authors have general statements such as a 'common finding' or a 'high prevalence'.

Potassium

A similar account can be given for disorders of potassium homeostasis. It is known that total body potassium falls with age (Lye, 1981), and that hypo- and hyperkalaemia increase in incidence with age (Lye, 1985). Following injury, even though it is known that the neurohumoral changes would influence potassium homeostasis, there are no studies which have quantified the scale of the problem in old people.

Water

Plasma osmolality (pOsm) is the most direct measure of water homeostasis. We have shown that the mean pOsm and variance increased with advancing years in subjects living in the community (McLean *et al.*, 1992), and there was a high prevalence of hyperosmolar states in both acutely ill elderly subjects (McLean *et al.*, 1990) and also those residing in continuing care (O'Neill *et al.*, 1990) with an associated high mortality. There have been no surveys of disorders of water homeostasis following injury or surgery in elderly people, including the prevalence of volume overload or depletion.

Neurohumoral response to injury

This section is confined to a description of those hormonal changes that may impinge on electrolyte and water homeostasis (see Fig. 15.1); fuller accounts of humoral responses are given elsewhere (Chapter 16).

Plasma increases are observed in several hormones, but the effect of these should be interpreted in the light of possible changes in degradation and clearance together with alterations in target organ responsiveness (Davis, 1979).

Arginine vasopressin

AVP is the hormone most closely related to water homeostasis. There have not been any studies examining the change in AVP following accidental physical trauma and, in particular, relating it to the magnitude of the injury using the Trauma or Injury Severity Score (Champion *et al.*, 1981) or physiological disturbance using the APACHE system (Knaus *et al.*, 1985).

It is known that, using elective surgery as a model of trauma, AVP rises rapidly following operation and returns to normal over the next 72 hours (Moran *et al.*, 1964; Haas & Glick, 1978); for cholecystectomy baseline values were reached within 24 hours (Cochrane *et al.*, 1981). The time course of the response is consistent with AVP being a major neurohumoral component of the ebb phase (Cuthbertson *et al.*, 1939), if this can be regarded as a distinct period (Chapter 14). The major influences on the magnitude of the response are probably nociceptive afferent fibres (Le Quesne *et al.*, 1985), although the type of anaesthetic employed may also modulate the response (Philbin, 1983). In addition, changes in blood volume may also influence the vasopressin levels attained (Le Quesne *et al.*, 1985), as may plasma osmolality. The reaction to a fall in blood volume is considered below.

There have been only a few reported studies concerning particular forms of injury. Patients with burns have a very high level of AVP in the immediate aftermath, particularly if severe (Hauben *et al.*, 1980; Morgan *et al.*, 1980), and persistent hormone concentrations have been found for several weeks even with a low plasma sodium (Shirani *et al.*, 1983).

After head injury a syndrome of inappropriate secretion of AVP may occur in up to 10% (Doczi *et al.*, 1982; Born *et al.*, 1985), but although these studies included large numbers of subjects, interpretation of the data is difficult as the 'inappropriate' secretion of the hormone was by inference as it was not actually measured. In animal studies of the syndrome, i.e. a moderately high urine osmolality in the face of a low plasma osmolality, a renal mechanism has been proposed rather than continued AVP secretion (Nelson *et al.*, 1984).

The possible consequences of the heightened AVP secretion immediately following trauma are considered below in terms of water, sodium and volume disturbance.

Adrenocorticotrophic hormone and cortisol

Other stress hormones may influence fluid and electrolyte balance. Adrenocorticotrophic hormone (ACTH) and cortisol increase following trauma and, as discussed

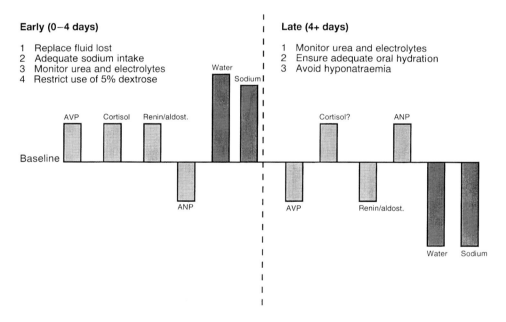

Figure 15.1. Schematic representation of the neurohumoral, sodium and water changes in the early and late stages following trauma. Aldost.: aldosterone; ANP: atrial natriuretic peptide; AVP: arginine vasopressin.

elsewhere, there is evidence of a prolonged response in elderly people (Frayn *et al.*, 1983). The pituitary adreno–cortical axis is important in water homeostasis in that cortisol has a permissive effect on water excretion and sodium retention whereby the presence of the hormone is required for it to take place (Ingle *et al.*, 1951).

The retention of sodium following trauma is not solely due to increased cortisol secretion as it still occurs in adrenalectomised patients (Forest *et al.*, 1957) on fixed doses of cortisol replacement, nor is it due to a reduction in cortisol degradation (Le Quesne, 1967). Furthermore, the retention of sodium persists for several days following abdominal surgery even though cortisol levels have returned to their preoperative levels (Le Quesne *et al.*, 1985).

Renin, angiotensin and aldosterone

The renin–angiotensin–aldosterone axis is one of the major systems for preserving sodium balance and it may also influence water homeostasis through stimulating thirst. In the elderly, basal plasma renin activity (PRA) is reduced but the response to tilt is preserved (Vargas *et al.*, 1986). There is, however, a decline in the renin response to sodium restriction (Crane & Harris, 1976) and diuretic administration (Nakamaru *et al.*, 1981), both of which may occur in the aftermath of injury and may predispose to electrolyte disturbance. The concentration of plasma renin substrate (Noth *et al.*, 1977) and inactive renin (Tsunoda *et al.*, 1986) does not decline with age.

In normal aging, Kala *et al.* (1974) and Skott *et al.* (1987) did not find any differences in angiotensin II levels despite lower PRA and aldosterone concentrations in the elderly groups. The absence of any demonstrable change may be due to a low sensitivity of the assay. Phillips *et al.* (1984) did not show any differences due to age in the angiotensin II response to prolonged dehydration, which may be of relevance in patients who are fluid restricted for any reason following trauma.

There are reductions in blood and urinary aldosterone levels with age, both under basal conditions and after salt restriction (Macias Nuñez *et al.*, 1987). In addition, the tubular response to administered aldosterone, shown from the reduction in sodium output, is reduced in the elderly (Macias Nuñez *et al.*, 1987). The implications of these observations are that an elderly person would have a reduced ability to preserve sodium when required, although other renal changes would influence the observed response.

Despite the apparent reduced aldosterone levels in old age, this hormone could be responsible for the sodium retention observed following surgery. The paper by Forest *et al.* (1957) referred to above is, however, against the hormone being a major factor, as is the continued sodium retention for several days despite the fall in aldosterone to preoperative levels within a few hours of surgery (Le Quesne *et al.*, 1985). It is known though that in the presence of hypovolaemia, aldosterone does promote a fall in urinary sodium excretion (Le Quesne *et al.*, 1985).

Atrial natriuretic peptide

Atrial natriuretic peptide (ANP) in physiological concentrations causes a natriuresis and a diuresis. The hormone level rises with age (Duggan *et al.*, 1991), but the effects of this may be mitigated by alterations at receptor and postreceptor sites (Duggan & O'Malley, 1990). During infusions of ANP, contradictory findings have been reported in the elderly (Heim *et al.*, 1989; Jansen *et al.*, 1990). There have been no studies, apart from burn injury, on the effect of trauma on ANP response and its interactions with age. Crum *et al.* (1988) reported that the admission levels of ANP decreased with increasing burn size. On day 4 the plasma concentrations then rose and remained elevated for several days, which coincided with the onset of a diuresis and natriuresis. It is difficult to intepret the subsequent rise in ANP and its relation to the initial trauma as the patients were resuscitated with hypertonic sodium lactate.

Water and electrolyte disturbance

Even allowing for the lack of epidemiological data on the scale of electrolyte, water and fluid volume abnormalities following trauma, generally it can be stated that there is an initial phase of water retention and a reduction in sodium excretion followed by natriuresis and a water diuresis. Gump *et al.* (1970) carried out detailed serial measurements of fluid and electrolyte balance in 20 trauma patients of varying severities and aetiologies. In the initial phase the positive water balance ranged from 3 to over 16 litres, reaching a maximum on the third day. The subsequent excretion of the retained water took up to 22 days in some patients. They observed a mild hyponatraemia during the study.

Water

The causes of the water retention are complex. At the time of trauma there may be significant blood loss which, even if only 5–10% of circulating blood volume, may promote the secretion of AVP by displacing to the left the threshold for its osmotic release and increasing the slope of the relationship (Robertson & Athar, 1976). If the trauma also causes a reduction in blood pressure of as little as 5% then this stimulates an AVP response (Robertson *et al.*, 1976), the magnitude of which is several times that produced by blood loss alone (Moran & Zimmermann, 1967). Rowe *et al.* (1982), however, demonstrated a reduced AVP response to standing in the elderly, which could point to a reduced hormonal response to hypovolaemia following trauma. Very high AVP concentrations were observed in hyperosmolar states in the sick elderly (Kirkland *et al.*, 1984), suggesting no decline in the osmotic response.

From the above, it can be seen that the secretion of AVP following trauma is due to several different mechanisms including osmotic, hypovolaemic, haemorrhagic and nociceptive stimuli (Le Quesne *et al.*, 1985). In combination these may have a synergistic effect causing a greater hormonal release than any one stimulus in isolation (Bie, 1980).

There is not a clear-cut relation, however, between the high circulating AVP levels and free water clearance (Le Quesne *et al.*, 1985). In one study of the effect of AVP on water excretion following major surgery (Fieldman *et al.*, 1985) there was no relation between variation in plasma AVP and urinary volume, with some patients exhibiting positive free water clearance when AVP was above a maximum antidiuretic concentration. It was found that the urine volume was closely related to the osmolar (solute) excretion.

In addition to any blood or fluid loss through trauma, which in the case of burns may be considerable (Carlson *et al.*, 1987), fluid may be sequestered within different spaces in the body. Over 60 years ago Blalock (1930) showed that trauma to a limb causes sequestration of fluid and electrolytes into that area. This 'third space' effect produces a reduction in effective circulating blood volume, the size of which is proportional to the severity of the trauma (Shires *et al.*, 1961). In burns patients the degree of fluid retention, after allowing for the losses through the burnt area, was predictive of survival in those over the age of 60 years (Carlson *et al.*, 1987).

Sodium

The aetiology of the sodium retention is similarly complex. The release of aldosterone and cortisol are influential as previously discussed. The reduction in effective extracellular volume will also promote sodium retention (Shires *et al.*, 1961; Zuidema *et al.*, 1985), which may be enhanced in elderly people with coexistent pathology such as cirrhosis or heart failure, causing a secondary hyperaldosteronism. Furthermore, sodium retention will be enhanced by the reduced circulating levels of ANP permitting a decrease in sodium excretion until several days have elapsed following injury (Crum *et al.*, 1988).

The decreased natriuresis may also be a result of alterations in renal function apart from those caused by the humoral response. Changes in renal perfusion may alter sodium excretion, through an increase in efferent arteriolar resistance. This increase maintains the total glomerular filtration rate (Early & Friedler, 1964) and produces a net increase in transfer of water and sodium from the proximal tubule. The changes are partially mediated by the renin–angiotensin system (Baer & McGiff, 1980) and also the sympathetic nervous system (Schrier, 1974). The latter may increase proximal tubular reabsorption of sodium directly (Schrier, 1974), so the apparent hyperadrenergic state in the elderly (Rowe & Troen, 1980) may enhance the retention of sodium in the initial post-trauma phase.

The effect of age on sodium retention following trauma is unknown. The described humoral, renal and autonomic nervous system changes that occur in the elderly make it difficult to predict any alteration in sodium handling with confidence and no definitive studies have been performed.

The retention of water slightly in excess of sodium produces a hyponatraemic state (Gump *et al.*, 1970), which in the case of some types of trauma may be extreme. It has been previously stated that the label of 'syndrome of inappropriate excretion of ADH' is often used without any measurement of the hormone levels, for example in the study of Steinbok & Thompson (1978), which inhibits any further analysis of the mechanisms involved.

Potassium

Changes may also take place in the serum potassium levels and, other than the neurohumoral responses to trauma, these are dependent on the nature of any fluid lost, such as through a burnt area, and the presence of a deranged acid–base balance. The latter is discussed elsewhere (Chapter 20), but the presence of alkalosis is associated with an effective hypokalaemia as potassium moves into the cells, and acidosis with a hyperkalaemia. An increase in urinary potassium loss has been reported following experimental trauma (Cuthbertson *et al.*, 1939), and high circulating levels of aldosterone and cortisol will promote this. Hypokalaemia may also be caused by the high circulating levels of catecholamines immediately following trauma (Frayn *et al.*, 1985), which drive potassium into the cells, analogous to that observed following acute myocardial infarction (Nordrehaug *et al.*, 1985). The injudicious prescription of diuretics would exacerbate the problem.

Effects of treatment and the late trauma phase

Immediately following trauma, the hormonal, water and electrolyte changes observed are likely to be related to the event or the body's compensatory reaction to it. After this period it becomes increasingly difficult to unravel the effects of trauma from its management. For example, Bonnet *et al.* (1982) found that the expected rise in AVP following total hip replacement was abolished using epidural anaesthesia. Similarly, the provision of adequate analgesia may modulate the nociceptive stimulus to hormonal release.

The fluids used in the immediate aftermath of trauma and the following days are going to influence any changes in fluid homeostasis, as was clearly shown in the paper by Crum *et al.* (1988) where hypertonic (250 mmol/l) sodium lactate solution was used. In the elderly there appear to be large amounts of 5% dextrose used in the management of trauma victims, although no data exist on the prevalence of its use. Similarly there is a paucity of any careful monitoring of the state of fluid balance other than that recorded on the anaesthetic record.

In the initial phase of the injury, the principal aim is the maintenance of intravascular volume through replacing the blood or fluid already lost and the ongoing leakage into the 'third space'. If the patient is hypotensive then the aim should be to use solutions which will remain within the intravascular compartment for a significant length of time. Both 5% dextrose and normal saline solutions fail to fulfil this requirement, although normal saline stays within the compartment for longer. Any fluid that leads to an increase in pulmonary extravascular water, either because of its properties or its overuse, will have deleterious effects on cardiorespiratory function (Van de Water *et al.*, 1970). This would particularly apply in an elderly population who are likely to have reduced homeostatic reserves. The value of invasive monitoring of fluid replacement is discussed elsewhere (Chapter 18), together with a more detailed review of perioperative management (Chapter 19).

The reliance on 5% dextrose as the principal fluid after operation is widespread and has a long history (Anonymous, 1969); it is attractive to a junior doctor in that water is regarded as being relatively safe, and is in keeping with the tendency to undertreat. In the face of water retention in excess of sodium retention (see above), it will promote the development of a significant hyponatraemia.

Towards better management

It is clear from the paper by Gump *et al.* (1970) that the excretion of any large fluid loads may be delayed, particularly in the presence of infection. Furthermore, the greater the initial sodium load then the larger the quantity retained (Le Quesne *et al.*, 1985). Both of these observations again highlight how the initial management of the patient is going to influence the ultimate outcome and the development of disturbances of fluid balance. In the immediate and subsequent post-trauma period, it is desirable to maintain an adequate urine volume, which is dependent on the solute (i.e. mainly sodium) load being presented to the kidney (Fieldman *et al.*, 1985). In the elderly, due to reduced concentrating ability, the obligate urine output approaches 1 litre/day (Dontas *et al.*, 1972), so allowance must be made for this plus any increase in insensible losses, for example due to fever (Chapter 8). It has already been commented that urine volume is not simply increased by increasing water intake (as 5% dextrose) due to the lack of relation between urine volume and AVP concentrations (Fieldman *et al.*, 1985). In the first few days, water should be restricted relative to sodium, until an adequate urine flow is achieved. Any water restriction may be helped by the reported reduction in thirst in the elderly (Phillips *et al.*, 1984), which would be compounded by the effects of any anaesthetic, sedative and analgesic drugs. Care needs to be taken to ensure that a water depleted, hypernatraemic state does not develop, which would lead to a downward spiral of increasing confusion coupled with decreasing fluid intake (Seymour *et al.*, 1980).

The complexity of management can be seen from the above. There is no standard fluid regime for treating trauma patients. What is lacking currently is adequate monitoring of requirements by accurate fluid balance recording, and, in particular, regular measurements of the blood chemistry and osmolality. It is only by adopting a more systematic approach that improvements can be made through regular audit of trauma management in the elderly.

References

Albert, S. G., Nakra, B. R. S., Grossberg, G. T. & Caminal, E. R. (1989). Vasopressin response to dehydration in Alzheimer's disease. *J Am Geriatr Soc*, **37**, 843–7.

Anonymous. (1969). Fluids for intravenous infusion. *Br Med J*, **4**, 670–1.

Arieff, A. I. & Guisado, R. (1976). Effects on the central nervous system of hypernatremic and hyponatremic states. *Kidney Inter*, **10**, 104–16.

Baer, P. G. & McGiff, J. C. (1980). Hormonal systems and renal haemodynamics. *Ann Rev Physiol*, **42**, 589.

Barton, R. N., Stoner, H. B. & Watson, S. M. (1987). Relationships among plasma cortisol, adrenocorticotrophin, and severity of injury in recently injured patients. *J Trauma*, **27**, 384–92.

Bevilacqua, M., Norbiato, G., Chebat, E., Raggi, U. & Cavaiani, P. (1987). Osmotic and nonosmotic control of vasopressin release in the elderly: effect of metoclopramide. *J Clin Endocrinol Metab*, **65**, 1243–7.

Bhatnagar, D. & Weinkove, C. (1988). Serious hypernatraemia in a hospital population. *Postgrad Med J*, **64**, 441–3.

Bie, P. (1980). Omsoreceptors, vasopressin and control of renal water excretion. *Physiol Rev*, **60**, 961.

Blalock, A. (1930). Experimental shock: the cause of low blood pressure caused by muscle injury. *Arch Surg*, **20**, 959.

Bonnet, F., Harari, A., Thibonnier, S. & Vias, P. (1982). Suppression of antidiuretic hormone hypersecretion during surgery by extradural anaesthesia. *Br J Anaesth*, **54**, 29–36.

Born, J. D., Hans, P., Smitz, S., Legros, J. J. & Kay, S. (1985). Syndrome of inappropriate secretion of antidiuretic hormone after severe head injury. *Surg Neurol*, **23**, 383–7.

Carlson, R. G., Miller, S. F., Finley, R. K., Billett, J. M., Fegelman, E., Jones, L. M. & Alkire, S. (1987). Fluid retention and burn survival. *J Trauma*, **27**, 127–35.

Champion, H. R., Sacco, W. J., Carnazzo, A. J., Copes, W. & Fouty, W. J. (1981). Trauma score. *Critical Care Medicine*, **9**, 672–676.

Cochrane, J. P. S., Forsling, M. L., Menzies Gow, N. & Le Quesne, L. P. (1981). Arginine vasopressin release following surgery. *Br J Surg*, **65**, 744–7.

Crane, M. G. & Harris, J. J. (1976). Effect of ageing on renin activity and aldosterone excretion. *J Lab Clin Med*, **87**, 847–59.

Crowe, M. J., Forsling, M. L., Rolls, B. J., Philips, P. A., Ledingham, J. G. G. & Smith, R. F. (1987). Altered water excretion in healthy elderly men. *Age Ageing*, **16**, 285–93.

Crum, R., Borrow, B., Shackford, S., Hansborough, J. & Brown, M. R. (1988). The neurohumoral response to burn injury in patients resuscitated with hypertonic saline. *J Trauma*, **28**, 1181–7.

Cuthbertson, D. P., Shaw, G. B. & Young, F. G. (1939). The effect of fracture of bone on the metabolism of the rat. *Q J Exp Physiol*, **29**, 18–25.

Davies, D. F. & Shock, N. W. (1950). Age changes in glomerular filtration rate, effective renal plasma flow, and tubular excretory capacity in adult males. *J Clin Invest*, **29**, 496–507.

Davis, P. J. (1979). Ageing and endocrine function. *Clin Endocrinol Metab*, **8**, 603–19.

Doczi, T., Tarjanyi, R., Huszka, E. & Kiss, J. (1982). Syndrome of inappropriate secretion of antidiuretic hormone (SIADH) after head injury. *Neurosurgery*, **10**, 685–8.

Dontas, A. S., Marketos, S. G. & Papanayiotou, P. (1972). Mechanisms of renal tubular defects in old age. *Postgrad Med J*, **48**, 295–303.

Duggan, J. D. & O'Malley, K. (1990). Ageing and atrial natriuretic factor. *J Hum Hypertens*, **4**, 53–6.

Duggan, J. D., Kilfeather, S., Lightman, S., O'Brien, E. & O'Malley, K. (1991). Plasma ANP and platelet ANP binding site density in ageing and hypertension. *Clin Sci*, **81**, 509–14.

Early, L. E. & Friedler, R. M. (1964). Observations on the mechanism of decreased tubular reabsorption of sodium and water during saline loading. *J Clin Invest*, **43**, 1928.

Fieldman, N. R., Forsling, M. L. & Le Quesne, L. P. (1985). The effects of vasopressin on solute and water excretion during and after surgical operations. *Ann Surg*, **201**, 383–90.

Forest, A. P. M., Brown, D. A. P., Morris, S. A. & Hendry, E. B. (1957). Metabolic response to surgery in totally adrenalectomised women. *J R Coll Surg Edinb*, **3**, 33–5.

Frayn, K. N., Little, R. A., Maycock, P. F. & Stoner, H. B. (1985). The relationship of plasma catecholamines to acute metabolic and hormonal responses to injury in man. *Circ Shock*, **16**, 229–40.

Frayn, K. N., Stoner, H. B., Barton, R. N. & Heath, D. F. (1983). Persistence of high plasma glucose, insulin and cortisol concentrations in elderly people with proximal femoral fractures. *Age Ageing*, **12**, 70–6.

Gump, F. E., Kinney, J. M., Iles, M. & Long, C. C. (1970). Duration and significance of large fluid loads administered for circulatory support. *J Trauma*, **10**, 431–9.

Haas, M. & Glick, S. M. (1978). Radioimmunoassayable plasma vasopressin associated with surgery. *Arch Surg*, **113**, 597–600.

Hauben, D. J., Le Roith, D., Glick, S. M. & Mahler, D. (1980). Nonoliguric vasopressin oversecretion in severely burned patients. *Isr J Med Sci*, **16**, 101–5.

Heim, J. M., Gottmann, K., Weil, J., Strom, T. M. & Gerzer, R. (1989). Effects of a bolus dose of atrial natriuretic factor in young and elderly volunteers. *Eur J Clin Invest*, **19**, 265–71.

Helderman, J. H., Vestal, R. E., Rowe, J. W., Tobin, J. D., Andres, R. & Robertson, G. L. (1978). The response of arginine vasopressin to intravenous ethanol and hypertonic saline in man: the impact of aging. *J Gerontol*, **33**, 39–47.

Hodkinson, H. M. (1980). In *Common Systems of Disease in the Elderly*, 2nd edn, p. 71. London: Blackwell.

Ingle, D. J., Meeks, R. C. & Thomas, K. E. (1951). The effects of fractures on urinary electrolytes in adrenalectomised rats treated with adrenal cortex extract. *Endocrinology*, **49**, 703–8.

Jansen, T., Tan, A., Smits, P., de Boo, T., Benraad, T. J. & Thien, T. (1990). Hemodynamic effects of atrial natriuretic factor in young and elderly subjects. *Clin Pharmacol Ther*, **48**, 179–88.

Kala, R., Fyhrquist, F. & Eisalo, A. (1974). Effect of short-term upright posture on plasma angiotensin II in man. *Scand J Clin Lab Invest*, **33**, 87–94.

Karlberg, B. E. & Tolagen, K. (1977). Relationships between blood pressure, age, plasma renin activity and electrolyte excretion in normotensive subjects. *Scand J Clin Lab Invest*, **37**, 521–8.

Kirkland, J. L., Lye, M., Levy, D. W. & Banerjee, A. K. (1983). Patterns of urine flow and electrolyte excretion in healthy elderly people. *Br Med J*, **287**, 1665–7.

Kirkland, J., Lye, M., Goddard, C., Vargas, E. & Davies, I. (1984). Plasma arginine vasopressin in dehydrated elderly patients. *Clin Endocrinol*, **20**, 451–6.

Kleeman, C. R. (1972). Water metabolism. In *Clinical Disorders of Fluid and Electrolyte Balance*, ed. M. H. Maxwell & C. R. Kleeman, p. 697. New York: McGraw-Hill.

Kleinfeld, M., Casimir, M. & Borra, S. (1979). Hyponatraemia as observed in a chronic disease facility. *J Am Geriatr Soc*, **27**, 156–61.

Knaus, W. A., Draper, E. A., Wagner, D. P. & Zimmerman, J. E. (1985). APACHE II: a severity of disease classification system. *Crit Care Med*, **13**, 818–29.

Le Quesne, L. P. (1967). The response of the adrenal cortex to surgical stress. In *Ciba Foundation. The Human Adrenal Cortex: Its Function Throughout Life*, pp. 65–78. London: Churchill.

Le Quesne, L. P., Cochrane, J. P. S. & Fieldman, N. R. (1985). Fluid and electrolyte disturbances after trauma: the role of adrenocortical and pituitary hormones. *Br Med Bull*, **41**, 212–17.

Ledingham, J. G. G., Crowe, M. J., Forsling, M. L., Phillips, M. L. & Rolls, B. J. (1987). Effects of aging on vasopressin secretion, water excretion and thirst in man. *Kidney Int*, **32** (Supppl. 21), S90–S92.

Lesser, G. T. & Markotksy, H. (1979). Body water compartments with human ageing using fat free mass as the reference standard. *Am J Physiol*, **R236**, 215–20.

Li, C.-H., Hsieh, S. M. & Nagai, I. (1984). The response of plasma arginine vasopressin to 14h water deprivation in the elderly. *Acta Endocrinol*, **105**, 314–17.

Ligthart, G. J., Corberand, J. X., Fournier, C., Galanaud, P., Hijams, W., Kennes, B., Muller-Hermelink, H. K. & Steinmann, G. G. (1984). Admission criteria for immunogerontological studies in man: The Senieur Protocol. *Mech Ageing Devel*, **28**, 47–55.

Lye, M. (1981). Distribution of body potassium in healthy elderly subjects. *Gerontology*, **27**, 286–92.

Lye, M. C. W. (1985). The milieu interieur and aging. In *Textbook of Geriatric Medicine and Gerontology*, ed. J. C. Brocklehurst, 3rd edn, pp. 201–29. London: Churchill Livingstone.

Macias Nuñez, J. F., Roman, A. B. & Commes, J. L. R. (1987). Physiology and disorders of water balance and electrolytes in the elderly. In *Renal Function and Disease in the Elderly*, ed. J. F. Macias Nuñez & J. S. Cameron, pp. 67–93. London: Butterworths.

Mahowald, J. M. & Himmelstein, D. U. (1981). Hypernatremia in the elderly: relation to infection and mortality. *J Am Geriatr Soc*, **29**, 177–80.

McLean, K. A., O'Neill, P. A. & Davies, I. (1990). Relationship of plasma osmolality to survival in acutely ill elderly patients. *Age Ageing*, **19**, P7.

McLean, K. A., O'Neill, P. A., Davies, I. & Catantia, J. (1991a). Changes in the response to a saline load with age. *Clin Sci*, **81**, 6P.

McLean, K. A., O'Neill, P. A., Catania, J. & Davies, I. (1991b). Changes in the response to a water load with age. *Clin Sci*, **81**, 6P.

McLean, K. A., O'Neill, P. A., Davies, J. & Morris, J. (1992). Influence of age on plasma osmolality: a community study. *Age Aging*, **21**, 56–60.

Miller, P. D., Krebs, R. A., Neal, B. J. & McIntyre, D. O. (1982). Hypodipsia in geriatric patients. *Am J Med*, **73**, 355–6.

Moran, W. H., Miltenberger, F. W., Shuayb, W. A. & Zimmermann, B. (1964). The relationship of antidiuretic hormone secretion to surgical stress. *Surgery*, **56**, 99–108.

Moran, W. H., Zimmermann, B. (1967). Mechanisms of antidiuretic hormone (ADH) control of importance to the surgical patient. *Surgery*, **62**, 639–44.

Morgan, R. J., Martyn, J. A. J., Philbin, D. M., Coggins, C. H. & Burke, J. F. (1980). Water metabolism and antidiuretic hormone (ADH) response following thermal injury. *J Trauma*, **20**, 468–72.

Mukherjee, A. P., Coni, N. K. & Davidson, W. (1973). Osmoreceptor function in the elderly. *Gerontol Clin*, **15**, 227–33.

Myers, J., Morgan, T., Waga, S. & Manley, K. (1982). The effect of sodium intake on blood pressure related to the age of the patients. *Clin Exp Pharmacol Physiol*, **9**, 287–9.

Nakamaru, M., Ogihara, T., Higaki, J. *et al.* (1981). Effect of age on active and inactive plasma renin in normal subjects and in patients with essential hypertension. *J Am Geriatr Soc*, **29**, 379–82.

Nelson, P. B., Seif, S., Gutai, J. & Robinson, A. G. (1984). Hyponatremia and natriuresis following subarachnoid hemorrhage in a monkey model. *J Neurosurg*, **60**, 233–7.

Nordrehaug, J. E., Johannessen, K.-A. & von der Lippe, G. (1985). Serum potassium concentration as a risk factor of ventricular arrhythmias early in acute myocardial infarction. *Circulation*, **71**, 645–9.

Noth, R., Lasmann, M., Tan, S., Fernandez-Cruz, A. & Mulrow, P. (1977). Age and the renin–aldosterone system. *Arch Inter Med*, **137**, 1414–17.

O'Neill, P. A., Faragher, E. B., Davies, I., Wears, R., McLean, K. A. & Fairweather, D. S. (1990). Reduced survival with increasing plasma osmolality in elderly continuing-care patients. *Age Ageing*, **19**, 68–71.

Philbin, D. M. (1983). Vasopressin and anesthesia. In *Endocrinology and the Anaesthetist*, ed. T. Oyama, pp. 81–94. Amsterdam: Elselvier.

Phillips, P. A., Rolls, B. J., Ledingham, J. G. G., Forsling, M. L., Morton, J. J., Crowe, M. J. & Wollner, L. (1984). Reduced thirst after water deprivation in healthy elderly men. *New Engl J Med*, **311**, 753–9.

Robertson, G. L. & Athar, S. (1976). The interaction of blood osmolality and blood volume in regulating plasma vasopressin in man. *J Clin Endocrinol Metab*, **42**, 613–20.

Robertson, G. L., Shelton, R. L. & Athar, S. (1976). The osmoregulation of vasopressin. *Kidney Int*, **10**, 25–37.

Rowe, J. W., Andres, R., Tobin, J. D., Norris, A. H. & Shock, N. W. (1976a). The effect of age on creatinine clearance in men: a cross-sectional and longitudinal study. *J Gerontol*, **31**, 155–63.

Rowe, J. W., Shock, N. W. & DeFronzo, R. A. (1976b). The influence of age on the renal response to water deprivation in man. *Nephron*, **17**, 270–8.

Rowe, J. W. & Troen, B. R. (1980). Sympathetic nervous system and aging in man. *Endocrinol Rev*, **1**, 167–79.

Rowe, J. W., Minaker, K. L., Sparrow, D. & Robertson, G. L. (1982). Age-related failure of volume-pressure mediated vasopressin release. *J Clin Endocrinol Metab*, **54**, 661–4.

Rowe, J. W. & Kahn, R. L. (1987). Human aging: usual and successful. *Science,* **237**, 143–9.

Schrier, R. W. (1974). Effects of adrenergic nervous system and catecholamines on systemic and renal haemodynamics, sodium and water excretion and renin secretion. *Kidney Int,* **6**, 291.

Seymour, D. G., Henschke, P. J., Cape, R. D. T. & Campbell, A. J. (1980). Acute confusional states and dementia in the elderly: the role of dehydration/volume depletion, physical illness and age. *Age Ageing,* **9**, 137–46.

Shirani, K. Z., Vaughan, J. M., Robertson, G. L., *et al.* (1983). Inappropriate vasopressin secretion (SIADH) in burned patients. *J Trauma,* **23**, 217–22.

Shires, T., Williams, J. & Brown, F. (1961). Acute changes in extracellular fluids associated with major surgical procedures. *Ann Surg,* **154**, 803.

Shock, N. W., Watkin, D. M., Yiengst, M. J., Norris, A. H., Gaffney, G. W., Gregerman, R. I. & Falzone, J. A. (1963). Age differences in the water content of the body as related to basal oxygen consumption in males. *J Gerontol,* **18**, 1–8.

Skott, P., Ingerslev, J., Neilsen, D. & Geise, J. (1987). The renin–angiotensin–aldosterone system in normal 85–year-old people. *Scand J Clin Lab Invest,* **47**, 69–74.

Steen, B., Lundgren, B. K. & Isakson, B. (1985). Body composition at age 70, 75, 79 and 81. A longitudinal population study. In *Nutrition, Immunity, and Illness in the Elderly,* ed. R. K. Chandra. New York: Pergamon Press.

Steinbok, P. & Thompson, G. B. (1978). Metabolic disturbance after head injury: abnormalities of sodium and water balance with special reference to the effects of alcohol intoxication. *Neurosurgery,* **3**, 9–15.

Sunderam, S. G. & Mankikar, G. D. (1983). Hyponatraemia in the elderly. *Age Ageing,* **12**, 77–80.

Tsunoda, K., Abe, K., Toshikazu, G. *et al.* (1986). Effect of age on the renin–angiotensin–aldosterone system in normal subjects: simultaneous measurement of active and inactive renin, renin substrate and aldosterone in plasma. *J Clin Endocrinol Metab,* **62**, 384–9.

Van de Water, J., Sheh, J.-M., O'Conner, N. E., Miller, I. T. & Milne, E. N. C. (1970). Pulmonary extravascular water volume: measurement and significance in critically ill patients. *J Trauma,* **10**, 440–9.

Vargas, E., Lye, M., Faragher, E. B., Goddard, C., Moser, B. & Davies, J. (1986). Cardiovascular haemodynamics and the response of vasopressin, aldosterone, plasma renin activity and plasma catecholamines to head-up tilt in young and old healthy subjects. *Age Ageing,* **15**, 17–28.

Wolf, A. V. (1958). In *Thirst. Physiology of the Urge to Drink and Problems of Water Lack.* Springfield, Illinois: Thomas.

Woodhouse, K. W., Wynne, H., Baille, S., James, O. F. W. & Rawlins, M. D. (1988). Who are the frail elderly? *Q J Med,* **255**, 505–6.

Yamada, T., Endo, T., Ito, K., Nagata, H. & Izumiyama, T. (1979). Age-related changes in endocrine and renal function in patients with essential hypertension. *J Am Geriatr Soc,* **27**, 286–92.

Zuidema, G. D., Rutherford, R. B. & Ballinger, W. F. (1985). *The Management of Trauma,* 4th edn, pp. 76–103. Philadelphia: W. B. Saunders.

16

Endocrine responses to trauma in old age

R. N. BARTON

Introduction

The lethality of injury is increased in old age. This applies both to early deaths after major injury and to later deaths after less severe injury (Chapters 3 and 4). One of the factors that determine whether people live or die after trauma is the way in which their endocrine systems respond. Many of those hormones whose secretion increases rapidly after injury, the so-called stress hormones, together with the sympathetic nervous system, have actions that reduce fluid loss or help to compensate for it. Failure of these early responses could therefore reduce survival within the first few hours of injury. On the other hand, if these responses were to occur and then fail to be extinguished, they could have deleterious effects on muscle function, defences against infection, etc., contributing not only to the late high death rate but also to the poor recovery so characteristic of old people after injury.

The present chapter addresses these issues to the extent that information is available. The only endocrine system to have been investigated extensively after trauma in old people, and apparently the only one to have been studied at all after trauma in aging experimental animals, is the hypothalamic–pituitary–adrenal (HPA) axis. This is covered in detail starting with the mechanisms of initiation of the response, about which, again, much more is known than for any other hormone.

Other endocrine systems are then considered. For many there are no directly relevant data, and the best that can be done is to consider the possible implications of the effects of aging in uninjured people. No mention in this chapter will be made of the hormones with major influences on water and electrolyte movements – vasopressin, aldosterone, natriuretic peptides and the renin–angiotensin system – which are covered in Chapter 15.

Hypothalamic–pituitary–adrenal axis

Trauma may stimulate the HPA axis in a number of ways. If injury is not severe, stimulation is most likely to occur through the low-pressure baroreceptors in the atria, which detect a fall in blood volume; through nociceptors, which respond to tissue damage; and through awareness of injury, perhaps via the limbic system. In severe injury, the high-pressure baroreceptors, responding to a fall in blood pressure, and the arterial chemoreceptors responsive to hypoxia, may also be involved. This list is not exclusive; for example, under the controlled conditions of surgery only tissue damage is likely to occur but additional effects may be caused by anaesthesia, and after head injury none of these stimuli may be present but a substantial neuroendocrine response is still observed. Cytokines may play a role after head injury as well as in patients who develop sepsis as a result of trauma (Chapter 8).

The available information suggests that most of these stimuli should become less effective in old people. Input from the baroreceptors (which is tonically inhibitory) is reduced because of arteriosclerosis and this is probably responsible for a decrease in sensitivity of the baroreflex (Chapter 12). Hypoxia may also not be as effective a stimulus, as judged by its effects on respiratory drive (Freeman, 1985). In general, pain is also reduced in the elderly (Kligman *et al.*, 1985) but it must be stressed that the nociception responsible for the HPA response does not necessarily involve perception of pain (as shown by the responses in anaesthetised surgical patients) and travels via different pathways (Barton & Gann, 1997).

The centre controlling the HPA axis is the paraventricular nucleus (PVN) of the hypothalamus, which synthesises the 41–residue corticotrophin-releasing factor (CRF) and vasopressin. These peptides, and possibly other stimulatory substances, are released into the primary plexus of the median eminence where they enter the pituitary portal system and are carried to the adrenocorticotrophic hormone (ACTH)-secreting cells. Much work has been done on the routes by which the stimuli elicited by injury are transmitted to the PVN (Barton & Gann, 1997). As far as cardiovascular and nociceptive information is concerned, it appears that a large number of brainstem areas and ascending pathways are involved. Among these areas are the nucleus of the tractus solitarius, which acts as the first relay station for receptors in the cardiovascular system; centres in the ventrolateral medulla, where this information is integrated with that from nociceptors; and nuclei in the dorsal rostral pons, including the locus coeruleus, locus subcoeruleus, parabrachial nucleus and dorsal raphe nucleus. The identity of the ascending pathways is not certain but there is evidence that noradrenaline is a major neurotransmitter: several noradrenergic pathways connect relevant areas of the brainstem to the hypothalamus, noradrenergic neurons appear to be the only ones synapsing onto CRF-secreting neurons and the current consensus is that noradrenaline is stimulatory for the HPA axis. Moreover, increased activity of noradrenergic neurons has been demonstrated after trauma. There are also serotoninergic pathways providing possible connexions and 5–hydroxytryptamine (5–HT) is another stimulatory neurotransmitter, but there is not good evidence that these pathways are activated after trauma.

There have been many studies on the effects of aging on central neurotransmitters (Rogers & Bloom, 1985; Simpkins & Millard, 1987). The consensus is that there is a general decline in the activity of noradrenergic pathways. The noradrenaline content of the brainstem has usually been found to fall and, although the same may not be true of the hypothalamus, noradrenaline turnover decreases in both regions. In addition there is some evidence for lower activities of the enzymes of noradrenaline synthesis, tyrosine hydroxylase and dopamine β-hydroxylase. Little appears to be known of hypothalamic adrenergic receptors in old age, but other brain areas show a decline in both β- and α-receptors (Rogers & Bloom, 1985). The changes in serotoninergic neuron activity are much less consistent. While these findings might lead one to expect stimulation of the HPA axis via noradrenergic pathways to be impaired in the elderly trauma victim, this is clearly an oversimplification of a very complex picture. One complicating factor is that much of the work on aging has used the rat, whereas the mechanisms of HPA activation after trauma have mainly been explored in larger animals, and the possibility of species differences cannot be ignored.

The evidence available indicates that aging does not diminish the HPA response to stimuli such as laparotomy in the rat. On the contrary, aged rats are slower to switch off the response once the stimulus has ceased (Sapolsky *et al.*, 1986). This is taken to imply impairment of feedback inhibition and forms the basis of the 'glucocorticoid cascade hypothesis', formulated by Sapolsky *et al.* (1986) and subsequently modified by McEwen (1992). The hypothesis focuses on the hippocampus, whose density of corticosteroid receptors is higher than that of other brain areas but decreases with age. A vicious cycle is proposed, wherein continual stress causes secretion of corticosterone (the major glucocorticoid in the rat), which leads to loss of hippocampal neurons and thus a decreased capacity for feedback inhibition and potentiation of the response to stress. An element of the hypothesis is that hippocampal neurons are susceptible to damage by glucocorticoids, a finding that has been confirmed, at least in old animals (Landfield & Eldridge, 1991; Meaney *et al.*, 1995; Seckl & Olsson, 1995). The relevance of this to persistence of HPA responses has been questioned (de Kloet *et al.*, 1991). One reason is that the receptor subtype whose density is particularly high in the hippocampus (type I) is unlikely to be essential for terminating stress responses because its affinity is so high; thus, it may be close to saturation even in an unstressed animal near the peak of the nyctohemeral rhythm. Moreover, there may be species differences in the effects of aging. In the dog, which, like humans, has cortisol as its main glucocorticoid, aging does not cause loss of type II receptors, which have a lower affinity than type I and are probably responsible for feedback inhibition after stress; the cortisol response to stress is also not prolonged, although it is enhanced acutely (Reul *et al.*, 1991).

As Sapolsky *et al.* (1986) recognise, not all the changes in HPA function in the aged rat are seen in humans. There is no consistent effect of aging on basal plasma cortisol or ACTH (Seeman & Robbins, 1994). Moreover, there is only slight, if any, impairment in the ability of dexamethasone to suppress plasma cortisol in normal old people (Sharma *et al.*, 1988; Seeman & Robbins, 1994). Sapolsky *et al.* (1986), however, have argued that disturbances in feedback inhibition only become apparent when old people are exposed to stress. There is evidence that this is so in major depression and dementia (Sharma *et al.*, 1988; Seeman & Robbins, 1994), and the same may well be true after trauma.

Like in the rat, aging does not impair the early HPA response to trauma in humans. The initial rise in plasma cortisol and ACTH was similar in elderly and younger patients undergoing either minor or major elective surgery (Blichert-Toft, 1975; Blichert-Toft & Hummer, 1976; Blichert-Toft *et al.*, 1979). Several other studies (for a review see Horan *et al.*, 1988) which have not included young controls have also shown a substantial cortisol response to surgery in old people. Within 2 hours of accidental injury plasma cortisol tended to be higher in patients aged more than 65 years than in those aged 17–40 years, although the difference was usually not significant (Frayn *et al.*, 1983; Barton *et al.*, 1987; Horan *et al.*, 1992). It should be pointed out that although some workers have found an advancement of the nyctohemeral rhythm of cortisol and ACTH in old age (Seeman & Robbins, 1994), this is not likely to hinder interpretation of the early effects of injury which overrides the rhythm (Barton *et al.*, 1987). However, plasma cortis as measured may conceivably underestimate the concentration of active, unbound cortisol as there is some tendency for plasma corticosteroid-binding globulin to decrease with age (Wagner, 1978; Pavlov *et al.*, 1986).

The abnormalities of HPA function after trauma in old people lie not in the initial response but in its persistence. Although Jeevanandam *et al.* (1993), taking morning blood samples 2–3 days after severe accidental injury, have shown similar cortisol concentrations in old and young patients, most studies of less severe injury have shown differences. A few hours after elective surgery plasma cortisol was higher and more variable in old than in young people (Blichert-Toft, 1975; Blichert-Toft *et al.*, 1979) and, in the case of major surgery, the difference continued for 4 days, samples being taken in the evening (Blichert-Toft, 1975). These findings have recently been confirmed with morning sampling (Langer *et al.*, 1992), although Watters *et al.* (1993) found that urinary free cortisol excretion declined as rapidly in the old as in the young. Frayn *et al.* (1983), studying accidental injury, showed that plasma cortisol was higher in elderly women 1 week after proximal femur fracture than in young patients at the same time after injuries of similar or greater anatomical severity. At 2–3 weeks the difference persisted and, while the values in the young were not significantly different from those in uninjured control subjects, those in the elderly were higher than in active, reasonably healthy old people. The comparison was complicated by another group of elderly controls in whom plasma cortisol was similarly raised, and because these were all relatively inactive inmates of an old people's home the persistence of the effect of injury was tentatively attributed to immobility. In a subsequent study (Roberts *et al.*, 1990), elderly women with proximal femur fracture were compared with two groups of elderly control women, at opposite ends of the spectrum as regards mobility, age and general health: subjects who had passed a stringent health screen and immobile patients in a continuing-care ward. Plasma cortisol 2 weeks after injury was higher than in either of the two control groups, which did not differ from each other. Blood samples were also taken 8 weeks after injury and the same differences were found. At neither time was there any relation between plasma cortisol and an index of mobility potential in the injured patients. These results contrast with others showing no difference in plasma cortisol between patients 3–4 days after hip fracture and healthy elderly subjects undergoing the same nutritional regimen (Nelson *et al.*, 1995).

To confirm that the persistently raised morning cortisol concentration 2 weeks after proximal femur fracture did not merely represent a change in rhythm, urinary free cortisol excretion was measured (Barton *et al.*, 1993). This index, which is thought to reflect the concentration of unbound plasma cortisol over the 24–hour collection period, was higher than in healthy elderly control women. The same experiments showed a rise in cortisol production rate measured by an isotopic method. This is consistent with the results of Blichert-Toft (1975) in elderly surgical patients, whose 17–ketogenic steroid excretion (an approximation to cortisol production rate) had still not returned to preoperative values by four days after surgery whereas it had done so by 3 days in younger patients. In the hip fracture patients there was a tendency for the metabolic clearance rate (MCR) of cortisol to be lower than in healthy elderly women, although this may merely have reflected the somewhat greater age of the patients (Horan *et al.*, 1991). From these data and from the cortisol production rate and corticosteroid-binding globulin concentration, which was unchanged, approximate calculation of the plasma free cortisol concentration averaged over 24 hours gave values nearly threefold higher in the injured patients, in line with the increase in urinary free cortisol excretion (Table 16.1).

The mechanism of the persistent increase in cortisol production is not clear. Feedback inhibition of the HPA axis, as indicated by the overnight dexamethasone suppression test, was impaired both 2 and 8 weeks after upper femur fracture, by comparison with healthy elderly women (Roberts *et al.*, 1990; Doncaster *et al.*, 1993; Table 16.1); totally immobile geriatric patients showed no such change (Roberts *et al.*, 1990). Another way of studying feedback inhibition is to give metyrapone, which inhibits conversion of 11–deoxycortisol to cortisol in the adrenal and thereby removes the inhibitory signal. Results with this test 5 days after major elective surgery were

Table 16.1. *Indices of hypothalamic–pituitary–adrenal function in healthy elderly women and in elderly women about 2 weeks after proximal femur fracture*

	Control women	Injured women	P[a]
Plasma cortisol[b] (μmol/l)	0.35(0.21–0.49)	0.59(0.27–0.95)	<0.01
Urinary free cortisol excretion (nmol/day)	40(10–170)	110(70–300)	<0.001
Cortisol production rate (μmol/day)	32(24–52)	48(27–76)	<0.01
Cortisol metabolic clearance rate (ml/min)	106(76–120)	82(54–142)	n.s.
Post-dexamethasone cortisol[c] (μmol/l)	0.04(0.03–0.07)	0.08(0.04–0.73)	<0.001
Plasma ACTH[b] (ng/1)	14(4–28)	16(10–24)	n.s.
Cortisol response to ACTH[d] (μmol/l)	0.29(0.16–0.50)	0.27(0.10–0.41)	n.s.

Note: All subjects were aged more than 65 years.
Data are given as medians with ranges in parentheses, and are for 9–16 subjects per group.
[a] Level of significance by Wilcoxon's rank-sum test; n.s., not significant.
[b] Mean from mid-morning blood samples on two successive days.
[c] Plasma cortisol at 08.00 after an oral dose of 1 mg dexamethasone at 23.00 the previous day.
[d] Increase in plasma cortisol 20 minutes after intravenous injection of 150 ng ACTH after suppression of endogenous cortisol production with dexamethasone.
The data have previously been reported by Roberts *et al.* (1990), Horan *et al.* (1991), Barton *et al.* (1993) and Doncaster *et al.* (1993).

equivocal. Although there was no significant difference in the ACTH response between elderly and young patients, many of the values were off-scale (Blichert-Toft & Hummer, 1976); and while the increase in plasma 11–deoxycortisol was greater in the elderly patients than in both young postoperative patients and elderly control subjects, there was no age-related difference in urinary 17–ketogenic steroid excretion (Blichert-Toft, 1975).

The impairment of feedback inhibition after hip fracture is reminiscent of the findings in aged rats. However, in injured elderly people, unlike in rats (Sapolsky *et al.*, 1986), there was no increase in plasma ACTH corresponding to that in cortisol (Roberts *et al.*, 1990; Doncaster *et al.*, 1993; Table 16.1). This could not be explained by heightened sensitivity of the adrenal cortex to ACTH as the rises in plasma cortisol when graded doses of ACTH were given 2 weeks after upper femur fracture were similar to those in healthy elderly control subjects (Doncaster *et al.*, 1993; Table 16.1). Discrepancies between cortisol and ACTH have been reported in various other experimental and clinical circumstances and a number of alternative explanations have been proposed (see discussion in Doncaster *et al.*, 1993). In particular, ACTH precursor peptides have been reported to stimulate cortisol production; however, there was only a small increase in their plasma concentration after upper femur fracture (Doncaster *et al.*, 1993). It may be that the pulsatile nature of ACTH secretion makes it difficult to detect the relatively small changes that would be sufficient to cause the raised cortisol secretion rate seen 2 weeks after injury in old people.

In contrast to cortisol secretion by the adrenal zona fasciculata, production of androgens by the zona reticularis is decreased after injury, as shown by falls both in the plasma concentrations of adrenal androgens and in urinary 17–ketosteroid excretion (for a review see Barton, 1987). A marked decline in adrenal androgen production also occurs in old age (Vermeulen, 1980; Pavlov *et al.*, 1986; Parker, 1991). It is not known whether these changes share a common mechanism and whether the lower baseline values in old people enhance or diminish the response to injury. Elderly women in hospital for other types of illness show no decrease in concentration of dehydroepiandrosterone or its sulphate and an increase in that of androstenedione compared with elderly control women (Rozenberg *et al.*, 1990; Spratt *et al.*, 1993). Injury also has similar effects to aging in decreasing the concentrations of testosterone and triiodothyronine, as will be discussed below.

Other pituitary hormones

Growth hormone and prolactin

Trauma usually causes a rise in plasma growth hormone (GH), although of variable duration (Barton, 1987). The influence of aging on this response seems to have been the subject of only two studies. Blichert-Toft (1975) showed that the increase in GH was smaller in old than in younger patients during the first few hours after major elective surgery, but there were no consistent differences between the age groups during the next 4 days. Jeevanandam et al. (1993) found no change in plasma GH 2–3 days after severe accidental injury in elderly patients compared with healthy elderly subjects; however, trauma caused a fall in GH in young patients studied under the same conditions. In both age groups plasma GH increased after a further 4 days on total parenteral nutrition (Jeevanandam et al., 1992).

There are problems in interpreting both these studies because the bulk of GH secretion occurs during the early stages of sleep. In normal elderly people the size of these nocturnal secretory peaks decreases, but the difference is not detectable by taking blood samples during the daytime (Minaker et al., 1985; Blackman, 1987; Corpas et al., 1993). Since only daytime samples were taken from the patients, the effect of trauma on total GH secretion in the elderly is not known. The GH response to arginine in elderly patients did not change between the preoperative state and 5 days after surgery (Blichert-Toft, 1975), but the interpretation of arginine stimulation tests is uncertain. GH secretion is controlled not only by GH-releasing hormone (GHRH) but also by a release-inhibiting hormone, somatostatin. Arginine may act by inhibiting somatostatin secretion; old people tend to have a decreased GH response to GHRH (Minaker et al., 1985; Blackman, 1987; Corpas et al., 1993) and it has been suggested that this is due to excessive somatostatin secretion as the response to combined GHRH and arginine stimulation is normal (Ghigo et al., 1990).

The effects of GH are mediated through the production in various tissues of an insulin-like growth factor (IGF-I), previously known as somatomedin C. Its plasma concentration sometimes provides a better index of overall GH activity than that of GH itself; in particular, it reflects the fall in basal GH secretion and increase with GH administration in the elderly (Hammerman, 1987). Injury leads to a fall in plasma somatomedin activity (for a review see Barton, 1987). It has recently been shown that in old as well as young people plasma IGF-I is decreased 2–3 days after severe injury (Jeevanandam et al., 1993) and subsequently rises when total parenteral nutrition is given (Jeevanandam et al., 1992).

The interpretation of IGF-I concentrations, however, is difficult because circulating IGFs are strongly bound to plasma proteins. The major one is IGFBP-3, whose constitution is altered in old age (Donahue et al., 1990). Seriously ill patients after major surgery, most of them elderly, were found to have low plasma concentrations of both IGF-I and the GH-independent IGF-II, and this was associated with loss of IGFBP-3 by proteolysis (Davies et al., 1991). This binding protein is thought to function as a reservoir for IGF-I and the effect of its degradation on IGF-I availability for tissues is uncertain. Similar patients had raised concentrations of IGFBP-1, which were greatly decreased by parenteral feeding (Ross et al., 1991). Although this protein has a much smaller binding capacity than IGFBP-3, it is thought to play a role in tissue uptake, raised concentrations preventing IGF-I from causing hypoglycaemia under conditions of starvation. A study of elderly women with hip and vertebral crush fractures showed no change in the concentrations of IGFBP-1 or IGFBP-3 from those in elderly control women, but the time after injury varied widely and overall the IGF-I concentration was unchanged (Rosen *et al.*, 1992). The authors' main interest was in IGFBP-4, an osteoblast product.

Plasma prolactin usually rises transiently after trauma (for a review see Barton, 1987). There is one report that the increase in concentration immediately after starting elective surgery was smaller in elderly than in young patients; in both groups the concentration had returned to normal the next day (Arnetz, 1985). There have been several studies of prolactin in normal elderly people but no agreement over the results. Some have shown that plasma prolactin falls with age in women and rises in men (Blackman, 1987); interpretation of the data may be complicated by alterations in the secretory pattern (Greenspan *et al.*, 1990). There is also disagreement over whether there is an enhanced response to thyrotrophin-releasing hormone (TRH), which stimulates prolactin secretion although it probably does not act as its main hypothalamic releasing factor (Blackman, 1987).

Thyroid hormones

Injury results in a pattern of change in plasma thyroid hormone concentrations that is characteristic of the 'euthyroid sick syndrome': a considerable fall in triiodothyronine (T3), a decrease in thyroxine (T4) which is substantial only if the patient becomes critically ill, a raised reverse T3 (rT3) concentration and a normal concentration of thyroid-stimulating hormone (TSH), both basally and in response to TRH administration (Barton, 1987). The mechanism of these changes, which may be protracted, is largely unknown (Barton & Gann, 1997). There are apparently only two studies of thyroid function in injured old people. Blichert-Toft *et al.* (1979) showed no significant difference from young people in plasma T4, T3, rT3 or T3 resin uptake (an index of T4 binding to thyroxine-binding globulin, which, however, may not be valid after injury). The injury was minor (elective herniorrhaphy), however, and the patients were followed for only 6 hours after the start of surgery. At longer periods after a more major operation (cholecystectomy), T4, T3, rT3 and TSH again responded essentially similarly in old and young women (Langer *et al.*, 1992). In this study plasma T3 tended to be higher throughout in the elderly patients. Usually aging itself leads to a small fall in plasma T3; although the secretion rate of T4 falls, its plasma concentration is maintained by a commensurate fall in MCR (Minaker *et al.*, 1985; Spaulding, 1987). As the euthyroid sick syndrome is not peculiar to injury, but common to many forms of illness, it has been suggested that the fall in plasma T3 is due to the greater prevalence of disease in old people. The consensus is that it is due rather to aging per se as the rT3 concentration is not raised concomitantly; in addition, most studies also show a decreased TSH response to TRH in old people, which is not seen in general illness. The mechanism of these age-related changes and their interaction with the effects of injury are unknown. Simons *et al.* (1990), studying elderly patients in hospital for a variety of illnesses, found independent negative correlations of plasma T3 with both severity of illness and age, the former being much the stronger. They concluded that the main effect of aging in such patients was to increase the prevalence of primary hypothyroidism.

Sex hormones

In men, injury results in an equally complex pattern of change in reproductive hormones. There is a fall in plasma testosterone which can persist for a substantial period, like in many other forms of non-endocrine illness. There is usually no change in sex steroid-binding globulin (SSBG), so plasma-free testosterone also decreases. Basal gonadotrophin concentrations tend to fall, but not nearly as consistently as testosterone; the reported responses to gonadotrophin-releasing hormone (GnRH) vary (Barton, 1987). The mechanisms of these changes are not known with certainty and there may be abnormalities at all three levels of the hypothalamic–pituitary–gonadal axis (Barton & Gann, 1997). The effects of aging on the responses to injury are apparently not known. Most studies have shown that plasma testosterone is lower in old than in young men and it has again been suggested that this is due to inclusion of unhealthy subjects. However, the consensus is that, at least in some communities, there is an inherent tendency for testosterone to decrease with age (Tsitouras, 1987). Most studies have also shown an increase in plasma SSBG so there is at least as great a fall in free as in total testosterone. Old men have a diminished testosterone response to stimulation with human chorionic gonadotrophin. Their gonadotrophin concentrations tend to be higher basally but respond subnormally to GnRH, indicating again changes at more than one level which make the implications for injury responses hard to predict.

   In women, aging is of course accompanied by much more dramatic changes than in men as a result of the menopause with its associated large decrease in plasma oestrogens and rise in gonadotrophins. There are reports of lower gonadotrophin concentrations after injury in premenopausal women (for a review see Barton, 1987) and after elective surgery in middle-aged postmenopausal women (Charters *et al.*, 1969). A number of studies have shown decreased plasma gonadotrophins in elderly women in hospital for other illnesses, mostly sufficiently serious to require intensive care, the lowest concentrations being seen in the most severely ill (Warren *et al.*, 1977;

Quint & Kaiser, 1985; Gebhart *et al.*, 1989; Spratt *et al.*, 1993). The results of tests with GnRH suggested a defect primarily at the pituitary level (Gebhart *et al.*, 1989).

Catecholamines and pancreatic hormones

Sympathoadrenal system

The sympathoadrenal system is central to the neuroendocrine response to injury. Not only does it have manifold circulatory, metabolic and other effects but it also influences the secretion of other hormones, notably the pancreatic hormones (discussed below) and the renin–angiotensin system (discussed in Chapter 14). Adrenaline is a true hormone secreted by the adrenal medulla; circulating noradrenaline, on the other hand, is only partly derived from the adrenal, the remainder representing noradrenaline released at sympathetic nerve terminals and not reabsorbed ('spillover'). The activity of the sympathetic outflow is not uniform; its distribution between tissues depends upon the nature of the stimulus, limiting the usefulness of plasma noradrenaline measurements.

The effects of injury on plasma catecholamines depend on its severity (Barton, 1987). Shortly after accidental injury both noradrenaline and adrenaline concentrations rise rapidly and more than proportionally to the severity of the injury. Elective abdominal surgery causes only a small rise in plasma adrenaline and not always an increase in noradrenaline. The duration of the responses also depends on injury severity and can vary from a few hours after surgery to several days after severe accidental injury or burns. Jeevanandam *et al.* (1993) found that the increases in concentration of both catecholamines 2–3 days after multiple injury were similar in old and young patients. Their elderly control subjects had higher noradrenaline but not adrenaline concentrations than young ones, in agreement with more detailed studies on the effects of aging (Morrow *et al.*, 1987), and this difference was maintained after injury. Håkanson *et al.* (1984), studying patients undergoing elective cholecystectomy, likewise found that the adrenaline response was unaffected by age. The increase in plasma noradrenaline, however, was larger and lasted longer in old (more than 55 years) than in younger patients, in keeping with studies showing exaggerated noradrenaline responses to other stimuli in the elderly (Rowe & Troen, 1980). In contrast, the minor operation of inguinal herniorrhaphy elicited responses that were unaffected by age for either catecholamine (Blichert-Toft *et al.*, 1979).

Insulin and glucagon

Insulin secretion is so sensitive to glucose that other influences on it can only be evaluated in the light of the prevailing glucose concentration (Chapter 14). On this basis, injury has opposite effects at different stages. Early on, when the patient is hyperglycaemic, there is little change in plasma insulin (Barton, 1987), implying an inhibitory influence counteracting the stimulation by glucose. The sympathoadrenal system is capable of inhibiting insulin secretion, acting both through the pancreatic nerves and through circulating adrenaline which binds to α_2 receptors (at low adrenaline concentrations there is a stimulatory β_2 effect). There is evidence that adrenaline is responsible for the inhibition after injury (Barton & Gann, 1997). Later, during the flow phase when the glucose concentration has fallen towards normal, the concentration of insulin rises (Barton, 1987). The reason for this is unknown. A number of factors are capable of enhancing the effect of glucose, but some of these, such as vagal efferents and gastrointestinal hormones, are mainly concerned with the insulin response to feeding and are unlikely to be relevant after injury. Other potentiators are amino acids and possibly cytokines. It is possible that amino acids play a role in the raised insulin concentration in the flow phase but this does not seem to have been tested.

Aging seems to have little effect on the early inhibition of insulin secretion after injury. There is little difference in plasma insulin or glucose between old and younger patients shortly after accidental injuries of varying severities (Desai *et al.*, 1989; Horan *et al.*, 1992) or elective surgery (Blichert-Toft *et al.*, 1979; Håkanson *et al.*, 1984; Watters *et al.*, 1990). About 2 days after severe accidental injury, there was still no difference in plasma insulin or C-peptide between old and young patients (Jeevanandam *et al.*, 1993), and the insulin concentration rose similarly after 4 days of parenteral nutrition in both groups (Jeevanandam *et al.*, 1992). Several studies have been carried out in elderly patients with proximal femur fracture. When such patients were given a day's total parenteral nutrition starting 2–3 days after surgery, neither glucose nor insulin differed from those in controls submitted to the same regimen, although plasma noradrenaline was still raised (Long *et al.*, 1992; Nelson *et al.*, 1995). Later, at one or 2–3 weeks, elderly women with proximal femur fracture had similar insulin concentrations to younger patients with other musculoskeletal injuries (Frayn *et al.*, 1983). As the aged patients had higher glucose concentrations, this was interpreted to indicate greater insulin resistance in the old people, but it could also be concluded that their insulin response to glucose was less potentiated by injury.

The glucagon response to injury is not fully understood. Although the rise in plasma glucagon is attributed to the sympathoadrenal system, which can stimulate glucagon secretion through both its neural and humoral arms, it usually occurs after a delay which has not been explained, and other stimuli such as amino acids may possibly be involved. In apparently the only study of the effects of aging on this response, glucagon concentrations were found to be similar in elderly and young patients 2–3 days after multiple injury (Jeevanandam *et al.*, 1993). Studies in healthy subjects have also shown no effect of aging on fasting concentrations, stimulation by amino acids, inhibition by glucose or insulin or clearance rate (Minaker *et al.*, 1985).

Conclusion

One of the questions initially posed was whether failure of the early neuroendocrine response to injury could impair the ability of elderly people to compensate for the effects of fluid loss and thus to survive the injury. From the limited information available, this seems unlikely. Despite some evidence for deterioration of the systems by which the body recognises that injury has occurred and transmits that information to the hypothalamus, those early neuroendocrine responses that have been studied appear to be intact in old age. The other question was whether hormone concentrations could contribute to the morbidity and high late mortality rate observed in injured old people. There is strong evidence that aging prolongs the cortisol response to injury. One would predict that this would exacerbate muscle protein catabolism and reduce resistance to infection after injury, losses the elderly can ill afford. No attempts to test this prediction have yet been reported, but this is clearly an area that would repay study as it is open to therapeutic intervention. Whether the persistence of early responses is confined to the HPA axis is not known. Indeed, no general conclusions can be drawn about the effects of aging on the endocrine changes that accompany the flow phase of injury because the available data are too fragmentary. For some hormones observations are confined to a single type of patient or a single time point, for some there are problems of interpretation and for others no data have been published at all. More research is needed into this increasingly important area.

References

Arnetz, B. B. (1985). Endocrine reactions during standardized surgical stress: the effects of age and methods of anaesthesia. *Age Ageing*, **14**, 96–101.

Barton, R. N. (1987). The neuroendocrinology of physical injury. *Baillière's Cl Endocr Metab*, **1**, 355–74.

Barton, R. N. & Gann, D. S. (1997). The response of the endocrine system to injury. In *Scientific Foundations of Trauma*, ed. G. J. Cooper, H. A. F. Dudley, D. S. Gann, R. A. Little & R. L. Maynard, pp. 643–65. Oxford: Heinemann Medical Books.

Barton, R. N., Stoner, H. B. & Watson, S. M. (1987). Relationships among plasma cortisol, adrenocorticotrophin, and severity of injury in recently injured patients. *J Trauma*, **27**, 384–92.

Barton, R. N., Weijers, J. W. M. & Horan, M. A. (1993). Increased rates of cortisol production and urinary free cortisol excretion in elderly women 2 weeks after proximal femur fracture. *Eur J Clin Invest*, **23**, 171–6.

Blackman, M. R. (1987). Pituitary hormones and aging. *Endocr Metab Clin North Am*, **16**, 981–94.

Blichert-Toft, M. (1975). Secretion of corticotrophin and somatotrophin by the senescent adenohypophysis in man. *Acta Endocr*, (Suppl.) **195**.

Blichert-Toft, M., Christensen, V., Engquist, A., Fog-Moller, F., Kehlet, H., Nistrup Madsen,

S., Skovsted, L., Thode, J. & Olgaard, K. (1979). Influence of age on the endocrine-metabolic response to surgery. *Ann Surg*, **190**, 761–70.

Blichert-Toft, M. & Hummer, L. (1976). Immunoreactive corticotrophin reserve in old age in man during and after surgical stress. *J Gerontol*, **31**, 539–45.

Charters, A. C., Odell, W. D. & Thompson, J. C. (1969). Anterior pituitary function during surgical stress and convalescence. Radioimmunoassay measurements of blood TSH, LH, FSH and growth hormone. *J Clin Endocr Metab*, **29**, 63–71.

Corpas, E., Harman, S. M. & Blackman, M. R. (1993). Human growth hormone and human aging. *Endocr Rev*, **14**, 20–39.

Davies, S. C., Wass, J. A. H., Ross, R. J. M., Cotterill, A. M., Buchanan, C. R., Coulson, V. J. & Holly, J. M. P. (1991). The induction of a specific protease for insulin-like growth factor binding protein-3 in the circulation during severe illness. *J Endocr*, **130**, 469–73.

de Kloet, E. R., Sutanto, W., Rots, N., van Haarst, A., van den Berg, D., Oitzl, M., van Eekelen, A. & Voorhuis, D. (1991). Plasticity and function of brain corticosteroid receptors during aging. *Acta Endocr*, **125** (Suppl. 1), 65–72.

Desai, D., March, R. & Watters, J. M. (1989). Hyperglycemia after trauma increases with age. *J Trauma*, **29**, 719–23.

Donahue, L. R., Hunter, S. J., Sherblom, A. P. & Rosen, C. (1990). Age-related changes in serum insulin-like growth factor-binding proteins in women. *J Clin Endocr Metab*, **71**, 575–9.

Doncaster, H. D., Barton, R. N., Horan, M. A. & Roberts, N. A. (1993). Factors influencing cortisol-adrenocorticotrophin relationships in elderly women with upper femur fractures. *J Trauma*, **34**, 49–55.

Frayn, K. N., Stoner, H. B., Barton, R. N., Heath, D. F. & Galasko, C. S. B. (1983). Persistence of high plasma glucose, insulin and cortisol concentrations in elderly patients with proximal femur fractures. *Age Ageing*, **12**, 70–6.

Freeman, E. (1985). The respiratory system. In *Textbook of Geriatric Medicine and Gerontology*, 3rd edn, ed. J. C. Brocklehurst, pp. 731–57. Edinburgh: Churchill Livingstone.

Gebhart, S. S. P., Watts, N. B., Clark, R. V., Umpierrez, G. & Sgoutas, D. (1989). Reversible impairment of gonadotropin secretion in critical illness. Observations in postmenopausal women. *Arch Intern Med*, **149**, 1637–41.

Ghigo, E., Goffi, S., Nicolosi, M., Arvat, E., Valente, F., Mazza, E., Ghigo, M. C. & Camanni, F. (1990). Growth hormone (GH) responsiveness to combined administration of arginine and GH-releasing hormone does not vary with age in man. *J Clin Endocr Metab*, **71**, 1481–5.

Greenspan, S. L., Klibanski, A., Rowe, J. W. & Elahi, D. (1990). Age alters pulsatile prolactin release: influence of dopaminergic inhibition. *Am J Physiol*, **258**, E799–E804.

Håkanson, E., Rutberg, H., Jorfeldt, L. & Wiklund, L. (1984). Endocrine and metabolic responses after standardized moderate surgical trauma: influence of age and sex. *Clin Physiol*, **4**, 461–73.

Hammerman, M. R. (1987). Insulin-like growth factors and aging. *Endocr Metab Clin North Am*, **16**, 995–1011.

Horan, M. A., Barton, R. N. & Little, R. A. (1988). Ageing and the response to injury. In *Advanced Geriatric Medicine* 7, ed. J. Grimley Evans & F. I. Caird, pp. 101–35. London: John Wright.

Horan, M. A., Fisher, R. & Barton, R. N. (1991). Effect of proximal femur fracture on cortisol kinetics in old people. *Circ Shock*, **34**, 57–8.

Horan, M. A., Roberts, N. A., Barton, R. N. & Little, R. A. (1992). Injury responses in old age. In *Oxford Textbook of Geriatric Medicine*, ed. J. Grimley Evans & T. Franklin Williams, pp. 88–93. Oxford: Oxford University Press.

Jeevanandam, M., Holaday, N. J., Shamos, R. F. & Petersen, S. R. (1992). Acute IGF-I deficiency in multiple trauma victims. *Clin Nutr*, **11**, 352–7.

Jeevanandam, M., Petersen, S. R. & Shamos, R. F. (1993). Protein and glucose fuel kinetics and hormonal changes in elderly trauma patients. *Metabolism*, **42**, 1255–62.

Kligman, A. M., Grove, G. L. & Balin, A. K. (1985). Aging of human skin. In *Handbook of the Biology of Aging*, 2nd edn, ed. C. E. Finch & E. L. Schneider, pp. 820–41. New York: Van Nostrand Reinhold.

Landfield, P. W. & Eldridge, J. C. (1991). The glucocorticoid hypothesis of brain aging and neurodegeneration: recent modifications. *Acta Endocr*, **125** (Suppl. 1), 54–64.

Langer, P., Balážová, E., Vician, M., Martino, E., Ježová, D., Michalíková, S. & Moravec, R. (1992). Acute development of low T_3 syndrome and changes in pituitary-adrenocortical function after elective cholecystectomy in women: some differences between young and elderly patients. *Scand J Clin Lab Invest*, **52**, 215–20.

Long, C. L., Geiger, J. W., Richards, E. W., Akin, J. M. & Blakemore, W. S. (1992). Plasma amino acid concentrations in geriatric control and hip-fracture patients. *Am J Clin Nutr*, **55**, 1135–41.

McEwen, B. S. (1992). Re-examination of the glucocorticoid hypothesis of stress and aging. *Prog Brain Res*, **93**, 365–81.

Meaney, M. J., O'Donnell, D., Rowe, W., Tannenbaum, B., Steverman, A., Walker, M., Nair, N. P. V. & Lupien, S. (1995). Individual differences in hypothalamic-pituitary-adrenal activity in later life and hippocampal aging. *Exp Gerontol*, **30**, 229–51.

Minaker, K. L., Meneilly, G. S. & Rowe, J. W. (1985). Endocrine systems. In *Handbook of the Biology of Aging*, 2nd edn, ed. C. E. Finch & E. L. Schneider, pp. 433–56. New York: Van Nostrand Reinhold.

Morrow, L. A., Linares, O. A., Hill, T. J., Sanfield, J. A., Supiano, M. A., Rosen, S. G. & Halter, J. B. (1987). Age differences in the plasma clearance mechanisms for epinephrine and norepinephrine in humans. *J Clin Endocr Metab*, **65**, 508–11.

Nelson, K. M., Richards, E. W., Long, C. L., Martin, K. R., Geiger, J. W., Brooks, S. W., Gandy, R. E. & Blakemore, W. S. (1995). Protein and energy balance following femoral neck fracture in geriatric patients. *Metabolism*, **44**, 59–66.

Parker, L. N. (1991). Control of adrenal androgen secretion. *Endocr Metab Clin North Am*, **20**, 401–21.

Pavlov, E. P., Harman, S. M., Chrousos, G. P., Loriaux, D. L. & Blackman, M. R. (1986). Responses of plasma adrenocorticotropin, cortisol, and dehydroepiandrosterone to ovine corticotropin-releasing hormone in healthy aging men. *J Clin Endocr Metab*, **62**, 767–72.

Quint, A. R. & Kaiser, F. E. (1985). Gonadotropin determinations and thyrotropin-releasing hormone and luteinizing hormone-releasing hormone testing in critically ill postmenopausal women with hypothyroxinemia. *J Clin Endocr Metab*, **60**, 464–71.

Reul, J. M. H. M., Rothuizen, J. & de Kloet, E. R. (1991). Age-related changes in the dog hypothalamic–pituitary–adrenocortical system: neuroendocrine activity and corticosteroid receptors. *J Steroid Biochem Mol Biol*, **40**, 63–9.

Roberts, N. A., Barton, R. N., Horan, M. A. & White, A. (1990). Adrenal function after upper femur fracture in elderly people: persistence of stimulation and the roles of adrenocorticotrophic hormone and immobility. *Age Ageing*, **19**, 304–10.

Rogers, J. & Bloom, F. E. (1985). Neurotransmitter metabolism and function in the aging central nervous system. In *Handbook of the Biology of Aging*, 2nd edn, ed. C. E. Finch & E. L. Schneider, pp. 645–91. New York: Van Nostrand Reinhold.

Rosen, C., Donahue, L. R., Hunter, S., Holick, M., Kavookjian, H., Kirschenbaum, A., Mohan, S. & Baylink, D. J. (1992). The 24/25–kDa serum insulin-like growth factor-binding protein is increased in elderly women with hip and spine fractures. *J Clin Endocr Metab*, **74**, 24–7.

Ross, R. J. M., Miell, J. P., Holly, J. M. P., Maheshwari, H., Norman, M., Abdulla, A. F. & Buchanan, C. R. (1991). Levels of GH binding activity, IGFBP-1, insulin, blood glucose and cortisol in intensive care patients. *Clin Endocr*, **35**, 361–7.

Rowe, J. W. & Troen, B. R. (1980). Sympathetic nervous system and aging in man. *Endocr Rev*, **1**, 167–79.

Rozenberg, S., Ham, H., Caufriez, A., Bosson, D., Peretz, A. & Robyn, C. (1990). Sex and adrenal steroids in female in- and outpatients. *Ann New York Acad Sci USA*, **592**, 466–8.

Sapolsky, R. M., Krey, L. C. & McEwen, B. S. (1986). The neuroendocrinology of stress and aging: the glucocorticoid cascade hypothesis. *Endocr Rev*, **7**, 284–301.

Seckl, J. R. & Olsson, T. (1995). Glucocorticoid hypersecretion and the age-impaired hippocampus: cause or effect? *J Endocr*, **145**, 201–11.

Seeman, T. E. & Robbins, R. J. (1994). Aging and the hypothalamic–pituitary–adrenal response to challenge in humans. *Endocr Rev*, **15**, 233–60.

Sharma, R. P., Pandey, G. N., Janicak, P. G., Peterson, J., Comaty, J. E. & Davis, J. M. (1988). The effect of diagnosis and age on the DST: a metaanalytic approach. *Biol Psychiatry*, **24**, 555–68.

Simons, R. J., Simon, J. M., Demers, L. M. & Santen, R. J. (1990). Thyroid dysfunction in elderly hospitalized patients. Effect of age and severity of illness. *Arch Intern Med*, **150**, 1249–53.

Simpkins, J. W. & Millard, W. J. (1987). Influence of age on neurotransmitter function. *Endocr Metab Clin North Am*, **16**, 893–917.

Spaulding, S. W. (1987). Age and the thyroid. *Endocr Metab Clin North Am*, **16**, 1013–25.

Spratt, D. I., Longcope, C., Cox, P. M., Bigos, S. T. & Wilbur-Welling, C. (1993). Differential changes in serum concentrations of androgens and estrogens (in relation with cortisol) in postmenopausal women with acute illness. *J Clin Endocr Metab*, **76**, 1542–7.

Tsitouras, P. D. (1987). Effects of age on testicular function. *Endocr Metab Clin North Am*, **16**, 1045–59.

Vermeulen, A. (1980). Adrenal androgens and aging. In *Adrenal Androgens*, ed. A. R. Genazzani, J. H. H. Thijssen & P. K. Siiteri, pp. 207–17. New York: Raven Press.

Wagner, R. K. (1978). Extracellular and intracellular steroid binding proteins. Properties, discrimination, assay and clinical applications. *Acta Endocr*, Suppl. **218**.

Warren, M. P., Siris, E. S. & Petrovich, C. (1977). The influence of severe illness on gonadotropin secretion in the postmenopausal female. *J Clin Endocr Metab*, **45**, 99–104.

Watters, J. M., Clancey, S. M., Moulton, S. B., Briere, K. M. & Zhu, J.-M. (1993). Impaired recovery of strength in older patients after major abdominal surgery. *Ann Surg*, **218**, 380–90.

Watters, J. M., Redmond, M. L., Desai, D. & March, R. J. (1990). Effects of age and body composition on the metabolic responses to elective colon resection. *Ann Surg*, **212**, 213–20.

17

Perioperative management

F. CARLI and H. T. DAVENPORT

Introduction

As the proportion of elderly persons in the population has increased so injury to the elderly has become more common. Most authors have reported that older people are more vulnerable to injury and have a reduced capacity for recovery compared with younger individuals (Lauer, 1959; Hogue, 1982; McCoy *et al.*, 1989). Although this age group comprises approximately 10–13% of the population, they represent 25% of all injury fatalities. While the death rate from accidental injury per 100000 persons has been reported to be approximately 40–50 for all ages combined, it rises to 80–90 for persons aged 65–74 years, 200 for those aged 75–84 and over 500 for persons aged 85 years or older (Iskrant & Joliet, 1968).

As trauma has become increasingly sophisticated, more attention has focused on the potential for rehabilitation after injury. Some authors have raised questions about the quality of life after serious trauma, particularly among elderly patients. Few studies have examined the long-term outcome of injured patients in this age group. Oreskovich *et al.* (1984) analysed the injury patterns and the outcome in 100 consecutive patients aged over 70 years with multiple injuries, and they found that the mortality for the group was 15%. While 85% of the injured patients survived, 88% of these did not return to their previous level of independence, and 72% required continuous nursing home care 1 year after discharge.

A second report, from a different American centre, studied 63 survivors of blunt trauma over the age of 65 years between 9 and 38 months after hospital discharge (DeMaria *et al.*, 1987a). In contrast to the previous study these authors reported that immediately after discharge 33% were independent, 37% were dependent but living at home and 30% required nursing home care. The last group of patients were older, more severely injured and requiring surgery more frequently. On the basis of these findings, these authors therefore supported the contention that aggressive treatment of the elderly trauma victim appears justified, as few patients require nursing home care and the majority can return to independent living after trauma.

Marx *et al.*, in 1986, in a well-designed study comparing over 70 years old patients who sustained polytrauma with a group of younger patients matched for similar pattern of injuries, showed that the greater mortality in the older patients was due to pre-existing medical disorders. Nevertheless, most of the older patients who survived could be satisfactorily rehabilitated. This reiterated the concept that adequate intensive treatment may improve the outcome even in the aged population.

Among the body regions injured the low extremities appear to be the most commonly involved. In this context, femoral fractures are relatively frequent with fall being the commonest mechanism of injury (Brocklehurst *et al.*, 1978; Boyce & Vessey, 1985). A working party on fractured neck of femur, set up in 1987 by the Royal College of Physicians, reported high mortality both perioperative and subsequently, with only a minority of the oldest old patients being able to regain their former mobility. Using current age- and sex-specific incidence rates for hip fracture in England and Wales, the probability that a woman will suffer a fractured hip before the age of 85 years is 12%; for a man it is 5%. The number of cases expected will almost double in 20 years' time, from 46000 to 94000 (Boyce *et al.*, 1985). Analysis of the figures from Northwick Park Hospital, a district general hospital in the North London area, over a period of 2 years in a population of elderly patients admitted with fracture of femur shows a hospital death rate of 1% in ages between 65 and 74 years, about 10% in ages between 75 and 84 years and 15–20% in ages between 85 and 94 years. Overall in 75% of deaths cardiopulmonary disease was the cause. Hospital stay varied between 3 and 200 days and only 10% of all the deaths occurred within the first week following surgery.

The increase in patients admitted with fractured hips will put considerable strain on the service available and needs careful planning of staff and facilities required.

A review of the literature on post-hip fracture mortality reveals a mortality rate higher than that of the general population in all studies. In those studies based on survival of at least 1 year following hip fracture, the mortality rates ranged from 14 to 36% (DeMaria *et al.*, 1987a). Mortality rates based solely on in-hospital postoperative deaths are inadequate as deaths continue to occur after hospital discharge at an increased rate above the general population.

Factors considered significant in influencing patient mortality are age, pre-existing medical conditions, postoperative level of ambulation and rehabilitation (Sixson & Lehner, 1988; Mahul *et al.*, 1991). In all studies reported the mortality rate for different age groups was 5–10% for the 60–69 years old, 12–15% for the 70–79 years old, 14–17% for the 80–89 years old and 30–37% for the 90–99 years old. Amongst the pre-existing medical conditions cerebral dysfunction (organic brain syndrome, senile dementia and severe Parkinson's disease) and chronic cardiorespiratory disorders contributed significantly to the high mortality rate. Postoperative complications such as pneumonia, wound infections and cardiovascular disorders are implicated in the cause of early death.

While it may appear that mortality rate in the aged following accidental injury cannot be reduced substantially more than has been achieved, further epidemiological studies are needed to investigate the role of intensive management in rehabilitation and quality of life in this particular group of individuals. It has been emphasised in many studies, including the report by the Royal College of Physicians, that besides prevention of trauma in the elderly subjects, a high standard of perioperative care must be ensured. This needs a team-orientated approach with involvement of senior medical, nursing and paramedical staff able to produce an effective therapeutic strategy and the monitoring of standards of care and outcome.

The aim of the authors of this article is to consider some of the most relevant aspects of perioperative management of accidental injury in the aged patients, which should help clinicians to formulate a care plan.

Assessment and preparation before operation

The perioperative period is not clearly defined and thus any available data are rarely comparable. It is clear that assessment and preparation before operation are doubly important in patients who may have reduced reserves. Also without careful follow-up for postoperative complications there will be little likelihood of progressive improvement of care. In all recent studies of morbidity and mortality in relation to anaesthesia it is evident there has been a considerable reduction in the past two decades (Buck *et al.*, 1987). Also anaesthesia plays a less important part in these figures than the surgery and acute medical state of the patient, although in many instances it is a combination of factors.

The most consistent reported correlation between postoperative complications and death is the American Society of Anesthesiology grading of the patient's medical state before operation (Keats, 1978). With accident patients who undergo emergency surgery which entails a twofold increase of morbidity this is not grossly increased by the poor medical condition of the patient. The optimal time for operating must allow for stabilisation of the patient, without which it is obvious that there is uncontrollable bleeding or vital organs are in jeopardy. Conversely, undue delay will lead to the gamut of ills that arise from enforced bed rest (Kenzora *et al.*, 1984).

It is widely accepted that emergency surgery in elderly patients is associated with a markedly higher incidence of intraoperative and postoperative complications and/or death compared with younger patients. When examining the role that the patient's age plays as a risk factor for aged individuals undergoing anaesthesia and surgery, the distinction between physiological age and chronological age becomes important. The greater risk of perioperative morbidity and mortality as a result of anaesthesia and surgery appears to be related to two separate factors: first, an increased prevalence of age-related concomitant diseases, and second, a decline in basic organ function. Tiret and colleagues (Tiret *et al.*, 1986) in a French survey on 198103 anaesthetics demonstrated that the rate of complications related far more closely to the number of associated diseases with which the patients presented rather than patients' age.

Elderly people can mount an adequate response to injury, but they are not equipped with the best of reserves capable of sustaining a prolonged insult to body functions. A large majority of patients with accidental injuries undergo surgery in a very short time and this may cause further stress on the whole organism. In planning a therapeutic rationale for perioperative management the clinician has to be aware of the major changes in cardiovascular and metabolic functions occurring with aging. Similarly, in pharmacokinetic and pharmacodynamic responses and changes in body compartments to a variety of anaesthetic drugs help in the design of an optimal anaesthetic technique which should aim at minimising the insult associated with surgery.

Recognising that acute disease in these patients with varying degrees of chronic disability is the crucial risk factor, every patient coming for operation after injury requires careful medical assessment. In emergency situations there may be a very limited period of time for preparation consequent upon the assessment but it does allow tailoring of postoperative management. It must also be accepted that in some instances cancellation or postponement of operations may be in the patient's best interest.

In the case of head injury for example mortality predictors include the Glasgow score (Teasdale & Jennett, 1974), the presence of inoperable haematoma, the cause of injury and presence of other damage as well as age. Obviously a most satisfactory perioperative course is probable if the patient has sound cardiopulmonary function. Disease and complication can be anticipated with these systems in the presence of a history of chest disease or any cardiovascular problem, smoking, limited mobility, effort intolerance and extreme obesity or thinness (i.e. a high ASA (American Society of Anesthesiology) score).

Pre-existing cardiorespiratory diseases predispose the elderly injured to severe risks of further cardiovascular dysfunction and mortality. When time is allowed, it is essential that unstable angina, cardiac failure and hypertension are treated by delaying surgery for 24–48 hours. There is now good evidence from several studies that treatment of these conditions in the elderly with fractured hip prior to surgery is associated with less mortality and morbidity (Schnets *et al.*, 1985).

Systolic blood pressure control is essential during surgery as arterial pressure may be responsible for an acute loading of the left ventricle with the risk of compromising the balance of oxygen supply and demand. Particular attention must be paid to avoid any reduced ventricular compliance as this increases the sensitivity of the cardiovascular system to changes in preload; even a modest decrease of the circulating volume may cause a large reduction in cardiac output. The pulmonary problems most likely to be encountered by anaesthetists caring for aged patients are: (1) an impairment of gas exchange with more frequent and profound hypoxaemia due to prolonged dependent lung atelectasis, (2) a greater degree of airway resistance, and (3) impaired control of ventilation and (4) respiratory muscle fatigue.

When using controlled ventilation, particular attention must be given to limiting the mean intrathoracic pressure (Editorial, 1987) but providing 'appropriate' distension of the bronchi (Campbell *et al.*, 1962). From the history the extent of preoperative testing is decided. As stated this is variable and limited by the urgency of the operation. It is salutary to note that eliciting the patient's subjective account of dyspnoea or sputum production (Nunn *et al.*, 1988), careful respiratory rate counting (McFadden *et al.*, 1982) and palpating the pulse strength or temperature of a digit can be highly informative (Joly & Weil, 1969). Sophisticated tests have in no study as yet been proven invaluable in old patients. Any patient with evidence of cardiac failure from whatever cause clearly needs any extra means of preparation and monitoring that may permit survival (Chapters 12 and 18).

Thromboembolism

For every patient immobilised by injury or major operation over the age of 40 years there is a considerable risk of thromboembolism. International multicentre trials have long since proven the value of low dose subcutaneous heparin as a prophylaxis. The newer low molecular weight heparin which is less likely to cause bleeding complications and because of a longer half-life allows once daily injection may become a favoured routine with or without laboratory measurement of antifactor XA activity (Samama *et al.*, 1988).

Renal failure

Of the various biological decrements due to age, creatinine clearance is one of the most common through diminished glomular filtration rate. This is protected most by ensuring good blood supply and meticulous fluid and electrolyte balance, both of which can be in serious jeopardy in the injured patient. The older patient's inability to concentrate or dilute urine will also make deficiencies and excesses of fluid balance poorly tolerated. Although renal insufficiency is often apparent, failure is not common perioperatively in older patients, but when it does occur mortality is high (Seymour & Vaz, 1989). If the routine use of balance charts and bladder catheterisation shows a urine output of less than 30 ml per hour prophylactic use of mannitol or dopamine should be considered and a nephrologist involved in the management to produce a better understanding of the older patient's kidney action in stress.

The aged diabetic

It is widely accepted that decreased glucose tolerance is evident with aging. Ten per cent of those over 65 years old are said to be suffering from diabetes mellitus. In emergency conditions a random blood sugar of 11 mmol/l (or fasting blood sugar higher than 7.2 mmol/l) is usually diagnostic. The aged are more likely to develop non-ketotic hyperosmolar coma, even those that are non-insulin dependent. As this can happen rapidly it is advisable to measure blood sugar frequently, including during long operations, and by titrating of glucose and insulin, the blood sugar should be maintained within a range of 6–12 mmol/l (Alberti & Thomas, 1979).

Pressure sores

With older immobile injured patients lying on hard surfaces perioperatively there is a considerable risk of pressure sores developing (Vershnysen, 1986). This may well be related to hypotension (Schubert, 1991). The effect of shearing or folding of skin can also initiate damage, thus resting on a hard surface should be of minimal duration and sliding or lifting undertaken with extreme care.

Other considerations

Drug handling

Elderly patients frequently present with multiple pathology together with a variety of medications. Distribution of drugs into fat soluble and water soluble compartments is therefore very variable. In the presence of hypovolaemia the dose has to be chosen with care. Anaesthetic agents are cardiovascular depressants except for ketamine which could be the drug of choice for the injured elderly who are also hypovolaemic.

As the minimal alveolar concentration for all inhalational anaesthetic gases and vapours is decreased with age (Stevens *et al.*, 1975), it follows that the initial induction will be easier when it is carried out with an inhalational agent or following a small dose of an intravenous induction agent. The use of small doses of opioid has the advantage over inhalational agents of providing cardiovascular stability, but this has to be done with care because of the serious risk of postoperative respiratory depression in a spontaneously breathing subject. The reversal of a neuromuscular blocking agent in the elderly is best carried out with neostigmine and glycopyrrolate which is less likely to cause central nervous system effects such as delayed awakening, confusion, hallucinations and memory loss or the arrhythmias produced by atropine (Muravchick *et al.*, 1979).

Heat balance

Hypothermia, defined as a core temperature of less than 36 °C, is common in severely traumatised patients, and its aetiology is multifactorial; heat loss is increased partly as a result of the immobilising effect of injury and the administration of cold fluids during resuscitation (Luna *et al.*, 1987), and partly as a result of impaired thermoregulation (Little & Stoner, 1981). In the elderly, this can be accentuated by the fact that they have reduced activity, they lack thermogenic nutrients in the diet and they have less lean body and muscle mass. These can contribute to a reduced metabolic and vasomotor response to a cold stimulus (Collins, 1987).

During the ebb phase shivering in traumatised patients can be absent despite having a body temperature below the normal threshold for shivering. The rate of fall in body temperature is directly related to the severity of injury. When their core temperature reaches normal values (flow phase) traumatised patients act as if they were cold and select an environment with a temperature that would be too warm for an uninjured patient.

Although a cold environment can aggravate hypothermia, it is not essential for it to develop. Hypothermia in elderly trauma victims is generally considered an ominous sign with increased morbidity and mortality. The study reported by Jurkovich *et al.* (1987) appears to identify a critical temperature in the trauma patient at admission of 32 °C below which no one in his series survived. This critical temperature, identified as an ominous predictor of mortality, was independent of the Injury Severity Score, presence of shock and volume of resuscitation fluids.

A plan of care is of paramount importance during the period of resuscitation and subsequently if surgery is needed. Monitoring body temperature at admission in casualty is often limited to an occasional measurement of axillary temperature. This site not only gives inaccurate readings of core temperature, but does not provide continuous monitoring during the rewarming phase. Aural canal/tympanic membrane (brain temperature) and oesophagus (myocardial temperature) are suggested sites for continuous measurement of core temperature. These sites are more reliable than oral, axillary and rectal ones (Cork *et al.*, 1982). The treatment of hypothermic patients is dependent on the extent of the lowered temperature: the more compromised the circulation, respiration and metabolism, the more urgent the treatment should be (Carli, 1989). Shivering must be avoided as this represents a major stress in the already compromised situation; the increase in oxygen consumption and lactic acid can precipitate respiratory failure and myocardial ischaemia (Roe *et al.*, 1966; Bay *et al.*, 1968).

A warming environment must be provided soon after arrival in the casualty department and continued throughout the perioperative period. A microclimate around the patient has been suggested by using a hot water mattress for skin surface warming and humidified warmed gas and warmed intravenous fluids for core warming. Radiant heat (thermal ceiling) applied to the torso and blush area has been shown to be effective in attenuating shivering, causing vasodilatation with less likelihood of a hypertensive crisis (Sharkley *et al.*, 1987). This piece of equipment has the advantage of maintaining a microclimate around the patient when resuscitative manoeuvres are in process, but it is expensive and occupies much space.

During surgery the warming device should continue to be applied because during operation patients also lose body heat. At the end of surgery the hypothermic elderly patient (core temperature less than 34 °C) who has a history of severe cardiorespiratory disorders should not be allowed to regain body heat at the expense of compromising the cardiovascular system. There is ample evidence of increased secretion of catecholamines and raised metabolic rate when no precaution is taken to maintain normothermia (Carli *et al.*, 1992). On the contrary, the use of either morphine and/or muscle relaxants combined with ventilatory support not only prolongs the rewarming time but also abolishes the increase in energy expenditure and production of lactic acid (Rodriguez *et al.*, 1983).

It is not clear whether hypothermia per se is a cause of mortality or is a response to the severity of injury (Steinemanns *et al.*, 1990). In the latter case it could represent a protective response to the major metabolic demands of injury. Aggressive rewarming techniques in the injured elderly are recommended while more controlled trials on this important aspect of trauma care need to be conducted (Gentinello *et al.*, 1990). The patient most at risk is perhaps the one who suffers hyperthermia.

Regional or general anaesthesia?

In this context we should consider the interactions between anaesthesia, the metabolic response to injury and the outcome. Regional anaesthetic techniques for the aged have attracted considerable interest in the past 10–15 years for the following reasons. They can provide profound analgesia, preservation of consciousness, effective muscle relaxation and good sympathetic blockade. In addition, regional anaesthesia blocks the afferent stimuli and therefore inhibits the metabolic response to injury and the metabolic consequence of it (Kehlet, 1984). This could be beneficial in the sense that the sustained increased demands on vital organs such as heart, lung and circulation as a result of the injury would be attenuated. Several studies have examined the influence of regional anaesthesia on surgical morbidity and mortality in elective surgery, and the overall consensus appears to be that complications such as postoperative hypoxaemia, bronchopneumonia and thromboembolic complications have all been shown to be decreased compared with general anaesthesia (Modig *et al.*, 1983; Scott & Kehlet, 1988). Some papers have reported quite remarkable differences in mortality, with the advantages being with regional anaesthesia (Yaeger *et al.*, 1987); however, these major differences have not been confirmed (Seeling *et al.*, 1990).

Outcome studies on the effect of regional anaesthesia for accidental injury have been limited to fracture of the hip, and it has been shown that this technique appears to reduce early postoperative mortality, but long-term survival of patients is, not surprisingly, dependent on factors other than the choice of anaesthetic (McKenzie *et al.*, 1984; Valentin *et al.*, 1986; Davis *et al.*, 1987). The use of local anaesthetic techniques in the presence of abdominal or thoracic trauma in elderly patients is sporadic and no extensive epidemiological studies on the beneficial effects of regional anaesthesia have so far been conducted. This might be due to several reasons, such as the risk of severe hypotension in the presence of hypovolaemia and an unstable cardiovascular condition, presence of clotting defects, technical difficulties in achieving a satisfactory blockade and to some extent the limitations of the local anaesthetic agents available at the present time.

While there has been a tendency to regard regional blockade as a more suitable technique for the less fit patient than general anaesthesia, the advent of new drugs together with a better understanding of their effects has enabled anaesthetists to use general anaesthesia in patients with accidental injuries. This technique is often chosen by the anaesthetist because it is the quickest way of achieving satisfactory conditions for the surgeon to start work. The conventional wisdom of using light general anaesthesia has been replaced by a well-balanced technique which attempts to attenuate nociceptive stimuli and catecholamine secretion. The already high circulating concentration of these hormones, as a result of the accidental injury, can have profound ill effects on the cardiovascular and metabolic systems.

Adjustments of ventilation, adequate myocardial filling pressure and optimisation of tissue blood flow are essential prerequisites for the maintenance of an oxygen supply to the aged brain and myocardium. Scott & Kehlet (1988), in a review article on the effect of regional anaesthesia on surgical morbidity, have pointed out that morbidity appears to be reduced only when procedures below the umbilicus are concerned. Evidence of the beneficial effect of regional blockade appears less convincing for upper abdominal and thoracic procedures. Few articles have been published on major surgery and epidural blockade, however, with special reference to immediate and late morbidity. Yaeger *et al.* (1987) showed that the use of regional blockade in high risk patients undergoing major thoracic or abdominal surgery makes a major impact on the outcome. These results are striking, and even though the sample sizes are not large, the findings suggest that significant improvement in outcomes might be made by using epidural anaesthesia and analgesia in high risk subjects. We are not aware of studies of this category of patients undergoing major surgery for accidental injuries. It might also be appropriate to establish a regional analgesia regimen as soon as the patients arrive in the accident department with potential beneficial effect on peripheral circulation and pain control. Controlled clinical trials are needed in the near future to identify the role of regional blockade, established throughout the perioperative period, in immediate and late outcome. While mortality cannot be to a great extent further reduced attention should be directed to the effect of anaesthetic administration on rehabilitation, convalescence, mental status and muscle fatigue.

Monitoring (Figure 17.1)

In general terms there are special considerations required during monitoring of older subjects. This includes simple technical matters such as careful application or removal of electrodes because of the thin, easily damaged skin and recognition of the tortuous easily damaged vessels which constrict poorly and can cause haematomas. In the case of arteries, plaques or sclerosis may lead to vessel fracture and emboli during cannulation. In functional terms there is great difficulty in interpreting results obtained by routine monitoring of heart rate, blood pressure, respiration, metabolism or secretion of hormones. This is because physiological, pharmacological and even mechanical stimuli may not produce the same response in the old as in the young. Thus in the case of the heart rate with stress the increase is on average 20% less than it would be in the young subject. With hypoxia the increase in heart rate will be a third of that experienced with younger patients and most dramatically hypercarbia can cause no increase of heart rate in the old but a consistent small increase in the young. Blood pressure changes from whatever cause are inclined to be more sudden and larger through reduced compliance and autonomic control of the vascular system (Charlson *et al.*, 1990). With significant arteriosclerosis a sphygmomanometer cuff will not compress the vessels easily and may produce a misleadingly high recording, hence the suggestion that the periphery of the arm or leg may be a better area to apply the cuff. If there is no valvular heart disease and no likelihood of a reduced ejection fraction then central venous pressure is helpful. Otherwise for the serious 'at risk' patient more central measurements are required (Chapter 18). Although the Swan Ganz catheter has been used for this purpose for two decades the indications and interpretation of this monitoring technique in the old are still unclear (Nadeau & Noble, 1986).

The external jugular or the femoral vessels is preferable as a route of entry because of the fear of covert damage: the majority of serious complications with this technique reported to date have been in older patients. Two purely age-related changes of heart function are an increase of left ventricular diastolic pressure and pulmonary artery wedge pressure, which have to be allowed for.

When monitoring the respiratory system it is recognised that during and after anaesthesia hypoxaemia commonly occurs in the old. Less well studied are important changes in the patency of the upper airway and central nervous respiratory and strong analgesics. While the respiratory distress syndrome after trauma can have an up to 60% mortality, with renal failure it is much greater especially in the old. While creatinine clearance is a good indicator of the lack of concentration power of the kidneys one again must allow for this occurring naturally with age to a marked extent (Rowe *et al.*, 1976). Fluid and electrolyte balance charting is most important together with acid–base studies as indicated.

In this regard two important factors are maintaining urine output at 0.5–1 ml per kg per hour and recognition that a rise of pH in the blood leads to a drop of potassium. The recent increased use of the oximeter and capnograph should markedly improve the care of older patients, particularly if not limited to the period of operation. When patients are mechanically ventilated it is crucial to remember that the unanaesthetised and the young can compensate by changing the vascular capacity for the effects of compression on the venous return vessels whereas others cannot, particularly the old. Temperature

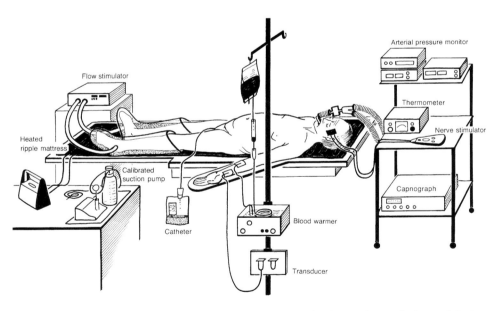

Figure 17.1. Additional aids to perioperative care in the aged. Routinely used devices such as the electrocardiograph, automatic BP and pulse oximeter have been omitted.

monitoring as explained elsewhere in this chapter is crucial but poorly perfused skin is an unsuitable site for measurement and the oesophagus or external ear is preferred. The clinical need to measure neuromuscular function when relaxants are used in old patients is paramount but not widely applied owing to the poor development of a suitable apparatus. Electroencephalography monitoring has to allow for a 30–40% abnormal wave pattern prevalence in older patients and this must be also allowed for in the imminent wider use of evoked potentials for anaesthesia depth measurement. As heart pacemakers are common in older patients the effect of widely used cautery on their activity must be countered by applying the ground plate and active cautery as far away from the pacemaker as possible and accepting that electrocardiographic monitoring is mandatory (Simon, 1977). Metabolic and hormone system monitoring is still experimental. As a low albumin clearly indicates a poor prognosis perhaps its control, as one would sugar in a diabetic, would be worth exploring.

Fluid and electrolyte balance is discussed in detail in Chapter 15. For anaesthetists the most dramatic occurrence is acute hyponatraemia which in the aged will present mostly as mental impairment and confusion. While it may be due to polypharmacy and multiple pathology in the case of the syndrome of inappropriate secretion of antidurietic hormone (Thomas *et al.*, 1978), it is most commonly caused by an acute respiratory infection. In the injury situation, both surgical and accidental trauma and psychological stress may be aetiological. It appears frequently in the second or third day after operation when the staff's attention is less intense.

Premedication

Sedation and anxiolysis are rarely indicated in older patients undergoing urgent surgery. Pain relief should be obtained through intermittent or continuous parenteral narcotics in very small doses (particularly in the presence of renal insufficiency). Anticholinergic drugs are now unnecessary and indeed unacceptable due to their side-effects (Bartus *et al.*, 1982). Ranitidine and metoclopramide may be used to reduce the risk of aspiration although this is rare in injured patients. Steroid supplementation may be required for those treated with steroids within 2 months of the operation. While there are a variety of regimens for the older vulnerable patient needing variable monitoring, it may be sensible to administer intramuscular hydrocortisone for 2–3 days. Antihypertensive therapy is best continued as there are few interactions with modern anaesthetics and maintenance of treatment provides a more stable patient (Dagmino & Prys-Roberts, 1986). If hypertensive untreated patients are encountered, to prevent any associated tachycardia, pulmonary oedema or myocardial ischaemia, those with a diastolic pressure greater than 120 mmHg require intravenous use of hydralazine or labetalol.

Anaesthetic management

In the hurried conditions of emergency or urgent operations corrections of hypovolaemia, hypothermia and electrolyte or acid–base imbalance are not refinements but need unrushed attention however inconvenient. Of investigations the FEV I, systolic blood pressure, creatinine clearance of blood and glucose tolerance correlate most with operative survival. Rapid sequence induction is indicated with hiatus hernia, obesity, obstruction, etc. and the dose of succinylcholine and thiopentone (and particularly the more potent propofol) must be carefully chosen because hypotension following their use is commoner in older patients. There is no clear information to indicate a preference between volatile and intravenous agents for maintenance of anaesthesia in older patients.

With controlled ventilation it is important to avoid overventilation with consequent decrease of $PaCO_2$ and possible reduction of cerebral blood flow and tissue oxygen affinity. Peak inspiratory pressure should be as low as possible to prevent cardiovascular effects and increase in the incidence of postoperative deep vein thrombosis. Blood loss requires meticulous replacement but the usual complications of a massive transfusion may be of more consequence in the old. Reduction of temperature, 2,3, DPG, calcium and magnesium and raised potassium may be important as are thrombocytopenia and reduced factors v and viii. Ultrafiltration of transfusions is recommended but adult respiratory distress syndrome seems more related to the injury experienced. Local anaesthetic management should be as complete as with general anaesthesia including the same monitoring, preparation for any complication and ensuring patient comfort. Various forms of autonomic block have the advantage of preventing heart rate and pressure increases with associated myocardial ischaemia. The only problems are prolonged clearance of agents, and therefore an increased risk of accumulation, and a marked sensitivity to supplementary drug administration, for example sedatives (Wildsmith, 1988). One must remember that a sympathetic block will increase vasodilation and may make the patient more prone to hypothermia and/or tissue damage.

Postoperative management

As previously indicated much of the excess postoperative morbidity in the aged relates to pre-existing medical problems. Therefore planning postoperative management should be arranged accordingly and high dependency nursing and rehabilitation organised as needed. Problems will present atypically and need more awareness of their likelihood. Oxygen should be given postoperatively to all patients. A concentration of 36% is most suitable. While prolonged artificial ventilation after major surgery or injury should be freely used the difficulty is deciding when to wean the patient.

While judgement regimens using blood gases are available simpler clinical judgements concerning the general well-being of the patient, including an active autonomic system as indicated by the presence of bowel sounds, and the intermittent use of a trial weaning and careful counting of respiration subsequently can be used. This can be refined by the use of assisted ventilation systems such as the mandatory minute volume device. Patients with lung or chest wall injury and, of course, tetanus will require prolonged ventilation and substitution of the nasotracheal tube by tracheotomy. Whenever tracheal toilet is difficult, a mini-tracheotomy can be desirable.

Relief of pain

Relief of pain in the old injured patient requires understanding of three general facts. Initial perfection of pain relief immediately postoperatively will markedly reduce the total pain experience. A preoperative explanation of the pain liable to be experienced and its management will reduce anxiety and diminish the overall need of analgesia even more than in younger patients (Egberg *et al.*, 1964) and, most important, whatever method is employed must not represent an added danger. Patient controlled analgesia and continuous epidural block applied by a pain control team is at present advocated as ideal in 1990 by the Royal College of Surgeons of England. We believe that continuous intravenous or subcutaneous administration with a pump-driven syringe by ward staff that are 'pain conscious' and suitably documented audit of treatment are the most widely useful and safe method (Davenport *et al.*, 1985). This may be supplemented by wound infiltration with long-acting local anaesthetics, rectal or other parenteral use of non-steroidal anti-inflammatory drugs, and even the application of a transcutaneous electrical nerve stimulator, which can be miraculous with bowel stasis and is innocuous. When narcotics are administered continuous use of doxapram has been shown to be protective of respiratory complications and needs further trial (Jansen *et al.*, 1990).

Mental changes

As in non-surgical situations a great majority of cases of acute confusional or delirium states are due to acute physical illness, particularly infection, metabolic upset or drugs, especially those with anticholinergic or sedative action. Anaesthetic emergency delirium can be due to pain, shock or hypoxia and may be aborted by intravenous physostigmine. It is also possible that such delirium is due to withdrawal from alcohol, benzodiazepines or other psychoactive drugs. If there is the converse delayed recovery of consciousness covert brain damage, drugs, hypothermia, hypoglycaemia or myxoedema must all be considered. A remoter or 'interval delirium' does occur on the second to seventh postoperative day (Seymour, 1986). This or more chronic changes are mostly observed in those with ventilation problems or myocardial infarction and in over the age of 80 years after very major surgery or injury. It could be related to subacute hypoxia and may indeed cause an alteration in memory, orientation and emotions which is only noticeable by close relatives or friends. For the management of the chronically mentally disturbed in hospital judicious use of diazepam or droperidol may be indicated.

Reliance, however, must be mostly on repeated simple explanation to the patient by the nursing staff of the circumstances and care required and encouragement by frequent visits of relatives and friends close to the patient. It is salutary to know that confusion after operation in elderly patients is four times as common in those who later become demented. Whether this is an inherent or a 'cause and effect' relation is unproven. This emphasises that much is unknown about older patients and by studying their care in detail we can learn a great deal that will benefit patients of all ages.

Conclusion

Geriatricians rightly stress the great disparity of old patients and the need to provide medical attention to patients always in relation to their pathophysiology not their age. The attention can be jeopardised by second-rate inappropriate anaesthetic or surgical actions perioperatively, especially in an emergency. Particularly in treating old or young patients the highest standard of care is necessary and this requires managers to provide superior staff and facilities.

Refences

Alberti, K. G. M. M. & Thomas, D. J. B. (1979). The management of diabetes during surgery. *Br J Anaesth*, **51**, 693–703.

Anonymous. (1986). Prevention of venous thrombosis and pulmonary embolism. National Institutes of Health Development Conference Consensus Statement. **6**, 1–8.

Bartus, R. T., Dean, R. L., Beer, B. & Lippas, A. S. (1982). The cholinergic hypothesis of geriatric memory dysfunction. *Science*, **217**, 408–14.

Bay, J., Nunn, J. F. & Prys-Roberts, C. (1968). Factors influencing arterial PO_2 during recovery from anaesthesia. *Br J Anaesthes*, **40**, 398–407.

Boyce, W. J. & Vessey, M. P. (1985). Rising incidence of fracture of the proximal femur. *Lancet*, **1**, 150–1.

Brocklehurst, J. C., Exton-Smith, A. N., Lempert Barber, S. M., Hunt, L. P. & Palmer, M. K. (1978). Fracture of the femur in old age: a two-centre study of associated clinical factors and the cause of the fall. *Age Ageing*, **7**, 7–15.

Buck, M., Devlin, H. B. & Lunn, J. H. (1987). *Confidential enquiry into perioperative deaths*. London: Nuffield Provincial Hospital Trust.

Campbell, E. J. M. & Howell, J. B. L. (1962). *Proprioceptive Control of Breathing in Pulmonary Structure and Function*, ed. A. V. S. de Rueck & M. O'Connor. Edinburgh: Churchill Livingstone.

Carli, F. (1989). Metabolic disturbances of hypothermia. *Clin Anaesthesiol*, **3**, 405–21.

Carli, F., Webster, J., Nandi, P., Pearson, J. & MacDonald, I. (1992). Thermogenesis after major surgery: the effect of perioperative heart conservation and epidural anesthesia. *Am J Physiol*, **263**, E441–E449.

Charlson, M. E., MacKenrie, C. R., Gold, J. P., Ales, K. L., Topkins, M. & Shires, G. T. (1990). Intraoperative blood pressure: what problems identify patients at risk of perioperative complications. *Ann Surg*, **212**, 567–580.

Collins, K. J. (1987). Effects of cold and old people. *Br J Hosp Med*, **37**, 506–14.

Cork, R. C., Vaughan, R. W. & Humphrey, L. S. (1982). Precision and accuracy of intraoperative temperature monitoring. *Anaesthesia Analgesia*, **61**, 284–7.

Covert, C. R. & Fox, G. S. (1989). Anaesthesia for hip surgery in the elderly. *Can J Anaesthesia*, **36**, 311–19.

Dagmino, J. & Prys-Roberts, C. (1986). *Anesthesia in the Hypertensive Patient in Geriatric Anesthesia: Principles of Practice*, ed. C. R. Stephens Association of R.A.E. Boston: Butterworth.

Davenport, H. T., Al-Khudairi, D., Cox, P. N. & Wright, B. M. (1985). Continuous subcutaneous pethidine for routine postoperative analgesia. *Ann R Coll Surg*, **67**, 379–81.

Davis, F. M., Woolner, D. F., Frampton, C., Wilikinson, A., Grant, A., Harrison, R. T., Roberts, M. T. S. & Thadaka, R. (1987). Prospective, multi-centre trial of morbidity following general or spinal anaesthesia for hip fracture surgery in the elderly. *Br J Anaesthesia*, **59**, 1080–8.

DeMaria, E. J., Kenney, P. R., Merriam, M. A., Casanova, L. A. & Gann, D. S. (1987a). Survival after trauma in geriatric patients. *Ann Surg*, **206**, 738–43.

DeMaria, E. J., Kenney, P. R., Merriam, M. A., Casanova, L. A. & Gann, D. S. (1987b). Aggressive trauma care benefits the elderly. *J Trauma*, **27**, 1200–5.

Editorial. (1987). Effects of ventilation on circulation. *Br Med J*, **1**, 283.

Egbert, L. D. (1964). Reduction of perioperative pain by encouragement and instruction of patients. *New Engl J Med*, **270**, 825–7.

Gentinello, L. M., Cortes, V., Moujaes, S., Viamonte, M., Malinin, T., Ho, C. H. & Gomez, G. A. (1990). Continuous arteriovenous rewarming experimental results and thermodynamic model simulation of treatment for hypothermia. *J Trauma*, **30**, 1436–49.

Hogue, C. C. (1982). Injury in late life. Part I. Epidemiology. *J Am Geriatr Soc*, **30**, 183–90.

Iskrant, A. P. & Joliet, P. V. (1968). *Accident and Homicide*, Cambridge: Harvard University Press.

Jansen, J. E., Sorensen, A. I., Naesh, O., Erichsen, C. J. & Pedersen, A. (1990). Effect of doxapram on postoperative pulmonary complications after upper abdominal surgery in high risk patients. *Lancet*, **335**, 936–8.

Joly, H. B. & Weil, M. H. (1969). Temperature of the great toe age as an initiation of the severity of shock. *Circulation*, **39**, 131–8.

Jurkovich, G. J., Greiser, W. B., Luteaman, A. & Curreri, P. W. (1987). Hypothermia in trauma victims. An ominous prediction of survival. *J Trauma*, **27**, 1019–24.

Keats, A. S. (1978). The A.S.A. classification of physical status: a recapitulation. *Anesthesiology*, **49**, 233.

Kehlet, H. (1984). The stress response to anaesthesia and surgery. Release mechanisms and modifying factors. *Clin Anaesthesiol*, **2**, 315–39.

Kenzora, J. E., McCarthy, R. E., Lowell, J. D. & Sledge, C. B. (1984). Hip fracture mortality, relation to age, treatment, preoperative illness, time of surgery and complications. *Clin Orthop*, **186**, 45–56.

Lauer, A. R. (1959). Age and sex in relation to accident. *Traffic Saf Res Rev*, **3**, 21–3.

Little, R. A. & Stoner, H. B. (1981). Body temperature after accidental injury. *Br J Surg*, **68**, 221–4.

Luna, G. K., Maier, R. V., Pavlin, E. G., Anardi, D., Copass, M. K. & Oreskovich, M. R. (1987). Incidence and effect of hypothermia in seriously injured patients. *J Trauma*, **27**, 1014–18.

McCoy, G. F., Johnstone, R. A. & Duthie, R. B. (1989). Injury to the elderly in road traffic accidents. *J Trauma*, **29**, 494–7.

McFadden, J. P., Price, R. C., Eastwood, H. R. & Briggs, R. S. (1982). Raised respiratory rate in elderly patients: a valuable physical sign. *Br Med J*, **284**, 626–7.

McKenzie, P. J., Wisharthy, S. & Smith, G. (1984). Long-term outcome after repair of fractured neck of femur. *Br J Anaesthesia*, **56**, 581–5.

Mahul, P., Perrot, D., Tempelhoff, G., Gaussorgues, P. L., Jospe, R., Ducreux, J. C., Dumont, A., Motin, J., Auboyer, C. & Robert, D. (1991). Short and long-term prognosis, functional outcome following ICU for elderly. *Intens Care Med*, **17**, 7–10.

Marx, A. B., Campbell, R. & Harder, F. (1986). Polytrauma in the elderly. *World Surg*, **10**, 330–5.

Modig, J., Borg, T., Karlstrom, G., Maripuv, E. & Sahlstedt, B. (1983). Thromboembolism after total hip replacement: rate of epidural and general anaesthesia. *Anesthesia Analgesia*, **62**, 174–80.

Muravchick, S., Owens, W. D. & Felts, J. H. (1979). Glycopyrrolate and cardiac arrhythmias in geriatric patients after reversal of neuromuscular blockade. *Can Anaesth Soc J*, **26**, 22–5.

Nadeau, S. & Noble, W. H. (1986). Misinterpretations of pressure measurement from the pulmonary artery catheter. *Can Anaesth Soc J*, **33**, 353–63.

Nunn, J. F., Milledge, J. S., Chen, D. & Dore, C. (1988). Respiratory criteria of fitness for surgery and anaesthesia. *Anaesthesia*, **43**, 543–51.

Oreskovich, M. R., Howard, J. D., Copass, M. K. & Carrico, C. J. (1984). Geriatric trauma: injury patterns and outcome. *J Trauma*, **24**, 565–72.

Rodriguez, J. L., Weissman, G., Damask, M. C., Askanazi, J., Hyman, A. T. & Kinney, J. M. (1983). Morphine and post-operative rewarming in critically ill patients. *Circulation*, **68**, 1238–46.

Roe, C. F., Goldberg, M. J., Blair, C. S. & Kinney, J. M. (1966). The influence of body temperature on early postoperative oxygen consumption. *Surgery*, **60**, 85–92.

Rowe, J. W. *et al.* (1976). The effects of age on creatinine clearance in man: a cross sectional and longitudinal study. *J Gerontol*, **31**, 155–63.

Royal College of Physicians Working Party (1989). Fractured neck of femur. Prevention and management. *J R Coll Phys Lond*, **23**, 8–12.

Samama, M., Bernard, P., Bonnardot, J. P., Comke-Tamzali, S., Lanson, Y. & Tissot, E. (1988). Low molecular weight heparin compared with unfractionated heparin in prevention of postoperative thrombosis. *Br J Surg*, **75**, 128–31.

Schubert, V. (1991). Hypotension as a risk factor for developing pressure sores in elderly subjects. *Age Ageing*, **20**, 255–61.

Schnets, R. J., Schultze, R. J., Whitfield, G. F., Lamura, J. J., Raciti, A. & Krishnamurthy, S.

(1985). The role of physiological monitoring for patients with fracture of the hip. *J Trauma*, **25**, 309–16.

Scott, N. B. & Kehlet, H. (1988). Regional anaesthesia and surgical morbidity. *Br J Surg*, **75**, 299–304.

Sharkley, A., Lipton, J. M. & Murphy, M. T. (1987). Inhibition of post-anaesthetic shivering with radiant heat. *Anaesthesiology*, **66**, 249–52.

Seeling, W., Bruckmooser, K. P., Hufner, C., Kneiturger, E., Rigg, C. & Rockermann, M. (1990). No reduction in postoperative complications by the use of catheterized epidural analgesia following major surgery. *Anaesthetist*, **39**, 33–40.

Seymour, D. G. (1986). *Medical Assessment of the Elderly Surgical Patient*. London: Croom Helm.

Seymour, D. G. & Vaz, F. G. (1989). A prospective study of elderly surgical patients. II. Postoperative complications. *Age Ageing*, **18**, 316–26.

Simon, A. B. (1977). Perioperative management of the pacemaker patient. *Anesthesiology*, **46**, 127.

Sixson, S. B. & Lehner, J. T. (1988). Factors affecting hip fracture mortality. *J Orthop Trauma*, **1**, 298–305.

Steinemanns, R. G., Shackford, S. R. & Davis, J. W. (1990). Implications of admission hypothermia in trauma patients. *J Trauma*, **30**, 200–2.

Stevens, W. C. *et al.* (1975). MAC of isoflurane with and without nitrous oxide in patients of various age. *Anesthesiology*, **42**, 197.

Teasdale, G. & Jennett, B. (1974). Assessment of coma and impaired consciousness: a practical scale. *Lancet*, **2**, 81.

Thomas, T. H., Morgan, D. B., Swaminathan, R., Ball, S. G. & Lee, M. R. (1978). Severe hyponatraemia: a study of 17 patients. *Lancet*, **1** (8065), 621–4.

Tiret, L., Desmonts, J. M., Hatton, F. & Vourc'h, G. (1986). Complications associated with anaesthesia – a prospective study in France. *Can Anaesth Soc J*, **33**, 336–44.

Valentin, N., Lonholt, B., Jensen, J. S., Hejgaard, N. & Kieiner, S. (1986). Spinal or general anaesthesia for surgery of the fractured hip? *Br J Anaesthesia*, **58**, 284–91.

Vershnysen, M. (1986). How elderly patients with femoral fracture develop pressures sores in hospital. *Br Med J*, **292**, 1311–13.

Wildsmith, J. A. W. (1988). The place of regional anaesthesia in the aged. In *Anaesthesia and the Aged Patient*, ed. H. T. Davenport, pp. 231–44. Oxford: Blackwell.

Yaeger, M. P., Glass, D. D., Neff, R. K. & Brick-Johnsen, J. (1987). Epidural anesthesia and analgesia in high risk surgical patients. *Anesthesiology*, **66**, 729–38.

18

Intensive care

J. D. EDWARDS

Introduction

In a classic paper Trunkey (1983) demonstrated the chronological patterns of deaths following trauma. Half of all deaths occur within minutes of the initial injury usually at the scene. About 30% occur several hours later and may be avoided by improved organisation of trauma care and more efficient resuscitation. Another 30% of deaths occur after an interval of days or weeks, usually on the intensive care unit from multisystem organ failure and sepsis. Only particular aspects of resuscitation can be addressed in this brief review. For more details the reader is referred to other reviews (Conn *et al.*, 1991) and the guidelines for Advanced Trauma Life Support (ATLS) published by the American College of Surgeons (ALTS, 1993). Intensive care unit (ICU) input can affect the outcome of the latter two types of death and possibly the first.

Intensive care of the trauma victim should begin as soon as possible after the incident: at the scene if necessary. There are two phases of management. First, the initial stage of resuscitation and assessment of injuries which have to take place simultaneously. The priorities are as always Airway, Breathing and Circulation. Both securing the airway and establishing venous and arterial access may be particularly technically difficult in the elderly patient. These aspects are discussed in some detail below. The initial management includes the correction of hypoxia and administration of intravenous fluids and/or blood as appropriate (Conn *et al.*, 1991). Apart from radiological assessment of obvious suspected injuries routine initial X-rays should include an erect film of the chest and films of the cervical spine. The latter can be difficult and tedious to obtain and a firm opinion on cervical bony or soft tissue injury may only be possible after computed tomography (CT) scanning. The next decision is whether immediate, as opposed to emergency, surgery is required. The patient may be transferred directly to the operating room or to the ICU for a period of stabilisation before surgery. Routine haematological and biochemical investigations will include

263

haemoglobin, coagulation studies, grouping and cross-matching of blood, urea and electrolytes, plasma glucose, serum creatinine and amylase, arterial blood gases and lactate. An increasing number of these investigations can be performed immediately using bedside laboratory technology, the so-called 'STAT LAB'.

After surgery, which should be as definitive as possible at the first visit to theatre, further stabilisation on the ICU will be required. After 24–48 hours two groups of patients will be identified. Some will recover rapidly with minimal support such as basic cardiovascular monitoring, attention to fluid balance, chest physiotherapy and analgesia. These will comprise patients with severe but isolated injuries such as a skull or serious long bone fracture without shock. A second group poses a much more challenging prospect. These are those victims who will require extended ICU support: prolonged mechanical ventilation, invasive cardiovascular monitoring and pharmacological support of the circulation. This group of patients is most at risk for development of the syndrome of multisystem organ failure (MSOF) (Fouler *et al.*, 1985; Montgomery *et al.*, 1985) which is closely, some might say inextricably, related to severe sepsis (Bell *et al.*, 1983). This aspect is discussed in more detail below.

In order for present day ICU approaches to trauma management to be put into context a brief review of the physiology involved is described.

Pathophysiology of circulatory and respiratory failure (shock)

Circulatory failure

The major function of the circulatory and respiratory systems is the effective transportation of oxygen (O_2) to the tissues. Oxygen is the most important single substrate carried by the circulation, is the most flow dependent and has the lowest body stores compared with demand. Traumatic shock is characterised by reduced oxygen supply but increased demand (Edwards *et al.*, 1988). The relation between oxygen delivery ($\dot{D}O_2$) and oxygen consumption ($\dot{V}O_2$) is termed oxygen transport (O_2T) (Edwards, 1990). These variables can be routinely measured and manipulated. The definition of oxygen delivery ($\dot{D}O_2$) is shown in equation 1 below and that of oxygen consumption (VO_2) in equation 2.

1 $\dot{D}O_2 = CO \times$ arterial O_2 content ml/min
2. $\dot{V}O_2 = CO \times$ arterial–mixed venous–oxygen content ml/min

(For explanations of these and other abbreviations and equations see the Appendix.) The original Fick equation:

$$CO = \frac{\dot{V}O_2}{CaO_2 - CvO_2}$$

was used to calculate cardiac output which was not measurable by other means in the days of the German physiologist. Cardiac output is now routinely measured at the bedside using a pulmonary artery flotation catheter and the thermodilution technique. A universally accepted definition of shock has yet to be produced; however, when considering victims of multiple trauma, and certainly those who require management on the ICU, the following definition provides a practical working basis for evaluation of the severity of the physiological disturbances present and a rational basis on which to proceed with resuscitation and continued management until recovery or death.

Shock is a state of inadequate $\dot{D}O_2$. The supply of oxygen to the tissues may be inadequate as a result of any combination of the following factors:

1. $\dot{D}O_2$ is too low in absolute terms to meet the demand for oxygen by the tissues.
2. There is maldistribution of the $\dot{D}O_2$ which is present.
3. Tissue perfusion pressure is too low for an adequate blood flow to vital organs.

These three factors will be considered in more detail.

$\dot{D}O_2$ too low to meet oxygen demand

If we were to substitute normal values in equation 1 we could calculate the $\dot{D}O_2$ of a healthy resting patient.

$$\dot{D}O_2 = CI \times CaO_2 \times 10 \text{ ml/min per m}^2$$

$$\text{where CI} = \text{cardiac index} = \frac{CO}{\text{Body surface area (BSA)}}$$

Assuming a haemoglobin of 150 g/l, resting CO of 5.0 l/min, arterial oxyhaemoglobin saturation (SaO_2) of 98% and arterial oxygen tension (PaO_2) of 13.3 kPa (100 mmHg) and BSA of 1.8 m^2 then

$$\dot{D}O_2 = 2.8 \times 19.5 \times 10 = 542 \text{ ml/min per m}^2$$

Using normal values for mixed venous blood, which assumes a mixed venous saturation (SvO_2) of 75% then VO_2 can be calculated from equation 2

$$\dot{V}O_2 = CI \times (CaO_2 - CvO_2) \times 10 \text{ ml/min per m}^2$$

$$\dot{V}O_2 = 2.8 \times (19.5 - 14.5) \times 10 = 140 \text{ ml/min per m}^2$$

The normal relation between $\dot{D}O_2$ and $\dot{V}O_2$ can be quantified by the oxygen extraction ratio (OER) which in many but not all circumstances, for example sepsis, will reflect the adequacy of supply to that of demand. The OER can always be calculated in any patient from either of two equations:

$$OER = \frac{CaO_2 - CvO_2}{CaO_2}$$

or

$$OER = \frac{\dot{V}O_2}{\dot{D}O_2}$$

The first equation is useful in that the calculation is technically independent of measurement of cardiac output. If the patient has a PaO_2 approaching or less than 13 kPa, i.e. the amount of dissolved oxygen is very small compared to that carried by haemoglobin, then an even more basic equation can be used:

$$OER = \frac{SaO_2 - SvO_2}{SaO_2}$$

This will obviate the need for measurement both of cardiac output and haemoglobin in the calculation of OER.

If the absolute level of DO_2 is inadequate to meet oxygen demand, and if the ability of the tissue to extract oxygen is maintained, then OER will rise, the normal arterial–mixed venous content difference of 50 ml/l will increase and SvO_2 will fall. If SvO_2 falls below 60%, then some tissues notably the liver will suffer from hypoxia as approximately 25–30% of oxygen bound to haemoglobin is unavailable at saturations toward the lower end of the oxyhaemoglobin dissociation curve. In trauma patients, especially the elderly with poor cardiorespiratory reserve, DO_2 is frequently globally inadequate, especially when oxygen demand is increased. This is discussed in more detail below.

A consideration of the variables in equation 1 will show that DO_2 can be reduced by a fall in cardiac output, a reduction in haemoglobin concentration (more precisely oxyhaemoglobin) and arterial hypoxaemia (which reduces SaO_2).

Cardiac output in turn is dependent on heart rate (HR) and stroke volume (SV). Stroke volume is dependent on cardiac preload, contractility and afterload. In trauma victims there may be abnormalities in any combination of these variables and frequently in all of them.

Maldistribution of available blood flow

The classic example of this is septic shock, which can in fact be a complication of trauma as early as the time of arrival of the patient in hospital (Border *et al.*, 1987). Septic patients may have normal or high cardiac index and therefore DO_2 but blood flow to vital organs is reduced or oxygen uptake is impaired. There have been many proposed explanations for this.

First, there may be a reduction in total systemic vascular resistance, i.e. generalised vasodilatation. Systemic vascular resistance (SVR) is calculated from the formula:

$$SVR = \frac{MAP - RAP}{CO} \times 80 \text{ dyne.s.cm}^{-5}$$

where MAP is mean systemic arterial blood pressure in mmHg and RAP is mean right atrial pressure in mmHg. Therefore under normal circumstances SVR can be calculated to be

$$SVR = \frac{90 - 70}{5.0} \times 80 = 1160 \text{ dyne.s.cm}^{-5}$$

The normal range is from 800 to 1200 dyne.s.cm^{-5}. If vasodilatation is profound then vital organs such as brain and kidney are unable to maintain autoregulation of blood flow. Of special importance is the microcirculation in the small bowel. Other explanations for the phenomenon of inability to utilise oxygen in the face of increased demand and higher than normal delivery that have been proposed include the opening up of arteriovenous fistulae at the periphery as a result of constriction of the precapillary metarteriolar sphincter, peripheral obstruction to capillary networks as a result of aggregates of leucocytes and/or platelets and a metabolic effect blocking mitochondrial uptake of oxygen. All of these proposed mechanisms are theoretical at the present time. Nevertheless the clinical scenario of high cardiac output, normal MAP, low SVR and defective oxygen extraction is well recognised in trauma patients. It may cause confusion as during the stage of spontaneous repair of injuries which begins approximately 48 hours after the initial trauma a similar pattern of delivery may be seen but of course there is no evidence of defective oxygen uptake: $\dot{V}O_2$ is high, not low, and arterial blood lactate levels are normal (see below).

Reduction in systemic arterial perfusion pressure

This is the classic textbook presentation of shock which was recognised prior to bedside measurements of cardiac output and calculations of $\dot{D}O_2$, and $\dot{V}O_2$. Blood pressure is dependent on cardiac output and SVR, i.e.

$$BP \propto CO \times SVR \text{ (normal range 90–105 mmHg)}$$

There is however another consideration and that is the adequacy of the perfusion pressure to individual organs, for instance for the centrilobular cells in the liver to which two-thirds of oxygen is supplied by the portal vein the perfusion pressure = portal venous pressure – hepatic venous pressure. In the case of cerebral perfusion pressure this equals mean internal carotid artery – jugular venous pressure and for the coronary circulation, coronary perfusion pressure (CPP) is given by the equation:

$$CPP = \text{aortic diastolic pressure} - RAP \text{ mmHg}$$

as the coronary sinus drains into the right atrium. For the subendocardial myocardium which is the most vulnerable in shock:

$$CPP = \text{aortic diastolic pressure} - LVEDP,$$

where LVEDP is left ventricular end diastolic pressure which is measured indirectly as the pulmonary artery occlusion pressure, popularly known as the 'wedge pressure' or WP. Because of differing ventricular function curves frequently found in the elderly and especially after trauma the WP is used as the clinical guide to preload of the left ventricle not the RAP or central venous pressure (CVP).

Aspects of respiratory physiology of relevance to intensive care of trauma victims

Of all the determinants of $\dot{D}O_2$, a lowered SaO_2 due to arterial hypoxaemia is the most important from the clinical and physiological point of view. Aspects of oxygen physiology are well reviewed by Nunn (1987). The relation between arterial PaO_2 and haemoglobin saturation is given by the oxyhaemoglobin dissociation curve (Figure 18.1). The points on this curve to note are: (1) the PaO_2 at which haemoglobin saturation begins to decline steeply (8 kPa, 60 mmHg), (2) the mixed venous PaO_2 (5.3 kPa, 40 mmHg) at which with normal position of the curve SvO_2 will be 75%, (3) the PaO_2 at which haemoglobin has a saturation of 50% (3.7 kPa, 28 mmHg), this known as the P_{50}. If there is a shift of the curve to the right P_{50} will increase and it is generally accepted that this would increase oxygen release to the tissues, and (4) the PaO_2 below which no oxygen is available for diffusion to the cells (2.7 kPa, 20 mmHg). There is an inevitable decline in 'normal' PaO_2 with age (Table 18.1). This can be calculated using the pragmatic equation:

$$\text{expected } PaO_2 = 13.6 - 0.44 \text{ (age in years) kPa.}$$

In acute respiratory failure of any aetiology various calculations are used to quantify the disturbance in the ability of the lungs to transfer oxygen to the arterial circulation. These include:

1. PaO_2/FIO_2 ratio (where PaO_2 is in mmHg). FIO_2 is fractional inspired oxygen concentration, e.g. 60% inspired oxygen is an FIO_2 of 0.6. The PaO_2/FIO_2 ratio should normally be more than 300.

2. Alveolar minus arterial oxygen tension difference $(A - aDO_2)$. Normally less than 5 kPa.
3. Respiratory index (RI). This is the alveolar – arterial oxygen gradient divided by PaO_2. If the patient is receiving an FIO_2 of 1.0 with adequate alveolar ventilation then alveolar $PO_2(P_AO_2)$ should almost equal inspired $PO_2(P_IO_2)$ minus water vapour pressure (P_{H2O}) and arterial carbon dioxide tension $(PaCO_2)$, corrected for body temperature and barometric pressure.

The most sensitive measure of ventilation/perfusion mismatch in severe acute respiratory failure is the calculation of the degree of pulmonary venous admixture or shunt fraction (Qs/Qt), i.e. the ratio of venous blood that is not effectively oxygenated as it passes through the pulmonary circulation (Qs) compared with the total blood flow (Qt).

$$\text{Shunt fraction} = Qs/Qt = \frac{CcO_2 - CaO_2}{CcO_2 - CvO_2}$$

where CcO_2 is ideal pulmonary capillary oxygen content, i.e. the content of oxygen in a capillary that has perfused a perfectly ventilated alveolus, i.e. V/Q = 1.0. This concept is theoretical but does have many advantages over other indices of pulmonary dysfunction. The shunt fraction may alter as a result of a change in cardiac output at constant VO_2 or vice versa. In these circumstances changes in SvO_2 will be seen.

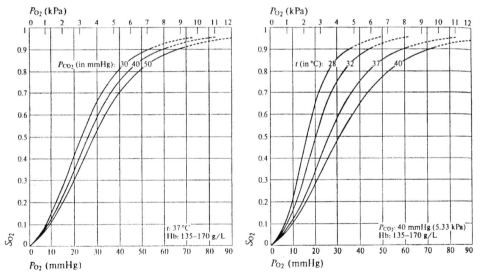

Figure 18.1 Oxygen-binding curves of haemoglobin, dependent on carbon dioxide pressure (PCO_2) and blood temperature (t) for adults more than 15 years of age.

Table 18.1. *Effect of increasing age on PaO$_2$*

Age (decades)	Average PaO$_2$(kPa) – on air
20s	12.5
30s	12.1
40s	11.7
50s	11.2
60s	10.8

Lactate measurements

Lactic acid is the byproduct of anaerobic glycosis. In laboratory experiments it is taken as an absolute indicator, some might say *sine qua non*, of tissue hypoxia. The clinical view is rather less dogmatic in that many patients have clinical and objective features of profound circulatory shock but no hyperlactataemia. Clinical aspects of lactate metabolism with reference to shock have recently been reviewed (Mizock & Falk, 1992). Normally lactate is produced by skeletal muscle, brain, gut and skin and metabolised by the liver (40–70%) and kidney. Thus hypoperfusion of either or both organs can be manifested by an increase in arterial blood lactate above the normal value (1.5 mmol/l). Reluctance to routinely measure lactate levels in clinical practice has been largely due to the inconvenience entailed in the past. There are now a variety of automatic bedside instruments which allow rapid, accurate and economic measurement of lactate. Also, the correlation between arterial and peripheral venous lactate is close obviating the need for an arterial puncture unless needed for other purposes. Persisting hyperlactataemia after trauma is an ominous sign and should lead to measurement of DO$_2$ and SvO$_2$ and manipulation if appropriate.

Practical aspects of the management of multiply injured patients

The aetiology of shock following trauma was the subject of fierce debate until the milestone study by Cournand published only in 1943 (Cournand *et al.*, 1943). He showed quite clearly in a group of 16 completely unresuscitated patients that hypotension was due to loss of circulating blood volume (falling cardiac preload) and haemoglobin. He also documented frequent reduction in SaO$_2$ in the absence of chest injuries. Cournand's clinical study confirmed laboratory experiments which demonstrated the presence of a lethal oxygen debt during controlled haemorrhage. Thus initial resuscitation is based on replacement of fluid and blood where necessary. In those elderly patients requiring intensive or high dependency therapy several patterns can be discerned, as of course many trauma victims can be dealt with without such facilities. These are:

1. Multiple long bone fractures.
2. Chest injury causing respiratory failure.
3. Head injury with impaired conscious level, Glasgow Coma Score (GCS) less than 10.
4. Pelvic or vertebral fractures.
5. Intra-abdominal injuries requiring laparotomy and more than 6 units blood transfusion.
6. Degloving of 10% or more skin surface area, crush injury or traumatic amputation.

In the elderly any one of the above injuries is an indication for ICU referral and certainly if they occur in combination. These are of course only general guidelines.

Respiratory support

All of the injuries listed above, not just chest injury, can be associated with hypoxaemia; therefore concurrent with volume expansion an adequate SaO_2 should be ensured. This may entail intubation of the trachea and commencement of mechanical ventilation. The use of continuous bedside pulse oximetry may be of value during initial resuscitation and assessment as well as during intubation. Indications for mechanical ventilation are both clinical and laboratory (Tables 18.2 and 18.3).

Blood gas data in elderly patients obviously have to be modified in view of the likelihood of pre-existing lung disease with chronic hypoxaemia or hypercarbia. The measurement of pH and standard and actual bicarbonate levels may be particularly useful under these circumstances as in chronic hypercarbia bicarbonate levels are elevated and pH is normal.

In order for mechanical ventilation to be implemented endotracheal intubation must be performed. The elderly may pose particular problems. First, diminished cardiovascular reserve, left ventricular dysfunction, coronary artery disease, peripheral vascular disease and autonomic neuropathy may enhance and prolong the effects of any sedative or anaesthetic agent used. Second, irrespective of any anatomical problems posed by the injuries themselves, for example maxillofacial fractures, there may be abnormalities of the cervical spine (shortening, lordosis, inability to flex or extend) due to cervical spondylosis. Rheumatoid disease may produce an unstable cervical spine. An additional technical problem is shortening of the cervical and upper thoracic spine due to degenerative disease of the vertebral bodies and discs. The modern practice is to use endotracheal tubes with high volume, low pressure cuffs to minimise trauma to the

Table 18.2. *Clinical indications for mechanical ventilation after major trauma*

Apnoea
Airway obstruction
Suspected aspiration of gastric contents
Head injury with GCS < 10
Paradoxical respiration
Flail segment
Respiratory rate < 4 or > 30/min

GCS: Glasgow Coma Score.

Table 18.3. *Laboratory indications for mechanical ventilation after major trauma*

Rising $PaCO_2$
SaO_2 < 90% despite supplemental inspired O_2
Falling SaO_2
Normal $PaCO_2$ with pH < 7.35

larynx and trachea. The cuff of the tube should be below the vocal cords but at least 2 cm above the carina. The normal distance between the vocal cords and carina is approximately 10–12 cm. This can be considerably reduced in the elderly, which makes it difficult to ensure a satisfactory position for the cuff as the distance from the proximal attachment of the cuff to the tip of the tube is 7–8 cm. This problem is occasionally insurmountable even by tracheostomy.

The methods and practicalities of intubation are crucial. An experienced anaesthetist must be consulted as the exact method used will vary enormously with circumstances. ATLS guidelines include use of awake blind nasal intubation but many operators will feel uncomfortable with this. Tracheostomy, cricothyroidotomy or fibreoptic techniques may be necessary.

The normal practice is to institute mechanical ventilation with a respiratory rate (RR) of 10 breaths per minute, tidal volume (TV) of 10–12 ml/kg and inspiratory to expiratory (I:E) ratio of 1:2. Initial FIO_2 is set at 0.6–1.0 and reduced rapidly according to measurements of PaO_2. The minute volume of ventilation is adjusted accordingly to estimates of adequacy of expired minute volume based on measurements of $PaCO_2$ or end expiratory CO_2 by capnography. In all patients but especially in the elderly peak inflation pressures are wherever possible kept below 50 cm of H_2O. One of the complications of intermittent positive pressure ventilation (IPPV), which may be particularly prevalent in the elderly with chronic obstructive pulmonary disease, is that of so-called intrinsic positive end expiratory pressure $PEEP_i$ (sometimes known as

Table 18.4. *Chronic lung disease which may be asymmetrical or unilateral in the elderly*

Bronchiectasis
Post-tuberculosis fibrosis
Previous plombage
Massive emphysematous bullae
Pleural thickening
Previous lobectomy/pneumonectomy

dynamic hyperinflation) (Iotti & Braschi, 1990). The use of extrinsic positive end expiratory pressure (PEEP$_e$) which is determined proactively by the clinician is discussed below. Different mechanical ventilators have differing levels of performance and versatility but the details are beyond the scope of this chapter.

Other problems related to pre-existing lung disease include those that produce asymmetrical or sometimes even totally unilateral lung disease. These can affect the distribution of ventilation when there is a sudden transition to IPPV. Some of these conditions are listed in Table 18.4.

Pulmonary injury

The concept of pulmonary insufficiency due to chest trauma has advanced far beyond the simplistic notion that multiple rib fractures at separate sites along the course of each rib or ribs lead to ventilatory failure because of a lack of integrity of the chest wall, the so-called 'flail segment'. Respiratory insufficiency, a term which encompasses both ventilatory failure and hypoxaemia, is multifactorial following trauma, and can occur with or without direct injury to the chest (Table 18.5).

A detailed account of the management of these problems is beyond the scope of this chapter, but the complexity of factors contributing to pulmonary insufficiency should highlight the need for specialist advice. With or without these initial problems after a latent interval of 12–72 hours the clinical picture of adult respiratory distress syndrome (ARDS) may develop.

Circulatory support

It is now widely accepted that the major cause of low cardiac output following trauma is a lack of sufficient venous return to the heart due to fluid loss and/or haemorrhage. This follows the milestone clinical study of Cournand *et al.* (1943) and the treatise of Guyton (Sheik, 1981). The first step is to secure adequate venous access. A short, large-bore cannula (at least 16 gauge) should be placed in a suitable peripheral vein.

Table 18.5. *Causes of early (<12 hours) respiratory insufficiency after trauma*

Pulmonary barotrauma
Pneumothorax
Pulmonary contusion
Blast lung
Intrapulmonary haemorrhage

Chest wall fractures
Ribs
Sternum
Clavicles
Scapulae
Thoracic vertebrae

Neurological
Cervical spine trauma
Head injury

Upper airway disruption
Maxillo-facial fractures
Lingual haematoma
Foreign body
Haematoma at base of neck
Ruptured trachea or main stem bronchus
Laryngeal injury

Miscellaneous
Massive blood transfusion
Ruptured diaphragm
Aspiration of gastric contents
Exacerbation of C.O.P.D.
Status asthmaticus
Cardiogenic pulmonary oedema
Early onset of bronchopneumonia

With multiple injuries access above and below the diaphragm may be needed to overcome disruption to the tributaries of the superior or inferior vena cava. Surgical cutdown to the long saphenous or percutaneous puncture of a neck vein may be required. In the latter circumstance the external jugular is the vessel of choice. The internal jugular may be inaccessible because of a cervical collar. Puncture of the subclavian vein may be difficult in the elderly because of disturbed anatomy at the base of the neck as a result of skeletal and vascular degeneration. Even when the Seldinger (guide wire) technique is used successful venepuncture may not guarantee access to the

Table 18.6. *Some indicators for insertion of a pulmonary artery flotation catheter*

1. Failure of initial volume replacement to reverse shock in the absence of obvious
      bleeding
2. Previous or recent cardiac disease including cardiac contusion
3. Suspected cardiogenic pulmonary oedema
4. Hypoxia or desaturation despite optimal ventilatory support
5. Use of positive end expiratory pressure (PEEP) ventilation

superior vena cava. A bladder catheter is inserted to check for possible urological injury but also to monitor urine output.

Fluids are given based on an estimate of the injuries and the clinical response, especially urine output NOT by monitoring central venous pressure which is notoriously misleading. If access to a central neck vein has been achieved a pulmonary artery introducer sheath (8.5 Fr gauge) provides excellent infusion characteristics. It is very unusual to overload even an elderly trauma victim. Under-resuscitation is much more common. Frequent bedside estimation of haemoglobin and lactate is helpful at this stage. Prior to, or immediately after, ICU admission an arterial cannula is inserted as when SVR is high non-invasive blood pressure measurements may be grossly inaccurate. A pulmonary artery flotation catheter (PAFC) may be indicated (Table 18.6).

Under no circumstances should PAFC insertion delay fluid replacement and other management priorities. It is not a procedure to be undertaken in the emergency department. The directly measured variables obtainable with a PAFC are summarised in Table 18.7.

Apart from inadequate volume replacement other causes of failure to resuscitate include unrecognised obstruction to the circulation such as pneumothorax and cardiac tamponade, myocardial contusion, non-viable crushed tissue or early onset of bacteraemia. In patients with pre-existing cardiac disease the influence of medication such as beta-blockers, calcium antagonists, antihypertensive agents or anticoagulants needs to be considered.

The classical view of the metabolic response to trauma was that of Cuthbertson (1942), who suggested an initial phase of reduced oxygen demand (the 'Ebb phase') merging after 24–48 hours into a prolonged period of increased oxygen demand (the 'Flow phase'). This gained widespread acceptance and may have influenced some resuscitation protocols; however, the original concept was based on inadequate and poorly interpreted data. A number of recent studied have shown that $\dot{V}O_2$ is usually increased within hours or minutes of trauma, even in elderly patients. A study of 16 patients with a mean time from injury to measurements of 1.6 hours showed that the majority had high levels of $\dot{V}O_2$ in the absence of hypothermia. Many patients had

Table 18.7. *Variables which can be measured with a pulmonary artery flotation catheter*

1. Right atrial pressure
2. Pulmonary artery pressures
3. Pulmonary artery wedge pressures
4. Cardiac output
5. Mixed venous oxyhaemoglobin saturation

high levels of OER leading to low levels of SvO_2 (Edwards *et al.*, 1988). These results are summarised in figures 18.2 and 18.3.

In a subsequent group of 24 chest trauma victims, again studied early (3.2 hours) (Rady *et al.*, 1992) after injury, it was possible to predict a high risk of death and MSOF. These results are summarised in Tables 18.8 and 18.9.

A recent study (Moore *et al.*, 1992) from a different group has confirmed these findings and demonstrated that development of MSOF was predicted most accurately by 12–hour values of $\dot{V}O_2$ and lactate. Trauma Score and Injury Severity Score were unhelpful. MSOF was much less of a problem in those with 12–hour $\dot{D}O_2$ of 750 ml/min per m^2 compared with those with values of 600 ml/min per m^2.

These contemporary studies are in agreement with results that can be extrapolated from older studies of Shoemaker *et al.* (1980), Shoemaker & Appel (1985), Stürm *et al.* (1979) and indeed those of Cournand *et al.* (1943). There seems little doubt that trauma victims have improved survival if they can maintain levels of $\dot{D}O_2$ at least in excess of normal resting values. In all studies where $\dot{D}O_2$ has been studied in the early stages of trauma there has been poor correlation between oxygen transport variables and the initial so-called vital signs: heart rate, blood pressure and CVP.

Multisystem organ failure and adult respiratory distress syndrome

Following the initial 48 hours or so after injury a new series of complications may set in which has traditionally been known as multisystem organ failure (MSOF). This was first described in the early 1970s by several authors, notably Tilney *et al.* (1973), in patients following ruptured aortic aneurysm and is now a well recognised sequel to trauma (Goris *et al.*, 1985). The features include failure of the neuromuscular, cardiovascular, gastrointestinal, haematological and immunological systems. Most notable is respiratory failure and this is a common complication of major trauma. Many of the pathophysiological features of this entity are similar to those seen in neonatal respiratory distress syndrome and it is now known as ARDS. Original descriptions

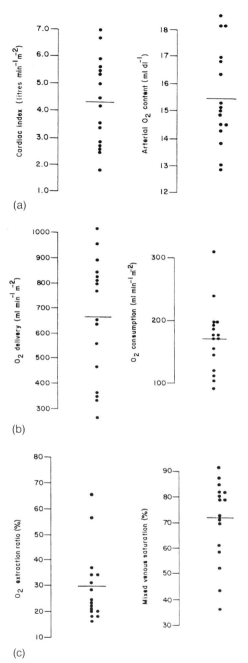

(a)

(b)

(c)

Figure 18.2. Oxygen transport variables in 16 acutely injured patients. (a) Cardiac index and arterial oxygen content. (b) Oxygen delivery and consumption. (c) Oxygen extraction ratio and mixed venous oxygen saturation.

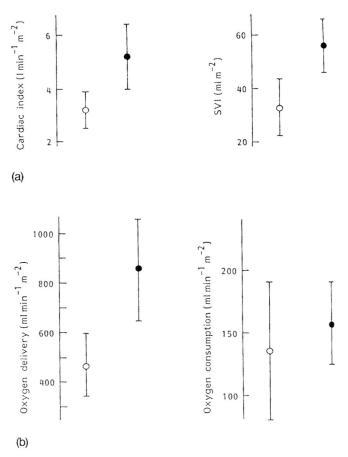

(a)

(b)

18.3. Oxygen transport variables measured acutely in 24 patients with severe blunt thoracic trauma. (a) Cardiac and stroke volume indices. (b) Oxygen delivery and consumption. Patients classified into two groups on basis of normal (●) or low (○) values of left ventricular stroke work index.

focused on its occurrence as a complication of trauma (Ashbaugh *et al.*, 1967; Hyers & Fowler, 1986) and earlier descriptions referred to 'Post Traumatic Pulmonary Insufficiency', 'Shock Lung', etc.

The clinical features are respiratory distress, tachypnoea and cyanosis with varying combinations of diminished air entry, crepitations and patchy bronchial breathing. Occasionally there may be rhonchi due to airflow limitation. Initial arterial blood gases reveal a respiratory alkalosis, hypoxaemia and hypocarbia. The hypoxaemia becomes progressive and responds poorly to an increase in FIO_2 with respiratory muscle fatigue and ultimately death unless IPPV is instituted. There is reduced

Table 18.8. (a) *Patient characteristics*

	Group 1 ($n=9$)	Group 2 ($n=15$)	P*
Age (years)	46(25)	35(17)	n.s.
Chest AIS	4(0.5)	4(0.6)	n.s.
Total Injury Severity Score	32(13)	26(8)	n.s.
ARDS	9	8	<0.05
Acute renal failure	3	0	<0.05
No. of deaths	7	2	<0.05

Note: Values are mean (s.d.). Chest AIS, Abbreviated Injury Scale score for the chest; ARDS: Adult Respiratory Distress Syndrome; n.s. not significant.
* χ^2 test

(b) *Associated abdominal, craniospinal and limb injuries*

Injury	Group 1		Group 2	
	n	Mean AIS	n	Mean AIS
Abdominal	5	3	7	3
Craniospinal	5	4	8	3
Limb	9	3	10	3

Note: Values are the number of patients with injuries and the mean Abbreviated Injury Scale (AIS) score for body regions
Source: Iotti & Braschi (1990).

pulmonary compliance, marked reduction in functional residual capacity (FRC), marked increase in Qs/Qt and a variable increase in extravascular lung water. It is tempting to consider ARDS as simply a form of non-cardiogenic pulmonary oedema but this is simplistic. The major cause of hypoxia is ventilation to perfusion (V/Q) mismatch with scattered areas of high V/Q (dead space) and low V/Q (shunt). Also pathologically there are abnormalities of the pulmonary vasculature and alveolar walls and ultimately hyaline membrane formation and progressive fibrosis in those patients whose lung injury fails to heal. In those who survive pulmonary function usually returns to normal.

The aetiology is multifactorial but the combination of multiple injuries, especially long bone fractures, multiple blood transfusions and any direct lung injury are agreed risk factors (Pepe *et al.*, 1982; Fowler *et al.*, 1983). Most cases occur in patients with Injury Severity Score (ISS) of greater than 30. Indeed in one study the ISS was the

Table 18.9. (a) *Haemodynamic data for groups 1 and 2 following controlled plasma volume expansion with modified fluid gelatin and blood*

	Group 1	Group 2	$P*$
Heart rate (beats min^{-1})	102(23)	94(18)	n.s.
Mean arterial pressure (mmHg)	82(9)	95(15)	n.s.
Central venous pressure (mmHg)	11(4)	11(5)	n.s.
Wedge pressure (mmHg)	14(7)	13(4)	n.s.
LVSWI (g m^{-2})	30(10)	62(14)	<0.001

Note: Values are mean (s.d.). LVSWI: left ventricular stroke work index

(b) *Oxygen transport data for groups 1 and 2 after controlled plasma volume expansion with modified fluid gelatin and blood*

	Group 1	Group 2	$P*$
Haemoglobin (g dl^{-1})	10.3(0.7)	12.1(1.7)	<0.001
Oxygen extraction ratio (%)	29(11)	19(6)	<0.001
S_vO_2 (%)	73(14)	82(5)	<0.02
Q_s/Q_t (%)	19(4)	22(11)	n.s.

Note: Values are mean (s.d.). S_vO_2: mixed venous oxygen saturation Q_s/Q_t: pulmonary venous admixture; n.s.: not significant.
* Student's paired t-test

strongest single correlate ($P<0.005$) along with early hypoxia (Pepe *et al.*, 1982). There is a strong correlation with systemic sepsis, as there is with MSOF in general. Some have developed predictive scoring systems such as the one by Goris (1987) which allocates a score ranging from 1 to 10 for high risk injuries, e.g. ruptured liver = 4 and flail chest = 10. In any patient with a score of 10 or more there is a 30% incidence of ARDS.

Prevention includes prompt recognition of all injuries and expeditious surgery to limit blood loss and tissue damage and hence blood transfusion. Ideally all blood should be filtered during transfusion. Early fixation of long bone fractures is now standard practice. Identification of any source of infection such as intraabdominal abscess is mandatory if respiratory failure persists for more than 10 days. This principle applies to all manifestations of MSOF.

Management of ARDS

This is essentially supportive with mechanical ventilation and optimisation of haemodynamic status. Mechanical ventilation is initiated as described above. As a result of reduced compliance and increased alveolar dead space a large tidal volume (15 ml/kg) may be required to produce normocapnia. This is associated with high inspiratory pressures, more than 50 cm H_2O, and sometimes approaching 100 cm H_2O. This causes an unacceptable incidence of pulmonary barotrauma. To minimise this a degree of elevation of $PaCO_2$ may be tolerated, so-called 'permissive hypercarbia'. Also improvement in V/Q mismatch can be achieved by adding Positive End Expiratory Pressure (PEEP) which usually improves oxygenation at least initially, allowing reduction in FIO_2 to less than 0.6, which traditionally has been thought to reduce the incidence of oxygen toxicity. If PEEP is used there is a danger of lowering the cardiac output and thereby $\dot{D}O_2$.

The cardiac output and thereby $\dot{D}O_2$ should be optimised to levels shown empirically to produce improved survival rates (Cryer *et al.*, 1989). This will entail the use of inotropes and/or vasopressors in the majority of cases. There is a growing amount of circumstantial evidence that this approach improves outcome and reduces the impact of MSOF.

Fluid balance and ARDS

There is continuing controversy concerning fluid therapy in trauma and ARDS. Opinions vary from active fluid loading (Shoemaker *et al.*, 1980; Shoemaker & Appel, 1985) to prophylactic use of diuretics to maintain negative fluid balance (Humphrey *et al.*, 1990). At the moment this debate is unresolved, indeed some may say unresolvable. Two points should be made. First, any active manipulation of fluid balance should not be made without appropriate monitoring of pulmonary artery wedge pressure and cardiac output. Second, one of the major aims of cardiovascular support is to prevent the onset of acute renal failure which when it complicates post-traumatic ARDS has a very high mortality rate even with dialysis (Kraman *et al.*, 1979).

Other manifestations of MSOF are shown in Table 18.10.

Unfortunately there is no agreement on the definition of the criteria used to confirm that an organ or system has failed. Recent proposals have suggested the use of the term 'multiple organ dysfunction' to describe partial organ failure not requiring artificial support.

Details of the management of all these problems are beyond the scope of this review. Some may have specific aetiologies such as *Clostridium difficile* infection as a cause of colitis, folate deficiency as a cause of acute megaloblastic anaemia, and aminoglycoside toxicity causing acute renal failure. Nutritional problems may be attenuated, but not totally prevented, by the early use of parenteral and more recently enteral nutrition by jejunal tube or jejunostomy if necessary.

There is a close link between MSOF and infection. Two major sources are trouble-

Table 18.10. *Some components of multi-system organ failure syndrome*

Neurological
Encephalopathy
Neuropsychiatric
Peripheral neuropathy

Musculoskeletal
Joint deformities
Muscle wasting
Proximal myopathy

Gastrointestinal
Gastric atony
Small bowel ileus
Stress ulceration
Diarrhoea
Pseudomembraneous colitis

Hepatobiliary
Cholestasis
Elevated transaminases
Coagulopathy
Acalculous cholecystitis

Haematological
Thrombocytopenia
Neutropenia
Anaemia

Nutritional/metabolic
Protein/calorie deprivation
Hypoalbuminaemia
Vitamin, trace element and haemotinic deficiencies
Electrolyte disorders

Renal
Oliguric and/or non-oliguric renal failure

some, namely nosocomial pneumonia and occult abdominal collections. Attempts have been made to reduce the former with the regimen of selective decontamination of the gastrointestinal tract (Stoutenbeek *et al.*, 1984; McLelland *et al.*, 1991). The rationale for this is that the majority of nosocomial pneumonias are due to Gram-negative bacteria aspirated from a colonised upper respiratory tract; however this approach has by no means gained universal acceptance (European Society of Intensive Care Medicine, 1992). A recent consensus conference has defined the systemic response to sepsis in an ICU population as:

Temperature $> 38\,^{\circ}\text{C}$ or $< 36\,^{\circ}\text{C}$
Heart rate $> 90/\text{min}$
Respiratory rate > 20 breaths/min or $PaCO_2 < 32$ mmHg (4.3 kPa)
WBC > 12000 or < 4000 or $> 10\%$ immature cells

Obviously sustained microbiological surveillance is mandatory. A major cause of difficultly is that many of the responses to injury can mimic those of sepsis, including high cardiac output and low systemic vascular resistance. The term systemic inflammatory response syndrome ('SIRS') has been coined to describe this phenomenon (American College of Chest Physicians, 1992).

The majority of late deaths in trauma victims are associated with MSOF with relatively few being due to progressive hypoxaemia. In general terms mortality increases exponentially with increasing numbers of failed organs or systems. The relatively limited organ reserve of elderly patients makes them particularly vulnerable to this syndrome.

Summary

The reader will no doubt have grasped the complexity of intensive care of trauma victims, the clinical aspects of which are in a constant state of flux. In this brief review one cannot hope to cover everything. Some of the problems associated with elderly victims are summarised below:

1. **Early**
   Anatomical variations posing technical problems.
   Prior organ dysfunction, especially cardiac and respiratory.
2. **Intermediate**
   Prior organ dysfunction
   Psychiatric disturbances, disorientation
   Drug toxicity; e.g. aminoglycosides, xanthine derivatives, anticonvulsants, digitalis
   Impaired fracture and wound healing
   Nutritional status
3. **Late**
   Poor mobilisation
   Delayed rehabilitation

Rehabilitation in particular can be a difficult and protracted process which is sadly sometimes neglected. Indeed there is a major deficiency in planned resources and facilities in this area.

Appendix

Equations: haemodynamic

$$SV = \text{stroke volume} = \frac{CO}{\text{Heart rate}} \text{ ml}$$

$$CI = \text{cardiac index} = \frac{CO}{BSA} \text{ l/min per m}^2$$

$$SVI = \text{stroke volume index} = \frac{CI}{\text{Heart rate}} \text{ ml/m}^2$$

$$\text{or } SVI = \frac{SV}{BSA} \text{ ml/m}^2$$

$$SVR = \text{systemic vascular resistance} = \frac{MAP - RAP}{CO} \times 80 \text{ dyne.s.cm}^{-5}$$

$$SVRI = \text{systemic vascular resistance index} = \frac{MAP - RAP}{CO} \times 80 \text{ dyne.s.cm}^{-5}\text{m}^{-2}$$

$$PVR = \text{pulmonary vascular resistance} = \frac{PAP - PAWP}{CO} \times 80 \text{ dyne.s.cm}^{-5}$$

$$PVRI = \text{pulmonary vascular resistance index} = \frac{PAP - PAWP}{CI} \times 80 \text{ dyne.s.cm}^{-2}\text{m}^{-2}$$

$$RVSWI = \text{right ventricular stroke work index} = SVI \times \frac{(PAP - RAP)}{CI} \times 0.0136 \text{ g.m.m}^{-2}$$

$$LVSWI = \text{left ventricular stroke work index} = RVI \times \frac{(MAP - PAWP)}{CI} \times 0.0136 \text{ g.m.m}^{-2}$$

Equations: oxygen transport

CaO_2 = arterial oxygen content = $Hb \times SaO_2 \times K$ + dissolved oxygen, ml/dl

CvO_2 = mixed venous oxygen content = $Hb \times SvO_2 \times K$ + dissolved oxygen, ml/dl

K is taken to be 1.34 or 1.39.

dissolved arterial oxygen content = PaO_2(mmHg) $\times$ 0.003 ml/dl or PaO_2(kPa) $\times$ 0.0225 ml/dl

dissolved mixed venous oxygen content = PvO_2(mmHg) $\times$ 0.003 ml/dl or PvO_2(kPa) $\times$ 0.0225 ml/dl

arterial $-$ mixed venous oxygen content difference = $CaO_2 - CvO_2$ ml/dl (sometimes abbreviated to $(a - v) \dot{D}O_2$)

DO_2 = oxygen delivery = $CO \times CaO_2 \times 10$ ml/min

$\dot{V}O_2$ = oxygen consumption = $CO \times (CaO_2 - CvO_2) \times 10$ ml/min

Fick equation $CO = \dfrac{\dot{V}O_2}{CaO_2 - CvO_2}$

$\dot{D}O_2$ I = oxygen delivery index = $CI \times CaO_2 \times 10$ ml/min per m^2

$\dot{V}O_2$ I = oxygen consumption index = $CI \times (CaO_2 - CvO_2) \times 10$ ml/min per m^2

In clinical practice the terms $\dot{D}O_2$ and $\dot{V}O_2$ are used to denote indexed values of oxygen delivery and consumption.

OER = oxygen extraction ration = $\dfrac{CaO_2 - CvO_2}{CaO_2}$ %

or OER = $\dfrac{SaO_2 - SvO_2}{SaO_2}$ %

Qs/Qt = pulmonary venous admixture = $\dfrac{CcO_2 - CaO_2}{CcO_2 - CvO_2}$ %

where CcO_2 is ideal pulmonary capillary oxygen content calculated from the alveolar gas equation solved for oxygen. (Pulmonary venous admixture is sometimes referred to as shunt fraction or degree of intrapulmonary shunting)

Other indices of oxygen exchange in popular use are

$A - a\dot{D}O_2$ = alveolar to arterial oxygen tension gradient = $P_AO_2 - P_aO_2$ mmHg or kPa (this should be abbreviated to $P(A - a)O_2$ but $A - a\dot{D}O_2$ is used by clinicians)

P_AO_2 is ideal alveolar oxygen tension calculated from the alveolar gas equation

P_aO_2/FIO_2 = the ratio of arterial oxygen tension to inspired oxygen concentration

P_aO_2/P_AO_2 = arterial oxygen tension to alveolar oxygen tension ratio

$$RI = \text{respiratory index} = \frac{P[A - a]O_2}{PaO_2}$$

References

Advanced Trauma Life Support (ATLS) programme for physicians (1993). *American College of Surgeons Committee on Trauma.* American College of Surgeons, Chicago.

American College of Chest Physicians/Society of Critical Care Medicine Consensus Conference. (1992). Definitions for sepsis and organ failure and guidelines for the use of innovative therapies in sepsis. *Crit Care Med*, **20**, 864–74.

Ashbaugh, D. G., Bigelow, D. B., Petty, T. L. & Levine, B. E. (1967). Acute respiratory distress in adults. *Lancet*, **ii**, 319–23.

Bell, R. C., Coalson, J. J., Smith, J. D. & Johanson, W. G. (1983). Multiple organ failure and infection in adult respiratory distress syndrome. *Ann Int Med*, **99**, 293–8.

Border, J. R., Hassett, J., La Duca, J., Seibel, R., Steinberg, S., Mills, B., Losi, P. & Border, D. (1987). The gut origin septic states in blunt multiple trauma (ISS = 40) in the ICU. *Ann Surg*, **206**, 427–48.

Conn, A. K. T., McCabe, C. J. & Warren, R. L. (1991). Initial management of trauma patients. In *Update in Intensive Care and Emergency Medicine*, ed. J.-L. Vincent, pp. 457–68. Berlin, Heidelberg, New York, Springer.

Cournand, A., Riley, R. L., Bradley, S. E. *et al.* (1943). Studies of the circulation in clinical shock. *Surgery*, **13**, 964–95.

Cryer, H. G., Richardson, J. D., Longmire-Cook, S. & Brown, C. M. (1989). Oxygen delivery in patients with adult respiratory distress syndrome who undergo surgery. *Arch Surg*, **124**, 1378–84.

Cuthbertson, D. P. (1942). Post shock metabolic response. *Lancet*, **i**, 433–37.

Edwards, J. D., Redmond, A. D., Nightingale, P. & Wilkins, R. G. (1988). Oxygen consumption following trauma: a reappraisal in severely injured patients requiring mechanical ventilation. *Br J Surg*, **75**, 690–2.

Edwards, J. D. (1990). Practical application of oxygen transport principles. *Crit Care Med*, **18**, S45–S48.

European Society of Intensive Care Medicine (1992). Consensus conference on selective decontamination in intensive care unit patients. *Intensive Care Med*, **18**, 182–8.

Fowler, A. A., Hamman, R. F., Good, J. T., Benson, K. N., Baird, M., Eberle, D. J., Petty, T. L. & Hyers, T. M. (1983). Adult respiratory distress syndrome. Risk with common predispositions. *Ann Int Med*, **98**, 593–97.

Fowler, A. A., Hamman, R. F., Zerbe, G. O., Benson, K. M. & Hyers, T. M. (1985). Adult respiratory distress syndrome: prognosis after onset. *Am Rev Respir Dis*, **132**, 472–8.

Goris, R. J. A. (1987). Can ARDS and MOF be prevented. In *Update in Intensive Care and Emergency Medicine*, ed. J.-L. Vincent, pp. 155–62. Berlin, Heidelberg, New York, Springer.

Goris, R. J. A., te Boeckhorst, T. P. N., Nuytinck, J. K. S. & Gimbrère, J. S. F. (1985). Multiple organ failure. Generalized autodestructive inflammation? *Arch Surg*, **120**, 1109–15.

Humphrey, H., Hall, J., Sznajder, I., Silverstein, M. & Wood, L. (1990). Improved survival in ARDS patients associated with a reduction in pulmonary capillary wedge pressure. *Chest*, **97**, 1176–80.

Hyers, T. M. & Fowler, A. A. (1986). Adult respiratory distress syndrome: causes, morbidity, and mortality. *Fed Proc*, **45**, 25–29.

Iotti, G. & Braschi, A. (1990). Respiratory mechanics. In *Update in Intensive Care and Emergency Medicine* 10, ed. J.-L. Vincent, pp. 223–60. Berlin, Heidelberg, New York, Springer.

Kraman, S., Khan, F., Patel, S. & Seriff, N. (1979). Renal failure in the respiratory intensive care unit. *Crit Care Med*, **7**, 263–6.

McClelland, P., Murray, A. E., Williams, P. S. *et al.* (1991). Reducing sepsis in severe combined acute renal and respiratory failure by selective decontamination of the digestive tract. *Crit Care Med*, **19**, 463–73.

Mizock, B. A. & Falk, J. L. (1992). Lactic acidosis in critical illness. *Crit Care Med*, **20**, 80–93.

Montgomery, A. B., Stager, M. A., Carrico, J. & Hudson, L. D. (1985). Causes of mortality in patients with the adult respiratory distress syndrome. *Am Rev Respir Dis*, **132**, 485–9.

Moore, F. A., Haenel, J. B., Moor, E. E. & Whitehill, T. A. (1992). Commensurate oxygen consumption in response to maximal oxygen availability predicts post-injury multiple organ failure. *J Trauma*, **33**, 58–67.

Nunn, J. F. (1987). *Applied Respiratory Physiology*. London: Butterworths.

Pepe, P. E., Potkin, R. T., Reus, D. H., Hudson, L. D. & Carrico, C. J. (1982). Clinical predictors of the ARDS. *Am J Surg*, **144**, 124–30.

Rady, M. Y., Edwards, J. D. & Nightingale, P. (1992). Early cardiorespiratory findings after severe blunt thoracic trauma and their relation to outcome. *Br J Surg*, **79**, 65–8.

Sheik, M. A. (1981). Respiratory changes after fractures and surgical skeletal injury. *Injury*, **3**, 489–94.

Shoemaker, W. C., Appel, P., Czer, L. S. C., Bland, R., Schwartz, S. & Hopkins, J. A. (1980). Pathogenesis of respiratory failure (ARDS) after hemorrhage and trauma. *Crit Care Med*, **8**, 504–12.

Shoemaker, W. C. & Appel, P. L. (1985). Pathophysiology of adult respiratory distress syndrome after sepsis and surgical operations. *Crit Care Med*, **13**, 166–72.

Stoutenbeek, C. P., van Saene, H. K. F., Miranda, D. R. *et al.* (1984). The effect of selective decontamination of the digestive tract on colonization and infection rate in multiple trauma patients. *Intensive Care Med*, **10**, 185–92.

Stürm, J. A., Lewis, F. R., Trentz, O., Oestern, H.-J., Hempelman, G. & Tscherne, H. (1979). Cardiopulmonary parameters and prognosis after severe multiple trauma. *J Trauma*, **19**, 305–16.

Tilney, N. L., Bailey, G. L. & Morgan, A. P. (1973). Sequential system failure after rupture of abdominal aortic aneurysms: an unsolved problem in post-operative care. *Ann Surg*, **178**, 117–22.

Trunkey, D. (1983). Trauma. *Sci Am*, **249**, 28–35.

19

Orthopaedic management

B. CLIFT and D. I. ROWLEY

Introduction

In considering the orthopaedic management of injury in the aged, we must ask the following questions. (1) Are there ways in which this management differs from that in the younger age groups? (2) Are there specific injuries that we regularly encounter in the elderly population compared with the population at large? The answer to both these questions is surely yes.

With fractures in this age group there are frequently predisposing factors other than the actual physical forces involved. Osteoporosis is the single biggest problem, but other pathologies such as metastatic tumour and Paget's disease are also common. Many of these injuries are therefore pathological fractures and are often 'low energy' injuries, as opposed to the much greater forces required to produce the same fracture in younger bone. Many old people break bones despite the absence of pathological bone and the frequency of injuries in the elderly may really be summarised as being due to the frequency with which they fall.

The perennial debate concerning operative or conservative management of fractures is particularly pertinent in the elderly. The early mobilisation permitted by internal fixation of a fractured neck of femur, thereby avoiding the dangers of prolonged recumbency, must be contrasted with the risks of anaesthesia and surgery, as well as the technical difficulties posed in dealing with comminuted, porotic bone. Although the evidence is now firmly on the side of surgery in that particular fracture, in other common injuries, such as ankle fractures, the debate continues.

Nearly all fractures and significant soft tissue injuries have specific complications. The elderly are as prone to these as everyone else. More important, however, in old age, are the general complications of injury and immobility, and their implications in management. All orthopaedic surgeons are familiar with the circumstance of an older patient, confined to bed for only a few days, developing a urinary infection, a deep venous thrombosis, a pulmonary embolus, severe confusion and so on. These relatively commonplace conditions carry with them a forbidding mortality and may greatly prejudice the chance of a successful return to the patient's previous environment.

In the elderly, the goals of treatment in a given injury may be much different to those in younger patients. The elderly tend to make fewer physical demands on their bones and joints and the needs of employment and sporting activities rarely have to be taken into account. Our guiding principles are to return the patient to their normal environment (a flat, sheltered housing, a residential home) and their normal state of dependency. These aims are only met by involving physiotherapists, occupational therapists, geriatricians and other members of rehabilitation teams.

Having made these points, our intention in this chapter is to describe the essentials of management of those particular injuries that are most commonly encountered in the aging population. The management of the general medical complications will not be discussed in detail here. We have confined ourselves to fractures, rather than soft tissue injuries, and in many relatively common injuries the management differs little from that in the younger patient. The interested reader is referred to the standard texts on trauma in such cases. The extremely important areas of epidemiology, osteoporosis, the response to injury and rehabilitation are covered elsewhere in this volume. In the following discussion, there are various references to eponymous classifications of fractures. These are currently in common usage, but it is likely that the AO classification of fractures will supersede these, as it is a logical system, based on first principles, with great relevance to treatment (Muller, 1991). The treatments described are for closed fractures. Open fractures all require some form of surgery in that wound excision and toilet are always needed and they may also require fixation techniques which go beyond the scope of this chapter.

Proximal femoral fractures

The 'fractured hip' is the commonest injury in the elderly that requires inpatient care. There are about 50000 such cases each year in the UK. It has been estimated that the annual cost to the National Health Service in 1990 would have been in the region of seven hundred million pounds (Bauer, 1990). In this more than any other injury, multidisciplinary management is essential for a satisfactory outcome. The description 'proximal femoral fracture' is used, as strictly speaking the trochanteric fractures do not involve the femoral neck. The distinction is relevant, as the treatment for the various fracture types may be very different.

Presentation

This fracture occurs between two and three times more often in women than in men, over the age of 65 years. In this age group the injury usually follows a fall, often of an otherwise trivial nature.

Pain is felt in the region of the hip and groin and weight-bearing is usually impossible. Some patients therefore reach hospital after many hours lying on the floor, before help arrives. This in itself carries complications such as dehydration, hypothermia and confusion. Clinical examination may reveal a shortened, externally rotated leg on the affected side, with pain on passive hip movement and tenderness on compression of the greater trochanter. Associated injuries such as vertebral and pelvic fractures should be looked for. Any serious underlying cause of the fall such as a stroke, transient ischaemic attack or myocardial infarction, needs to be excluded.

Diagnosis

Following clinical assessment, the key investigation is an anteroposterior (AP) radiograph of the whole pelvis, with a lateral view of the symptomatic hip joint. These will demonstrate the vast majority of hip fractures if present. Between 1 and 2% of patients with this injury will have normal radiographs at presentation. These patients should be admitted and repeat films taken after a few days. Normal radiographs are insufficient reasons for not admitting patients where there is a high index of clinical suspicion. If doubt persists, a radioisotope bone scan will settle the issue (Fairclough *et al.*, 1987). If a fracture is discovered, then all patients should undergo a thorough preoperative assessment (urea and electrolytes, full blood count, the cross-matching of three units of blood, electrocardiograph (ECG) and chest radiographs) as nearly all these fractures are treated surgically. Prior to surgery most patients are more comfortable if simple skin traction is applied to the affected leg. The bone biochemistry should be checked at this time to aid diagnosis in that small group of patients in whom their fracture is secondary to metastatic tumour, Paget's disease or osteomalacia.

These investigations should not delay surgery unnecessarily and many management problems can be identified but resolved subsequent to surgery. The anaesthetist is in the best position to arbitrate on whether the patient is yet fit for an operation, not a physician. In general, however, provided electrolyte balance is reasonable, and particularly potassium levels, then there are few contraindications to prompt surgical management. Delay is often counter-productive as nursing becomes increasingly difficult and new problems associated with prolonged immobility simply accumulate. The value of an excellent spinal anaesthesia service which is consultant led at every list is difficult to overestimate.

Surgery

Very few proximal femoral fractures are treated conservatively. Some form of traction and prolonged bed rest may allow bony union, but there is a high complication rate associated with the many weeks of inactivity and the end result may well be poor due to shortening and deformity. With modern techniques, particularly spinal anaesthesia, very few patients are completely unfit for surgery, so conservative treatment will not be discussed further.

The key question in evaluating the fracture and therefore to choose the correct operation, is to decide whether the femoral head has been rendered irreversibly ischaemic. This would lead inevitably to avascular necrosis and a hemiarthroplasty is required as a primary procedure. If the head is judged to be well vascularised, then some form of internal fixation, following reduction if necessary, is required. The blood supply to the femoral head is mainly via arteries along the superior aspect of the neck, which become intraosseous in the subcapital region. Intracapsular fractures high in the neck, if displaced, are likely to disrupt these vessels. In extracapsular fractures around the trochanteric region these vessels are unaffected and the head remains viable. On the preoperative radiographs one therefore looks for the level of the fracture and the amount of displacement. All fractures proximal to the greater trochanter should be regarded as at risk of ischaemia. The degree of displacement is commonly judged by Garden's criteria (Garden, 1976), based on the continuity in the AP film of the bony trabeculae in the proximal femur and acetabulum. Garden grades 1 and 2 are essentially undisplaced and grades 3 and 4 should be regarded as displaced. It is this latter group which requires hemiarthroplasty. The various surgical options are now presented.

Extracapsular fractures

These trochanteric injuries (Figure 19.1) may usefully be divided into stable and unstable groups according to the classification of Evans (1949). The key to stability is the integrity of the posteromedial cortex at the fracture site. About 70% are stable. These require reduction in theatre if displaced, using the image intensifier, and simple fixation using a telescoping screw or trifin nail in the femoral head and neck attached at 135° to a plate along the lateral cortex of the shaft. The telescoping allows the fracture to impact on weight-bearing, which promotes both stability and healing. Among the most popular such devices are the Dynamic Hip Screw and the Pugh nail and plate (Figure 19.2).

In unstable fractures the posteromedial bony cortex is disrupted. It is often possible to treat these in the same way as the stable fractures, but there is a significant risk that the lack of support will result in collapse in that area. This leads to varus angulation and leg shortening and the screw or nail may cut out of the femoral head. There are several operations designed to overcome these problems, the aim of which is to create a more stable valgus position by either 'over-reduction' or osteotomy of the upper femoral shaft (de Lee, 1984). As stated above, these unstable injuries may fare well with a 'routine' reduction and fixation and the question is whether the more difficult procedures are required as primary operations or whether they should be reserved as salvage procedures.

Intracapsular fractures

The undisplaced fractures are best treated with multiple compression screws inserted into the femoral head under image intensifier control (Figure 19.3). This can often be performed percutaneously. The aim is to get three screws, usually in a triangular configuration, parallel to each other.

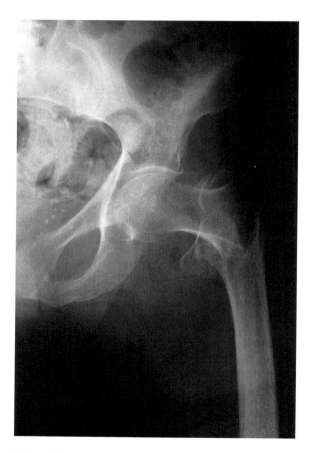

Figure 19.1 Comminuted intertrochanteric proximal femoral fracture.

Displaced fractures can also be treated in this way, following reduction, but the incidence of avascular necrosis and non-union is high. In the elderly there is little doubt that the femoral head should be replaced. The Austin–Moore and Thompson hemiarthroplasties have been the mainstay of this treatment for many years, but more recently bipolar prostheses have become popular (Bochner *et al.*, 1988). In these implants hip joint movement occurs at an inner bearing inside the main artificial head. They are thought to cause less postoperative pain and acetabular erosion than the older implants and as such are useful for the relatively young and active patient. A large scale prospective trial comparing the two is awaited. The actual surgery in both forms of implant is relatively quick and simple (Figure 19.4).

Very rarely, in an active, fit elderly person, a cemented total hip replacement may be

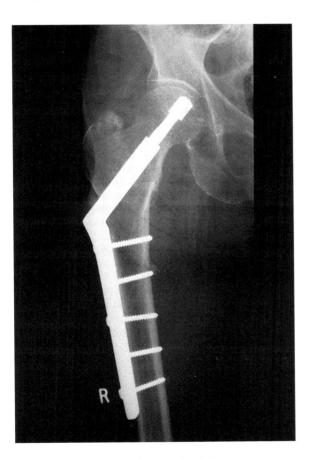

Figure 19.2. Extracapsular proximal femoral fracture treated with a Pugh nail and plate.

indicated as primary treatment. It remains the gold standard in terms of pain and function, but it is a much more demanding procedure in the context of acute trauma and carries a substantial morbidity. It may also be useful if a fracture occurs in the presence of a diseased hip joint, notably in rheumatoid arthritis, although bipolar prostheses are becoming increasingly popular in that situation.

Mobilisation and rehabilitation

Following surgery a check radiograph is required and the usual postoperative care is carried out. Many patients require transfusion. At 24–48 hours after surgery, the patient may sit out if all is well and commence weight-bearing as comfort allows. The active participation of the nurses and physiotherapists is essential. Most postoperative care takes place on orthopaedic wards, but it has been shown that a better outcome is achieved by early transfer to a geriatric rehabilitation ward, both in terms of length of inpatient stay and return to the patient's previous environment and level of function (Kennie *et al.*, 1988). This may be impractical in most units, but it stresses the need for a

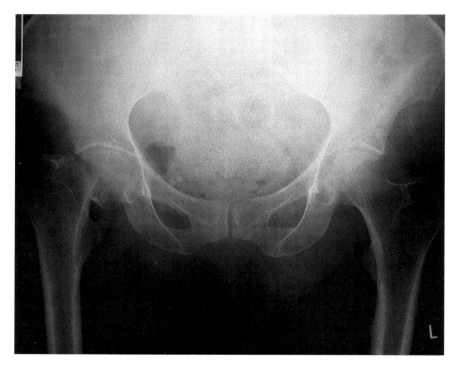

Figure 19.3. Displaced subcapital fracture of the right femur. There is a very high risk of avascular necrosis of the femoral head.

close working relationship with the geriatric service. The Hastings system is a prime example of this (Irvine & Strouthidis, 1977).

Many surgeons do not review these patients after discharge. Unless there have been specific problems in their fracture treatment, there seems to be no merit in outpatient follow-up.

Inoperative complications

These are the usual acute problems of surgery in the elderly, primarily metabolic and cardiovascular disorders. The best remedy is adequate preoperative assessment and correction of fluid balance, heart failure and the other common problems. The use of

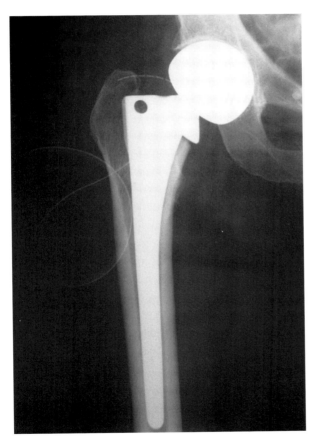

Figure 19.4. The fracture shown in Figure 19.3 has been treated with a Bateman bipolar hemiarthroplasty.

spinal anaesthesia has made this field of surgery much safer than in the past. Occasionally specific complications such as neurological and vascular damage occur, but these are rare. Minor femoral fractures are common with hemiarthroplasty, but major femoral shaft fractures are very rare.

Postoperative complications

General

Myocardial infarction, stroke and pulmonary embolism carry a 70% mortality in this situation (Jensen, 1984). The incidence of deep venous thrombosis and pulmonary embolism is minimised by the use of spinal anaesthesia, graduated compression stockings and early mobilisation. If mobilisation is delayed, other problems such as pressure sores, infections, confusion and chest infections rapidly appear and are often difficult to treat. Wound infection rates vary from centre to centre. In view of the disastrous consequences of deep infection in the presence of a fracture and an implant, we treat superficial infections aggressively with early wound excision and mechanical cleansing in the operating theatre. The use of prophylacticc preoperative antibiotics, usually a cephalosporin, is recommended.

Specific

(A) Extracapsular fractures

Failure of fixation Poor reduction, porotic bone and the wrong choice of operation may lead to the implant cutting out of the bone, or progressive deformity and breakage of the implant. This problem is more common in unstable fractures. Revision surgery is necessary.

Malunion Unstable fractures may unite in a varus position, often with malrotation. Revision is necessary only when symptoms are present. If left untreated, osteoarthritis of the hip is the eventual outcome.

Non-union This occurs in only about 1% of these fractures.

(B) Intracapsular fractures

Avascular necrosis of the femoral head This usually becomes apparent within 3 years of injury. The overall incidence following union of the fracture is between 30 and 40% (Butt, 1990). It is not seen this often as most displaced fractures are treated by hemi-arthroplasty. It presents as a painful hip, with characteristic radiological features. The treatment is hip replacement.

Non-union In Garden grades 1 and 2, which are normally treated by internal fixation of the femoral head, the radiological non-union rate at 1 year is around 10%. Treatment in the elderly patient is with either a hemiarthroplasty rf a total hip replacement, but only if it is symptomatic.

Complications of hemiarthroplasty Dislocation is a risk, minimised by using an anterior approach to the hip, when its incidence is 1%. It is commoner in confused patients and in those with strokes and Parkinson's disease. Only if it is recurrent does this complication warrant further open surgery. Pain is a significant problem in the more active patient. In the years following surgery acetabular and femoral erosion can occur, which both cause pain, maximal on weight-bearing. Revision to a cemented total hip replacement is the answer, or even excision of the joint. The tip of the femoral stem may produce an area of abnormal stress on weight bearing and femoral shaft fracture is an occasional consequence of this. Treatment then depends on the exact fracture type.

Mortality

The fracture type and the various operations do not in themselves influence mortality. The most important factors are undoubtedly the degree of independence before injury and the mental ability score (Ions and Stevens, 1987). Mortality is increased in specific conditions such as stroke and Parkinson's disease. The timing of surgery is important; there must be adequate pre-operative assessment and preparation, but delay beyond about forty eight hours increases the mortality. The majority of deaths occur in the two months following injury. An overall figure of about 22% has been quoted as the one year mortality (White *et al.*, 1987).

Fractures of the ankle

These fractures are due to indirect violence. They are slightly commoner in women than men and their incidence is said to be increasing in elderly osteoporotic women (Cedell, 1989). They highlight the continuing dilemma between conservative and operative fracture management in the elderly.

Presentation

The history is of a stumble or fall, usually with a twisting component. The pain is intense and bruising and swelling rapidly develop over the malleoli. Emergency treatment is often necessary to reduce the associated dislocation of the ankle joint before skin necrosis, due to local pressure, becomes inevitable and to restore the distal circulation. This should be carried out under sedation as soon as possible. The deformity is obvious and a radiograph is unwarranted delay at this stage.

Diagnosis

AP and lateral ankle films are required. Some medial malleolar fractures are associated with fractures of the proximal fibula and further radiographs may be required, depending on the clinical assessment. The films allow one to classify the injury and hence to plan treatment. Typically there is a fracture of the lateral malleolus. This may be associated with a medial malleolus fracture and also there may be a fracture of the posterior margin of the distal tibia (Figure 19.5).

Conservative or operative management?

It is difficult to be dogmatic about this. In active young people, very many of these injuries are treated by open reduction and internal fixation. In the correct hands a perfect reconstruction can usually be achieved, with obvious advantages to the long-term function of the joint. In the elderly, this may be less important. In addition, as in so many other fractures, the osteoporotic bone is not ideal for holding screws and plates. Prolonged anaesthetic times, coupled with the use of a tourniquet (often in the presence of some degree of cardiovascular disease), have the potential for a high morbidity. The decision must therefore be based on many factors: the previous activity and general health of the patient; the skill of the surgeon; the degree of osteoporosis and the stability of the fracture. Highly unstable fractures of any sort require surgery, as a successful closed reduction will almost certainly displace in a cast. It may be impossible to decide until the patient has been examined under an anaesthetic, in which case consent must have been obtained for both procedures.

The available evidence suggests that in elderly women, conservative measures should usually be attempted, due to the high morbidity and failure rate of internal fixation, but in men the bone is usually adequate for surgery if so desired (Beauchamp *et al.*, 1983). There have also been prospective studies demonstrating no difference in ankle function between patients over a wide age and sex range treated conservatively and operatively (Rowley *et al.*, 1986). It is proposed, therefore, that closed manipulation and cast fixation is in most cases the correct primary treatment of ankle fractures in the elderly.

Conservative management

Undisplaced fractures require only a simple plaster cast, extending initially above the knee to control rotation. Displaced fractures require manipulation under general or spinal anaesthesia. The principle is to reverse the forces which produced the fracture, hence the value of accurate classifications. Charnley's description of this technique has not been bettered, and should be available for reference (Charnley, 1950). Once reduced and in a cast, a check radiograph is needed. The difficulty is in holding the reduction. Further radiographs are necessary weekly for 2 or 3 weeks. Once the fracture is considered to be stable, the above-knee cast may be reduced to a shorter patellar-tendon-bearing cast, and the patient can put weight through it. The usual time in plaster is 6–8 weeks. If the reduction fails, a remanipulation or open reduction and internal fixation is performed.

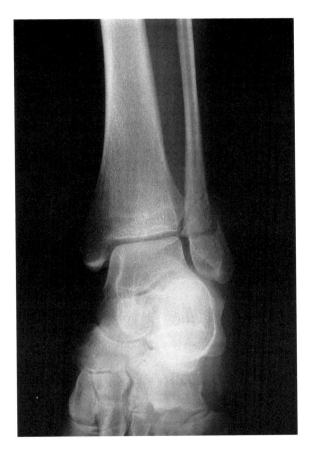

Figure 19.5. There is an isolated fracture of the lateral malleolus. This injury did well with conservative management.

Complications

Malunion can occur if the reduction has been inaccurate or inadequately monitored. It tends later to cause arthritis. Non-union is rare. Stiffness is common due to the prolonged immobilisation and is an inherent disadvantage of this technique. Physiotherapy is then needed.

Operative management

Surgery is ideally performed within 8 hours of injury. The principle is to reduce the fibular fracture and keep it out to length. A plate with screws is the usual technique. Further screws may be needed to fix the medial malleolus and to maintain reduction of the inferior tibiofibular joint. After surgery weight-bearing must be avoided for 6–8 weeks. In many patients, particularly the elderly, a cast is required for extra safety in this period and one of the advantages of surgery (early mobilisation to prevent stiffness) is therefore lost. A check radiograph is required with a further radiograph when mobile, usually at 1 week. Failure of fixation due to poor bone quality is a major risk. Unless it is causing problems, the current trend is to leave all metalwork in the ankle, thus avoiding a later operation.

Complications

The usual problems of infection, deep venous thrombosis and so on may occur, although they are not common. Failure of fixation manifest on the radiograph by loss of reduction and displacement of the metalwork is a potential problem within the first few weeks. Even in anatomically-reduced injuries post-traumatic arthritis may supervene within a few years following severe fractures. The only effective treatment is arthrodesis.

Fractures of the proximal humerus

These are common injuries in the elderly. The female:male ratio is 1:2 and the incidence is about half that of proximal femoral fractures.

Presentation

Following a fall, usually onto the outstretched hand, the patient has pain in the shoulder and upper arm with loss of shoulder movement. Occasionally deformity of the arm is evident.

Diagnosis

AP and axial, or lateral, radiographs are required of the affected shoulder. The standard classification of this injury is based on whether the fracture is displaced, the specific site of the fracture and the number of fragments (Neer, 1970). Ninety per cent of fractures are undisplaced or impacted two-part fractures at the surgical neck of the humerus. The remaining 10% are complex injuries and these two groups require different management. When the radiographs are scrutinised, the relation of the humeral head with the glenoid must be checked, as fracture dislocations or simple anterior and posterior dislocations can present similarly (Figure 19.6).

Goals of treatment

A full range of shoulder movement is in practice unnecessary and in older people almost always impossible to achieve. What is required finally is the ability to reach the mouth, hair and perineum for activities of daily living. Also, the patient should be pain free. These goals require the help of both physiotherapists and occupational therapists. The following treatment protocols are given with these points in mind.

Conservative treatment

This applies to 90% of these injuries. They are treated, often as outpatients, with analgesia and a collar and cuff to provide external support – although a broad arm sling may be more comfortable initially as this provides a little support. The crux of treatment is early mobilisation, often within a few days of injury. Patients must be quite clear about the need for this and about the recommended regimen. Early pendulum exercises and passive movement using the other arm are followed by active movements, as the symptoms permit. Physiotherapy supervision is often needed. Displaced two-part fractures may also be treated this way with satisfactory results, even when angulated, as this usually corrects in the collar and cuff.

Surgical treatment

This may be required for displaced two-part fractures, although only very rarely in the elderly. Three-part fractures, in which the greater or lesser tuberosity is fractured, often do well in the older patient if treated conservatively. Four-part fractures, which involve both tuberosities, nearly always require surgery in the elderly because of the very high incidence of avascular necrosis of the humeral head and pain and stiffness of the shoulder. The choice is between some form of reconstruction and internal fixation, and using screws, plates and wires, prosthetic replacement of the humeral head. In the elderly, a difficult and lengthy reduction and fixation is rarely worthwhile and the trend is now to perform a hemiarthroplasty in these situations. This also permits repair of the rotator cuff so optimising any residual shoulder function. The Neer prostheses are widely used and the results are generally good (Stableforth, 1984). The principle is similar to that in hip hemiarthroplasty for a fractured femoral neck. The most important operative point is correctly to repair the rotator cuff. Much of the postoperative morbidity may be traced to inadequate attention to this area.

Complications

Non-union is rare in these injuries. It is usually due to soft tissue interposition at the fracture site. Malunion of some degree is not uncommon, but only very rarely is it a problem. Axillary nerve damage may occur at the time of injury. The neuropraxia may

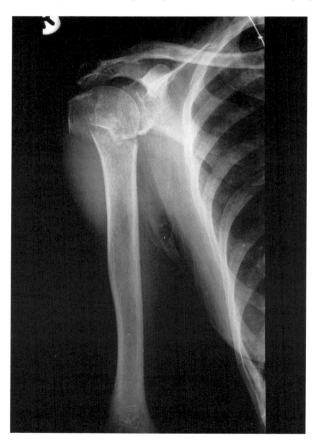

Figure 19.6. Typical impacted fracture of the surgical neck of the humerus.

take several months to recover, during which the deltoid component of shoulder abduction is lost. Avascular necrosis is now infrequently seen due to the trend towards primary hemiarthroplasty. The most common complications are pain and stiffness due to adhesions forming in the joint and subacromial bursa. These are minimised by early mobilisation, but when present, treatment may involve physiotherapy, steroid infiltration of the joint and bursa and very occasionally manipulation under anaesthetic.

Olecranon fractures

This is a relatively common injury in the elderly. It is due to a fall onto the point of the elbow. The fracture frequently enters the joint and the pull of the triceps tendon produces displacement of the fragment. For these reasons, even in very elderly patients, operative fixation is nearly always required. In the rare undisplaced fractures immobilisation in a long arm cast with the elbow in extension can be tried, but there may be considerable stiffness as a result (Figure 19.7). The ideal treatment is open reduction and internal fixation using a tension band wiring system. This is a quick procedure which allows mobilisation of the elbow within a few days. The accurate reduction minimises the risk of subsequent arthritis.

Fractures of the distal radius

There are several fracture patterns commonly occurring at this site. The Colles, and Smith's fractures will be discussed in some detail.

Colles' fractures

This is one of the commonest fractures in the elderly. It occurs three times as often as hip fractures. Fortunately most of these injuries can be treated on an outpatient basis. The classical injury was first described in 1814 by Abraham Colles of Dublin.

Presentation

There has been a fall on the outstretched hand. The wrist is painful, with loss of movement. Swelling is usual and the 'dinner fork' deformity may be obvious on inspection. The median nerve function in the hand should be checked and documented at this time.

Diagnosis

An AP and lateral wrist radiograph is required. The injury is a fracture of the distal radius; the distal fragment is angulated dorsally and radially and lies supinated. It is usually impacted and there may be considerable dorsal displacement. An estimate should be made of the degrees of angulation, whether the fracture extends into the joint and the amount of shortening of the radius in relation to the distal tip of the ulna. The degree of comminution on the dorsal aspect of the radius is perhaps the most important feature to note, as in combination with the other factors described, it has a great bearing on the stability of the reduced fracture (Figure 19.8) (Jupiter, 1991).

Management of stable fractures

A small number of fractures do not require reduction if the angulation and displacement are minimal. These should be immobilised in a forearm plaster slab extending over the extensor and radial surfaces as far as the metacarpophalangeal joints. The

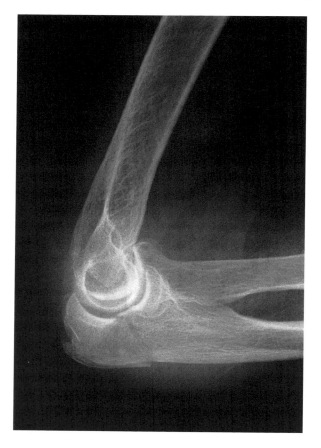

Figure 19.7. Undisplaced fracture of the olecranon. This injury was successfully treated in a cast, although most olecranon fractures require internal fixation.

majority of fractures require reduction. This is easily performed in a well-staffed casualty department, using a Bier's block to anaesthetise the whole forearm. The technique involves exsanguinating the forearm, maintaining this using a high pressure tourniquet and injecting the emptied veins with 30–40 ml of prilocaine. It is very effective and lasts for long enough to allow remanipulation if the first effort is unsuccessful. There are few absolute contraindications to this method, but hypertension is one, as it requires too high a tourniquet pressure. Reservations have been expressed about the safety of this technique, which is usually performed without the aid of an anaesthetist, but long experience has shown very little morbidity with good equipment and experienced nursing staff. The alternatives to Bier's block are either local anaesthetic injected into the fracture haematoma, or a general anaesthetic. The former can be useful, but the pain relief is often patchy and there is a risk of introducing infection directly into the fracture, as well as systemic absorption of the anaesthetic. General anaesthesia requires hospital admission with a full work-up and carries its own not insignificant risks, as well as its financial cost.

Management of unstable fractures

In the elderly even those fractures which are likely to be unstable are nearly all treated using the above protocol. If they have slipped by the time of the radiographs at 1 week

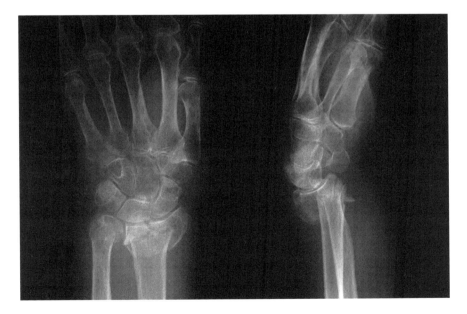

Figure 19.8. Typical Colles' fracture.

there are a number of options: remanipulation and another cast; remanipulation and percutaneous pinning of the distal fragment; remanipulation and external fixation using a special fixator or plaster; open reduction and internal fixation and simply accepting the position.

Most of these injuries are remanipulated and put back into plaster, but in the elderly, redisplacement is almost invariable (McQueen *et al.*, 1986) and a hazardous waste of time and resources. The simplest surgical option is to maintain reduction using percutaneous wires and a further cast. This is a straight forward procedure and the results have been good (Clancey, 1984). The other surgical options have mainly been used in younger patients with high energy injuries and are rarely needed in the elderly. There is a case to be made for leaving these unstable injuries in the 'poor' position, as even those fractures which appear stable at 1 week often slip at a later date. We are all familiar with patients who have an obvious deformity at the unit, but no appreciable disability. This was Colles' own view of the final outcome of the fracture. In the final analysis, the decision is unique to each patient, based on their individual needs; however, provided that sufficient length is maintained to prevent ulnar impingement then an acceptable functional result is likely.

Complications

Median nerve involvement

This manifests itself with sensory symptoms and occasionally weakness, which usually develops later. Its incidence is about 6% (Cooney *et al.*, 1980). It is an absolute indication for reduction of the fracture. If, following reduction, there is still a partial nerve lesion, it is usually safe to elevate the arm and observe the situation for a week. If there is then no improvement, surgical decompression is required. If, after reduction, there is a complete lesion of the nerve, immediate decompression is indicated (McCarroll, 1984). Occasionally patients present later with median nerve symptoms in association with a malunited Colles' fracture; again surgery is required.

Tendon rupture

Extensor pollicis longus ruptures in just under 1% of these injuries (Cooney *et al.*, 1980). The cause is either ischaemia or pressure from the bone fragments. It usually presents a few weeks after removal of the plaster and a tendon transfer procedure is required. Very rarely, flexor tendons may rupture in association with a Colles' fracture.

Reflex sympathetic dystrophy

This occurs only rarely, but leads to serious disability if not treated aggressively. There is intense local pain, swelling and tenderness, with thin shiny skin over the wrist and hand. If untreated the hand becomes cold and stiff, with atrophic skin. It is due to a local autonomic upset. Some consider it to be linked with median nerve compression, but the true pathogenesis is unknown. Radiographs have a patchy porotic appearance. The treatment consists of elevation, intense daily physiotherapy, analgesia and avoidance of extreme temperatures. Local sympathetic blocks may be needed to get this regimen under way.

Malunion

As suggested above, clinical malunion appears to be common, but usually asymptomatic. Radiological shortening appears to correlate with reduced grip strength and residual angulation and displacement are associated with a decreased range of wrist movement (Villar *et al.*, 1987). Although these findings may cause problems in the younger patients with jobs, driving and sporting activities, in the elderly there is very rarely real disability and corrective surgery is hardly ever required unless ulnar impingement is severe.

Arthritis

In those fractures which involve the joint surface, pain and stiffness may eventually develop but it is a surprisingly small problem and can usually be managed with anti-inflammatory agents and analgesics.

Smith's fracture

In this fracture the distal radius fragment is angulated and displaced towards the palmar or volar aspect of the wrist. It is much rarer than the Colles' fracture but it is also due to a fall on the outstretched hand, when in pronation, hence the impact is on the dorsal surface with the above deformity as a result. The diagnosis may be suggested clinically and radiographs confirm it. Holding is difficult and surgical fixation, even in the elderly is advisable (Figure 19.9).

Pelvic fractures

The pelvic bones fracture easily in the elderly. These are common injuries and are usually the result of a fall. The pubic and ischial rami are the usual sites of injury and normally both rami on the same side are fractured. The patient complains of pain, usually in the groin, and a fractured hip is often suspected. Examination may be unhelpful, but it is possible to palpate bony tenderness of the superior rami and pain is usually produced by bilateral compression of the pelvis. An AP radiograph of the pelvis usually reveals the injury, if in doubt a radioisotope scan confirms it. The pelvis, like the spine, is frequently a site of bony metastases. If there is any suspicion of malignancy in such fractures, a bone scan should be performed and any other relevant screening investigations.

These fractures do not compromise the stability of the pelvic ring and they are always managed conservatively. After a few days in bed the patient is gradually mobilised, as the discomfort allows. Patients are usually pain free within a few weeks. The only significant complications are the usual ones of enforced bed rest.

Less commonly seen are acetabular fractures. They occur in the same circumstances, but present with pain in the hip. The AP pelvis radiographs may show the fracture, but specific oblique views are sometimes required. Unlike in the young patient, these are low-energy fractures and again conservative treatment is indicated. Bed rest, with skin traction on the affected leg is required. The pain may take several weeks to settle enough for weight-bearing. Apart from the dangers of recumbency, these fractures may be complicated by late secondary arthritis of the hip, as the articular surface has been disrupted. A total hip replacement may therefore be the eventual outcome.

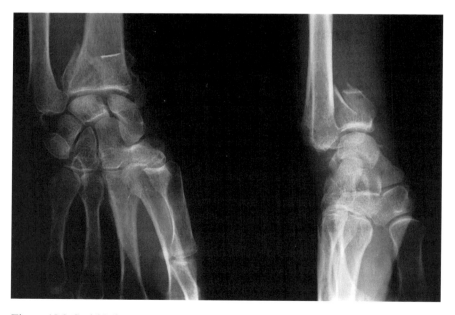

Figure 19.9. Smith's fracture. Compare with Figure 19.8.

Fractures of the thoracolumbar spine

The spinal fractures that commonly occur in the elderly are compression fractures of the vertebral bodies. It is important to realise that these are virtually all stable injuries with no risk to the spinal cord and cauda equina. They are low-energy injuries – the main aetiological factor is osteoporosis and frequently there is no history of trauma. They present with localised back pain and tenderness and a kyphotic deformity may be evident of loss of the lumbar lordosis. A neurological examination should be performed. As with pelvic fractures, this is a common site for metastases and appropriate vigilance is required.

Radiological findings

AP and lateral radiographs of the spine are required. The compression may affect the whole vertebral body but more commonly there is anterior wedging as these are flexion injuries. Occasionally, lateral wedging is visible on the AP view when nerve root compression can be a problem. If there is any doubt about the stability of these fractures (if the height of the anterior margin is less than half that of the posterior margin) then a computed tomography scan of that level will show whether the spinal canal is compromised.

Management

Patients may require admission. Bed rest and analgesia are employed, with gradual mobilisation as comfort allows. Persistent back pain is often difficult to manage, but a judicious deployment of analgesics, weight loss, moderation of activity and external orthoses usually controls the symptoms.

Pathological fractures

There are numerous causes of pathological fracture in the aged. The commonest is osteoporosis and reference has been made to the problems related to this in the above text. Two further categories that merit some specific attention are Paget's disease and metastatic bone tumours.

Paget's disease

This relatively common disorder is occasionally the underlying cause of long bone fractures, particularly of the femur. There are several potential pitfalls in obtaining good internal fixation, if this is indicated. First, the hypervascularity of the bone may cause profuse bleeding on reaming and deaths have been reported from this cause. Second, there are areas of bone which are abnormally hard which may be impossible to drill or ream and instruments can become jammed. Lastly, if the bone is considerably deformed, an intramedullary nail or a plate may be impossible to use without performing osteotomies and these can become formidable operations. With these points in mind, it is clear that the treatment of fractures in pagetoid bone requires careful planning. One possible advance is the use of disodium pamidronate in the immediate preoperative period which is thought to decrease the vascularity of the bone, but this has yet to be proven in clinical trials.

Metastatic bone tumours

Metastases are the commonest malignancies of bone and the commonest primary tumours are breast, prostate, kidney, lung and thyroid. Fractures are almost inevitable if the patient lives long enough and are the cause of considerable pain and disability. For these reasons, as a general rule, such pathological fractures should be treated with internal fixation even if the patient has only a short time to live. A stable fixation greatly helps with pain relief and nursing care and the fractures may even heal once stabilised if local radiotherapy is also given. Occasionally a pathological fracture may be the first sign of an occult primary and all suspicious fractures should therefore be biopsied if an operation is performed.

References

Bauer, G. C. H. (1990). Hip fracture in the elderly: a success story or a social problem? *Curr Orthop*, **4**, 147–9.

Beauchamp, C. G., Clay, N. R. & Thexton, P. W. (1983). Displaced ankle fractures in patients over 50 years of age. *J Bone Joint Surg*, **65B**, 329–32.

Bochner, R. M., Pellicci, P. M. & Lyden, J. P. (1988). Bipolar hemiarthroplasty for fracture of the femoral neck. *J Bone Joint Surg*, **70A**, 1001–10.

Butt, W. P. (1990). Mini-symposium: fractured neck of femur. (iii) Radiological evaluation. *Curr Orthop*, **4**, 156–64.

Cedell, C. A. (1989). Trauma (i) Ankle fractures. *Curr Orthop*, **3**, 244–50.

Charnley, J. (1950). The Pott's fracture. In *The Closed Treatment of Common Fractures*, ed. J. Charnley. Edinburgh: E & S Livingstone.

Clancey, G. J. (1984). Percutaneous Kirschner–wire fixation of Colles fractures. A prospective study of thirty cases. *J Bone Joint Surg*, **66A**, 1008–14.

Cooney, W. P., Dobyns, J. H. & Linscheid, R. L. (1980). Complications of Colles' fracture. *J Bone Joint Surg*, **62A**, 613–19.

de Lee, J. C. (1984). Fractures and dislocations of the hip. In *Fractures in Adults*, vol. 2, 2nd edn, ed. C. A. Rockwood & D. G. Green. Philadelphia: J. B. Lippincott.

Evans, E. M. (1949). The treatment of trochanteric fractures of the femur. *J Bone Joint Surg*, **31B**, 190–203.

Fairclough, J., Colhoun, E., Johnston, D. & Williams, L. A. (1987). Bone scanning for suspected hip fractures. A prospective study in elderly patients. *J Bone Joint Surg*, **69B**, 251–3.

Garden, R. S. (1976). Malreduction and avascular necrosis in subcapital fractures of the femur. *J Bone Joint Surg*, **58B**, 2–24.

Ions, G. K. & Stevens, J. (1987). Prediction of survival in patients with femoral neck fractures. *J Bone Joint Surg*, **69B**, 384–7.

Irvine, R. E. & Strouthidis, T. M. (1977). The geriatric orthopaedic unit. In *Geriatric Orthopaedics*, ed. M. Devas. London: Academic Press.

Jensen, S. S. (1984). Determining factors for the mortality following hip fractures. *Injury*, **15**, 411–14.

Jupiter, J. B. (1991). Current concepts review: fractures of the distal end of the radius. *J Bone Joint Surg*, **73A**, 461–9.

Kennie, D. C., Reid, J., Richardson, I. R., Kiaman, A. A. & Kelt, C. (1988). Effectiveness of geriatric rehabilitation care after fracturing of the proximal femur in elderly women: a randomised controlled trial. *Br Med J*, **297**, 1083–6.

McCarroll, M. R. Jr. (1984). Nerve injuries associated with wrist trauma. *Orthop Clin North Am*, **15**, 279–87.

McQueen, M. M., Maclaren, A. & Chalmers, J. (1986). The value of re-manipulating Colles' fractures. *J Bone Joint Surg*, **68B**, 232–3.

Muller, M. E. (1991). The comprehensive classification of fractures of long bones. In *Manual of Internal Fixation*, 3rd edn, ed. M. E. Muller, M. Allgower, R. Schneider & H. Willenegger. Berlin: Springer.

Neer, C. S. II. (1970). Displaced proximal humeral fractures. Part 1. Classification and evaluation. *J Bone Joint Surg*, **52A**, 1077–89.

Rowley, D. I., Norris, S. H. & Duckworth, T. (1986). A prospective trial comparing operative and manipulative treatment of ankle fractures. *J Bone Joint Surg*, **68B**, 610–13.

Stableforth, P. G. (1984). Four-part fractures of the neck of the humerus. *J Bone Joint Surg*, **66B**, 104–8.

Villar, R. N., Marsh, D., Rushton, N. & Greatorex, R. A. (1987). Three years after Colles' fracture: a prospective review. *J Bone Joint Surg*, **69B**, 635–8.

White, B. L., Fisher, W. D. & Laurin, C. A. (1987). Rate of mortality for elderly patients after fracture of the hip in the 1980s. *J Bone Joint Surg*, **69A**, 1335–40.

20

Burns in the elderly

G. M. WATKINS

Introduction

Bull classically defined elderly by Probit Analysis (Bull, 1972). In 1981, Watkins and colleagues first noted two or more pre-existing diseases resulted in a high mortality rate for elderly patients with less than 40% body surface area (BSA) burn. Pruitt *et al.* (1976) and Larson *et al.* (1992) used ages 50 and 45 years, respectively, as equivalent to 'elderly' because of increased mortality associated with burned individuals at those ages. Sixty years or older still remains a good measure of elderly because important physiological changes inevitably occur around that age: thinning of the skin, delay in wound healing and decreasing cardiovascular and pulmonary function. Muscle mass, bone density, visual acuity, body fat changes, hearing loss and multiple other problems detailed in other chapters of this volume inevitably occur around age 60 years.

Classification and causes

First degree burns at any age cause erythema and pain. These burns result from minimal contact with heat over a brief period of time. The damage does not extend beyond the epidermis. Second degree burns involve the dermis to variable degrees. Second degree is divided into superficial and deep. Blistering commonly occurs with the superficial second degree burn. Deep second degree burn may be impossible to distinguish from third degree by clinical examination. Third degree burn implies necrosis of the entire skin and loss of skin appendages. A zone of stagnation around a more deeply burned area causes enlargement of the third degree area by 24–36 hours after injury because of associated late venous thrombosis.

An increased incidence of house fires, inhalation injuries and scald burns occurs in the elderly. Burn abuse is being reported more frequently in the elderly (Watkins, 1988).

Treatment

Pre-hospital treatment consists of usual trauma diagnosis and care. An important exception is that burning or smouldering clothes should be removed from the individual as a first step. Protocols should require all elderly burned to be transported to a burn centre. An important pre-hospital treatment is prevention of hypothermia. Wet or cool applications are avoided. The patient is covered by sterile sheets and reflective blankets. During transport, 100% oxygen is used to counteract any effects of carbon monoxide poisoning and to increase oxygen delivery because blood volume and/or cardiac output may be low. In distant areas prophylactic intubation and resuscitation with fluids are part of the care. The former can be protocol guided alone. The latter must in part be under medical command.

At hospitals oxygen should be continued. Advanced burn life support protocols should be followed. Multiple injuries or illness may antecede or occur simultaneously with the burn. A complete history from a variety of sources as well as complete examination of the patient with all clothes, jewellery, etc. removed is essential. Oedema of the head and neck may occur more quickly in the elderly. With head and neck burns, prophylactic intubation is freely used. Controversy continues over the appropriate mode of resuscitative therapy in the elderly. Central lines should not be utilised before the patient arrives at the final treating facility. In the author's series of 47 elderly burns (Watkins, 1981), original intravenous lines were removed and a central line inserted on a semi-emergency basis. There were no cases of septic phlebitis at any site. No consensus exists about frequency of changing central venous lines. Frequent blood gases and continuous oximetry help monitor ventilation and oxygenation status. Continuous pulse oximetry helps monitor adequacy of oxygenation. Central venous catheter lines alone are of limited use in determining cardiac function. Combinations of a Swan–Ganz catheter plus blood gases, haemoglobin levels, arterial pressures, pulse and oxyhaemoglobin fraction are important for ongoing assessments, especially where pre-existing cardiovascular disease is present. One can also calculate oxygen available/oxygen extracted ratio (O_2 A/E). Mixed venous oxygen tension and/or reflective oximetry via Swan–Ganz catheter are usual monitoring adjuncts. Reflective oximetry does not account for shifts in oxyhaemoglobin dissociation, nor does it remain accurate over time. It allows observers to discover sudden changes in O_2 A/E.

Resuscitation formulae poorly estimate fluid resuscitation in the elderly patient. When burns are over 20% BSA or the individual has a complex series of illnesses, modifications of the formula may be appropriate. If burns encompass more than 15% BSA, there is a local and total body 'capillary leak' of fluid into the interstitial space. This leak begins to close 2–4 hours after injury, is 50–75% complete by 12 hours and is closed by 24 hours after injury. For this reason, the author's practice is to resuscitate those elderly with greater than 20% body surface area burns (formerly with a probability of dying of more than 0.9) using 2 ml of fluid/kg per %BSA burn; half is fresh frozen plasma, half is crystalloid. This resuscitation usually replaces lactated Ringer's by 4–6 hours after injury and continues for the first 24 hours.

Haemoglobin is maintained at 15–16 g for oxygen delivery (Watkins, 1988). The elderly may have a hidden anaemia especially when arteriosclerotic cardiovascular disease exists (Sharpey-Schaeffer, 1944). Watkins *et al.* (1974) confirmed that blood volume is low due to anaemia alone. Geha & Baue (1978) noted declination in cardiac function in animals with decreasing haematocrit where coronary artery stenosis was present. Most studies of 'enhanced oxygen delivery' with anaemia are short-term studies in animals where intravascular volume was kept at or higher than normal. The burn patient not only has a different response because of leaky capillaries but also has a markedly diminished peripheral vascular resistance in the burned area (Wilmore *et al.*, 1977). A majority of studies of traumatised individuals have shown both a continuing volume deficit and partial hidden red cell mass deficit during the flow stage. The author's choice for the patient at high risk has been to accept the small but definite risk of major transfusion reaction and long-term possibilities of infection because of the benefits of fresh frozen plasma (Alexander *et al.*, 1979) and normal red cell mass. The result is only a 15–20% increased use of blood products over that reported by others. In burn patients, most blood products are given because of loss during and after operative procedures or because haemoglobin has reached critical levels by any standards during prolonged intensive care unit (ICU) stays. Blood pressure and pulse are not reliable monitors in the elderly. The maximum effective pulse rate is much lower in the older individual. Blood pressures may vary widely for numerous reasons.

Urine output has been used as a guide for determining perfusion. Cioffi has recently shown that free water clearance in burns is reduced while urine output is normal (Cioffi *et al.*, 1991). A clinically unrecognised 20% blood volume deficit was thought to be the cause. In an elderly person with fragile renal function such diminished blood volume may not be acceptable. Different priority monitors need to be developed. Changes in the burn extremities are important indicators of total perfusion and any vascular compromise due to constricting eschar. Sensation, function and Doppler distal pulses of the hands and/or feet of affected areas are monitored hourly during the first 48–72 hours. All elderly burn victims are admitted to the hospital and usually the ICU. Exceptions to ICU care are when patients are otherwise healthy, have no inhalation injury, do not have critical body areas involved and have less than 5% BSA burn. After injury stress may uncover diseases that were not apparent on admission.

Metabolic changes

Ebb and flow response is blunted in the burned elderly. An elderly individual may become malnourished earlier and debilitatingly lose muscle mass earlier as a result of starting with less muscle mass and/or fat reserves. An elderly individual has the same increase in protein needs but less increase in total caloric needs than predicted by the Curreri formula. The elderly diabetic with a blood sugar greater than 200 mg/l has impaired burn wound healing. Earlier closure of the burn wound does not ameliorate the hypermetabolic response in younger patients and probably does not in the elderly.

The elderly become hypothermic quickly in the operating, resuscitation and recovery rooms. It is our practice to keep resuscitating and operating rooms at 29.5–31 °C. Liberal use of reflective thermal blankets, heating pads, heated intravenous fluids, heated and humidified ventilation, and radiant heat is all important in ameliorating temperature declination. Any open surfaces, especially those wet with moist pads, should temporarily be covered with sterile plastic film to cut down on heat loss during resuscitation, debridement or skin grafting.

Ventilation

In the elderly burn patient, tracheostomies are generally avoided until the wound is closed because of the fear of nosocomial infections. Elderly individuals who are on prolonged ventilator support still can be weaned. In the author's experience, one elderly burn patient was weaned after 310 days of ventilator therapy. The author's first series of elderly burns contained only a handful of patients who died from pneumonia. As burn wound sepsis was almost obliterated by early excision and grafting, overall survival improved dramatically. Pneumonia-related mortality rose to 50%, however (Watkins, 1988). Early extubation, frequent change in position, physical therapy, ambulating at the bedside even of intubated patients, etc., lowers the incidence of pneumonia and atelectasis.

Nutrition

During initial resuscitation a feeding tube should be passed under fluoroscopic control until it is beyond the ligament of Trietz. A nasogastric tube should also be passed. Since 1984, the following regimen has been utilised: 25% calories as protein, 10% as fat, 15% as carbohydrate, plus minerals and vitamins with food colouring added to the solution started. Half-strength formula is started at 75 ml/hour via the feeding tube. The concentration is increased and volume decreased every 6–8 hours until the calculated amounts per hour as derived from the Curreri formula are achieved. Charts are placed on the wall of the patient's room with a red line drawn showing the protein goal on one graph and the caloric goal on the other. The diet is changed in arrears one day to make up for any protein deficiencies from the previous one. If 75% of calculated caloric requirements are met, little attention is paid to total calories being made up.

Water is adjusted as clinically indicated. If nasogastric residue shows food colouring or there is more than 400 ml/hour nasogastric tube drainage, feedings are stopped or decreased for 1–2 hours and then begun again. If such occurs, radiographs usually show the tube feeding in the upper duodenum or stomach. Watery diarrhoea (more than 4–6 liquid stools/day) is treated by using half-strength tube feedings and giving 16 mg codeine every 4 hours through the feeding tube. If diarrhoea does not slow down or cease, tube volume feeding is reduced by 50%. Occasionally, tube feedings have to be diluted to half-strength or withheld for 6–8 hours.

Patients are encouraged to eat during the transition phase to oral regimen. Calculated protein needs are made up the next day by manipulating enteral feedings until the patient is able to sustain appropriate oral nutrition. Tube feedings experimentally reduce endotoxaemia and bacterial translocation. The earlier tube feedings start the more the gut mucosal barrier is preserved (McDonald *et al.*, 1991). Hyperalimentation has not been used by the author in the past 11 years for acute burns. Such therapy is increasingly being abandoned by other burn units. Enteral feedings are continued throughout surgical procedures when a patient is intubated and has a nasogastric tube without residual colouring, and the feeding tube is beyond the ligament of Trietz. No incidence of aspiration has been documented with such a regimen. Glutamine and proportions of 3–omega or 6–omega fatty acids may be important additives.

Other care

Low-flow airbags prevent bedsores and conversion of second degree burns to full thickness. 'Floating bead beds' have been associated with dehydration, hypothermia and mental disturbance. The remainder of burn care is no different from ordinary patients except for a higher index of suspicion of burn wound sepsis caused by local invasion. Areas of invasion may be treated in one of four ways: (1) tangential incision removing all contaminated areas, (2) excision to normal fat or fascia, (3) coring out penetrating ulcer clusters (best used for *Mucor*), or (4) subeschar injection of antimicrobials (such is fraught with hazard in the elderly as most effective antibiotics are nephrotoxic). Escharotomies are performed as discussed elsewhere (Watkins, 1988). A technique point concerning escharotomy: completeness is ascertained by running a finger down the escharotomy line. If no septa are felt and only normal fat, the escharotomy is complete. Compartment syndromes have rarely developed in unburned limbs. For electrical burns, fasciotomies and occasional carpal tunnel decompression may be necessary. The chest may require an escharotomy so that the ribs and/or abdomen may expand. The face is treated conservatively in the elderly. Sulfamylon or silversulfadiazine are not used because of potential eye irritation. Head and face dressings are not used routinely. Sulfamylon is used on potentially exposed ear cartilage or joints.

Early excision and coverage

An elder's skin thins increasingly with age. Most deep second degree burns should be considered third degree. The best wound therapy is to begin excision and coverage as a part of the resuscitation. The goal is to have the patient grafted before the onset of burn wound sepsis (5–10 days after a burn). The author's method is to begin excision at 24 hours after burn, using teams of two surgeons, two anaesthetists and two scrub nurses in a room at 31 °C with warm fluids, humidified and heated ventilation, and the body parts covered. The operations are staged one day apart and are ended 1.5 hours after surgery starts, if the patient's temperature drops below 35.8 °C or one-half of the patient's blood volume is estimated lost. For grafts of major burns in the elderly, 0.008 inch split thickness skin grafts from the sides, chest, abdomen and suprascapular areas of the back are taken. These grafts are meshed for 6:1 expansion, placed on the recipient bed and covered by a 1.5:1 meshed viable homograft placed at right angles to the inner graft. This complex is stapled into place. The lower half of the body is avoided as donor sites because of poor healing. Donor sites are covered with stapled viable pigskin ensuring a closed wound. The operative procedures are detailed elsewhere (Watkins, 1988). Recent clinical release of substitute dermis and experimental shortening of tissue culture time may make cultured skin/artificial dermis composites useful in clinical practice.

Rehabilitation

In hopeless cases, carrying out no treatment may be a humane option but the elderly with burns formerly considered lethal now may survive. Elderly trauma victims may take longer to recover but those survivors most often return to home care or normal environment, satisfied with the outcome (Manktelow *et al.*, 1987). This may be true even in an older person who develops prolonged no-stroke coma during the acute phase.

References

Alexander, J. W., Ogle, C. O., Stinnett, J. D. *et al.* (1979). Fresh frozen plasma versus plasma protein derivative as adjunctive therapy for patients with massive burns. *J Trauma*, **19**, 502–11.

Bull, J. P. (1972). The revised analysis of mortality due to burns. *Lancet*, **2**, 1133–4.

Cioffi, G. C., Vaughan, G. M., & Heironimus, J. D. (1991). Dissociation of blood volume and flow in regulation of salt and water balance in burn patients. *Ann Surg*, **214**, 213–18.

Geha, A. S. & Baue, A. E. (1978). Graded coronary stenosis and coronary flow during acute normovolemic anemia. *World J Surg*, **2**, 645–52.

Larson, C. M., Saffle, J. R. & Sullivan, J. (1992). Lifestyle adjustments in elderly patients after burn injury. *J Burn Rehab Med*, **13**, 48–52.

McDonald, W. S., Sharp, C. W. & Deitch, E. A. (1991). Immediate enteral feeding in burn patients; safe and effective. *Ann Surg*, **213**, 172–83.

Manktelow, A., Meyer, A. A., Heroz, S. R. *et al.* (1987). Analysis of life expectancy and living status of elderly patients surviving a burn injury. *J Trauma*, **29**, 203–7.

Pruitt, B. A., Mason, A. D. & Hunt, J. L. (1976). Burn injury in the aged or high risk patient. In *The Aged and High Risk Surgical Patient*, ed. J. H. Siegal & P. Chodoff, pp. 523–46. New York: Grune & Stratton.

Sharpey-Schaeffer, E. P . (1944). Cardiac output in severe anaemia. *Clin Sci*, **5**, 125–32.

Watkins, G. M.(1981). *Burn Care in the Elderly*. Presented at the Annual Meeting of the Am. Assoc. for the Surgery of Trauma

Watkins, G. M. (1988). Care of the geriatric individual who is burned. In *Surgical Care of the Elderly*, ed. J. L. Meakins & J. L. McClarin, pp. 455–72. Chicago: Yearbook Medical Publishers.

Watkins, G. M., Rabelo, A., Bevilaqua, R. G. *et al.* (1974). Bodily changes in repeated hemorrhage in normal man. *Surg Gynecol Obstet*, **139**, 161–75.

Wilmore, D. W., Aulick, L. H., Mason, A. D. *et al.* (1977). Influence of the burn wound on local and systemic responses to injury. *Ann Surg*, **186**, 444–76.

21

Principles and organisation of orthopaedic rehabilitation

C. T. CURRIE and W. J. MACLENNAN

Introduction

In a 1984 study (Robbins & Donaldson) the authors sought to develop a method to document extended acute hospital stay by hip fracture patients and analysed what they termed stages of care. Their 217 patients accumulated a total of 5167 bed-days, of which 10% were spent awaiting surgery, 51% recovering without complications and 28% awaiting discharge after the completion of surgical and medical care. The methodology is questionable. Is it likely that on each day every patient was engaged in only one of the above? Both the practices and attitudes revealed give cause for concern. If non-operated cases are excluded, the preoperative delay averaged 60 hours. Recovering without complications, even if abruptly ended by a terminological switch to waiting for discharge, conveys the assumption that hip fracture patients get better by themselves. Awaiting discharge likewise implies a degree of passivity, and even the stated aim of the work is so modest as to appear defeatist: patients given adequate surgical treatment stay so long in the ward that a method is required simply to document their unwelcome presence.

Yet it is worth citing this work in detail because, however inadvertently, it draws attention to three key issues in the rehabilitation of elderly fracture patients: (1) the importance of minimising preoperative delay, (2) the role of early and sustained functionally oriented rehabilitation, and (3) the potential of discharge planning in reducing length of stay.

A 50-year-old woman may now face over her remaining lifetime a 15% risk of a Colles' fracture, 16% risk of hip fracture and 30% risk of vertebral fracture (Cummings et al., 1989). Daunting enough in these individual terms, osteoporotic fractures now pose enormous challenges for hospital and community health services throughout the developed world as the very elderly grow in numbers and the age-specific incidence of the most significant injury, proximal femoral fracture (PFF), continues to rise. Although the evidence is complex and perhaps incomplete, it appears that many societies face substantial further increases in already high incidences of osteoporotic PFF as a late consequence of a secular downward trend in physical activity (Astrom *et al.*, 1987) and as a concomitant of mass survival, including that of the frail, to very old age (Finsen, 1988).

The service implications are formidable. A study from New South Wales (Lord & Sinnett, 1986) using projections from recent hospital statistics on acute care, secondary rehabilitation and long-term care outcomes, predicted an 83% rise in bed-day use by PFF patients between the years 1986 and 2011. Such predictions, however, assume unchanging practice and must be set alongside reports based on the experience of services developing in response to the substantial challenges of the last 30 years. Here there may be some grounds for optimism. Reports from a pioneering service in Lund, Sweden (Ceder *et al.*, 1987) describe how the local incidence of PFF doubled over the period 1966–83. Over the same period, by a combination of surgery directed at early mobilisation, vigorous rehabilitation and early and maximal involvement of community services, the proportion of patients returning directly home rose from 44 to 75%, mean hospital stay fell from 44 to 16 days and the total number of bed days used for hip fracture fell by one-third despite the doubling of its incidence.

This achievement reflects many local factors, including a comprehensive prepaid health care system, a highly developed provision of multidisciplinary primary health care and, not least, the Scandinavian orthopaedic tradition of self-critical enthusiasm. Around the world most orthopaedic services must make do with less, but few can avoid the clinical burdens imposed by osteoporotic fractures.

While new devices and surgical techniques for fracture management can be passed quickly from centre to centre, the same cannot often be said of advances in the rehabilitation of the elderly orthopaedic patient. Such innovations and service developments as have been described depend on a range of local conditions including resources, attitudes, systems of reimbursement and the nature of working relationships between the professionals involved. Inevitably they reflect these local conditions. A standard approach, even if one were to be validated and recognised, would be unlikely to prosper in widely varying circumstances. Similar considerations tend to complicate the evaluation of the effectiveness of different strategies adopted.

Nevertheless, as the pattern of fractures and other clinical, social and functional problems encountered in the elderly orthopaedic patient is broadly comparable across the developed world, a number of general principles of rehabilitation are worth examining. In addition this chapter reviews some of the common barriers to rehabilitation and describes the various patterns of service that have evolved. Many services have now been developed and reported and few orthopaedic surgeons whose patients have access to them would wish them to be discontinued. In the strictest methodological terms, however, the effectiveness of geriatric orthopaedic rehabilitation remains controversial. The evidence is discussed.

The over-riding imperative is one of urgency. If surgery is required for an elderly fracture patient it is best carried out with minimum delay and should have as its aim the quickest possible restoration of function in the affected limb. Thereafter management is directed to restoring mobility and independence in self-care with a view to returning the patient to his/her usual circumstances as soon as possible.

Inevitably hip fractures loom large in orthopaedic life and literature. The hip fracture is by far the commonest serious injury seen in the elderly, accounting for around half of elderly trauma admissions, with no other single diagnosis accounting for more than a few per cent of cases (Whitaker & Currie, 1988). Hip fractures are only rarely missed. Almost all cases are admitted to hospital. As a 'standard injury' hip fracture therefore offers a conveniently common and well-defined entity for epidemiological, surgical and rehabilitation studies. Specific studies on the rehabilitation of other fractures are comparatively rare. For practical purposes it can safely be asserted that service arrangements which cope with the surgery and rehabilitation challenges of hip fracture patients will suffice also to serve the needs of those suffering from the heterogeneous but mainly less severe range of other injuries encountered in the elderly. The same themes, namely a 'fix-it-and-forget-it' approach to the injury and 'whole-patient' approach to rehabilitation, apply; the same systems will be effective (Table 21.1).

Preoperative assessment and management

Many patients presenting with a fractured proximal femur have a complex premorbid history and may be on a multiplicity of drugs. It is essential, therefore, that the doctor referring the patient provides as much of this background information as possible. There often have been several previous hospital admissions, so that an efficient medical records system also plays an important part in the preoperative assessment of fracture patients (Table 21.2).

The referring doctor may also include details of social circumstances and previous support. These will be helpful in providing baseline information for further action at the stage of rehabilitation. It is important to know whether the patient lives alone, how many flights of stairs have to be negotiated, what the patient's pre-injury level of mobility was and what formal and informal supports were in place (community services such as home help, meals on wheels; community health input such as district nurse, day hospital attendance; family support such as help with shopping and cooking). Patients from sheltered housing with alarm systems and wardens in place may manage to go home more quickly than those from ordinary housing. Patients from residential care settings may require some rehabilitation before discharge, as nursing care is not normally provided. Patients from high dependency settings such as nursing homes and

Table 21.1. *Orthopaedic diagnoses in patients over 70 years of age admitted to an orthopaedic unit*

Orthopaedic diagnosis	Percentage of cases
Fractured proximal femur	52.8
Fractured pelvis	4.4
Fractured ankle	2.8
Fractured wrist	2.4
Fracture/dislocation of previous fractured proximal femur fixation	2.4
Fractured neck of humerus	2.0
Fractured shaft of femur	1.6
Fractured tibia and fibula	1.6
Fractured vertebral body	1.2
Multiple fractures	3.6
Soft tissue injury	6.0
Back pain (no body injury)	2.8
Other	16.8

Source: Whitaker & Currie (1989).

Table 21.2. *Concurrent medical problems identified in 50 women admitted to an orthopaedic unit with a fractured proximal femur*

Medical condition	Number of patients
Congestive cardiac failure	9
Cardiac arrhythmia	3
Dementia	18
Hemiparesis	4
Vertebrobasilar ischaemia/drop attack	9
Parkinson's disease	2
Chronic obstructive airways disease	5
Pneumonia	2
Restrictive lung disease	1
Dysphagia	2
Haematemesis	2
Malabsorption	1
Diabetes mellitus	3
Carcinoma of thyroid	1
Thyrotoxicosis	1

Note: Some patients had more than one concurrent medical problem.
Source: Campbell (1976).

long-term care wards may be assumed to require only a brief and essentially peri-operative stay in the orthopaedic unit, plans for a prompt return to familiar surroundings being made quite early.

Where possible, the patient's usual mental state should be determined. It is not always easy to do this when the patient is in pain, disoriented or frightened. Sympathetic enquiries from accompanying relatives should be informative. If a patient can normally manage their own affairs such as shopping and cooking, there will probably have been no serious mental problems. Difficulties arise in the previously slightly impaired, managing quite well at home in normal circumstances. They are likely to become more confused in relation to trauma and its management and their confusion may well be an important barrier to their rehabilitation. Early knowledge of previous mental state is important because of its prognostic significance.

Among the more common chronic conditions precipitating falls and fractures are dementia, Parkinson's disease, a previous stroke, visual impairment, muscle weakness, osteoarthritis, severe anaemia, congestive cardiac failure and postural hypotension. Although acute illnesses may precipitate falls, such falls cause only a small minority of hip fractures. Subsequent to the fall, however, patients may lie undetected at home for several hours developing a number of different disorders which include hypothermia, dehydration, bronchopneumonia, decubitus ulcers and acute confusion.

It clearly is important that, prior to surgery, all patients should have a thorough physical assessment including the measurement of temperature, using a low reading thermometer if necessary. Investigations should include a full blood count, blood urea and electrolytes, blood glucose, thyroid function tests, and a chest radiograph. An electrocardiogram should probably be reserved for patients with an arrhythmia or who have clinical features suggesting a myocardial infarction.

A fine judgement is required in balancing the advantages of treating associated medical disorders against the increased morbidity and mortality normally associated with delaying surgical intervention. Disorders requiring correction before surgery include dehydration, congestive cardiac failure, bronchopneumonia. hypothermia, poorly controlled diabetes mellitus and anaemia with, say, a haemoglobin of less than 100 g/l.

Preoperative delay

A brief and well-managed period of preoperative care will minimise risks to frail elderly patients and pave the way for their early rehabilitation. Even at that stage it is worth explaining the rehabilitation process and the prospects for early mobilisation and discharge. It should be remembered that the patient's expectations may have been formed decades ago when 3–4 months in hospital was the norm for hip fracture. Good pain control will promote confidence. Care of pressure areas is an essential investment of nursing time and expertise for patients unable to move around in bed because of injury.

A period of prolonged uncertainty and discomfort prior to surgery will quickly destroy morale. Confusion too is more likely. If theatre list planning is over-ambitious fasting may be unnecessarily long, with consequent dehydration, metabolic upset and risk to the skin. Repeated fasting is not unknown, and of itself can lead to further delay, for ostensibly anaesthetic or medical reasons, as the likelihood of electrolyte disturbance and intercurrent infection increases. Skin damage acquired in hours (though taking days to appear) may heal only over weeks or months and come to dominate management long after the fracture for which surgery was necessary has ceased to be a problem. An initial and unnecessarily prolonged period of uncertainty, discomfort, dehydration, sensory deprivation and helplessness will have a predictable and deleterious effect on subsequent confidence and progress. It is better that postoperative rehabilitation begins without the need for apologies about previous management.

Surgery will be delayed if operable fractures are not diagnosed. Hip fracture is more likely to be missed if the patient is confused or previously dependent or has an undisplaced fracture (Eastwood, 1987). Assuming the diagnosis, prompt surgical management of hip fracture has been shown to improve outcome. Immediate surgery (delay not exceeding 6 hours) for femoral neck fracture has been linked to quicker union and a lower incidence of subsequent collapse (Manninger *et al.*, 1989). Villar *et al.* (1986), in a series of patients managed by hemiarthroplasty and in which delay had occurred for administrative reasons only (i.e. unwell patients whose surgery had been delayed for medical reasons were excluded), showed that in those showing good rehabilitation at 3 months the median delay had been 29 hours and that in those showing poor rehabilitation it had been 57 hours. A Swedish series (Dolk, 1989) demonstrated a correlation between preoperative delay and increased length of stay and need for after-care.

Prognosis

The proportion of patients recovering mobility, with or without a walking aid, after a fractured proximal femur ranges from 62 to 83% (Barnes & Dunovan, 1987). Determinants of a poor outcome include extreme age, contractures involving the lower limb, weakness of hip abductors on the affected side, and the presence of a trochanteric rather than cervical fracture. Other adverse factors are mental impairment and a low level of premorbid mobility (Cheng *et al.*, 1989). In addition, patients whose fracture has been pinned are less likely to mobilise than those given a hip prosthesis (Barnes & Dunovan, 1987).

The factors which determine the likelihood of an individual eventually being discharged to his/her own home are similar in that they include age, presence or absence of multiple pathology, mental function, and premorbid mobility and self-care capacity (Broos *et al.*, 1988). In this situation the degree of mobility achieved after rehabilitation, and the availability of relatives at home also are extremely important.

The mortality from fractures of the proximal femur ranges from 17 to 36% at 1 year (Ions & Stevens, 1987). Factors having an adverse effect upon this include an advanced age, being male, and concurrent congestive cardiac failure or dementia (Clayer & Bauze, 1989). Also of importance are poor mobility prior to injury and an operative delay of more than 24 hours in previously healthy individuals (Sexson & Lehner, 1987).

Postoperative management

In the immediate postoperative period, a number of non-orthopaedic problems may arise. Ideally the orthopaedic unit should have access to the advice of a geriatrician, and the nursing staff have training and experience in the management of problems specific to elderly patients.

Confusion

In a review of confusion in patients with a fractured proximal femur, it was found that 33% were confused prior to surgery and that a further 28% developed the condition after operation (Gustafson *et al.*, 1991b). Concurrent disorders contributing to the confusion were dementia, cerebrovascular disease, parkinsonism and cardiovascular disease, and medications that might have contributed to the problem included antidepressants, neuroleptics, benzodiazepines, antiparkinsonian drugs and anticholinergic drugs. Patients with confusion often have biochemical evidence of thiamine deficiency, but a controlled trial of thiamine supplements demonstrated that these had no effect on mental status (Day *et al.*, 1988).

Unless medical and nursing staff in an orthopaedic unit focus their attention on the problem confusion is likely to be missed or misdiagnosed (Gustafson *et al.*, 1991a). A useful measure to increase diagnostic accuracy is to apply a simple mental test score to all admissions.

There has been a report on an intervention programme designed to reduce the incidence of confusion in fracture patients (Gustafson *et al.*, 1991b). Prior to surgery, all patients had a thorough medical assessment, usually by a geriatrician who recommended measures such as increased doses of diuretics in heart failure, and the use of dextran as prophylaxis against thromboembolic disease. An attempt was made to minimise any delay between the fracture and surgery. All patients had blood gas measurements made before, during and after surgery, and oxygen-enriched air given during the operation and for at least 24 hours after this. Anaesthetic measures included preventing hypotensive episodes, and using spinal anaesthesia in patients over the age of 75 years. Subsequent to surgery patients were regularly reviewed and treated for medical conditions by a geriatrician. The effect of this package was to reduce the incidence of postoperative confusion from 61.3 to 47.6%.

Particular attention has been given to the merits of spinal anaesthesia in elderly patients, but there is no evidence that this achieves a lower incidence of postoperative confusion than general anaesthesia (Berggen *et al.*, 1987).

Poor nutrition

A review of elderly women admitted with a fractured proximal femur established that, when assessed by anthropometric measurements and serum albumin levels, one-fifth were severely undernourished (Bastow *et al.*, 1983). The problem is compounded by the extra demands that trauma and surgery impose on energy and protein balance. Evidence for this is the observation that in the first 8 days after surgery 90% of elderly women with a fractured proximal femur were in negative calorie and nitrogen balance (Stableforth, 1986).

Oral supplementation, using sip feeding with supplements, is effective in increasing both energy and protein intakes, but rarely eliminates the negative balance (Stableforth, 1986). In one small study, these measures reduced the 6 month mortality in hip fracture patients from 37 to 24%, and the rate of complications at 6 months from 37 to 16% (Delmi *et al.*, 1990). There was the problem, however, that nurses often experienced difficulty in persuading patients to take adequate quantities of supplements.

An alternative approach in patients with evidence of particularly severe undernutrition is to give supplements by a fine-bore nasogastric tube (Bastow *et al.*, 1983). If given overnight rather than during the day, supplementation need not interfere with the intake of nutrients at normal mealtimes. A major side-effect is that a proportion of patients develop diarrhoea associated with the hyperosmolar nature of the supplement. When used in a small number of severely undernourished fracture patients, the technique was associated with a reduction in mortality from 22 to 8%, and a reduction in the time taken to regain independent mobility.

Immediate postoperative complications

Deep leg vein thrombosis

The increased risk of deep leg vein thrombosis and pulmonary embolism associated with surgery for fractures of the proximal femur can be reduced by treatment with low-dose heparin (Collins *et al.*, 1988). This is given subcutaneously as calcium heparin in a dose of 5000 units 8-hourly. Even greater prophylaxis can be achieved by adjusting the dose in relation to its effect on the activated partial thromboplastin time (Taberner *et al.*, 1989).

Pressure sores

In surveys, up to 30% of patients treated for fractures of the proximal femur have developed pressure sores (Hughes, 1986). A major cause is the immobility which follows the injury, but poor nutrition and, in some instances, a poor state of hygiene further increase the risk. Ulcers also are more likely to occur if sensation is impaired by analgesics or pre-existing neurological disease, while patients with cardiovascular or peripheral vascular disease are at particular risk.

The most important measure is to avoid prolonged pressure by turning patients regularly and protecting the heels with appropriate padding. Local massage of areas at risk also is practised widely by nursing staff but is of more doubtful value, as is the wide range of barrier, zinc and antiseptic creams used in conjunction with this. Patients with anaemia, hypoalbuminaemia, and ascorbic acid or zinc deficiency benefit from appropriate supplementation. There also are a number of mechanical devices which reduce pressure on the affected sites. These include large cell ripple mattresses, water beds and air beds, but these should be seen as an adjunct rather than a substitute for high quality nursing care.

With modern orthopaedic management designed to promote immediate mobilisation, only a few patients now require the prolonged periods of bed rest associated with the risk of pressure sores. Most elderly trauma patients mobilise quickly and satisfactorily. Good early rehabilitation is the mainstay of pressure sore prevention.

Infection

A recent review of patients requiring surgery for a fractured proximal femur revealed that the incidences of superficial and deep infections of the operative site were 11.5 and 2.2%, respectively (McQueen *et al.*, 1990). The incidence of infection can be reduced by giving cephalothin in regular doses for 72 hours, or by using nafcillin in a similar fashion for 48 hours. In the study in question, a single dose of cefuroxime was ineffective. It remains questionable whether the relatively low rate of infection justifies the use of comparatively expensive antibiotics.

Constipation

Limited mobility, dehydration, a low intake of fibre and treatment with morphine derivatives mean that a high proportion of fracture patients become constipated. In the immediate postoperative period the best way of treating this is with suppositories such as bisacodyl or with phosphate enemas.

Depression

Depression is common in the elderly and elderly trauma patients are not exempt. The diagnosis is easily missed, but is common particularly after major injury. A large study of elderly female hip fracture patients (Mossey *et al.*, 1989) found elevated depression scores in 51% following surgery. High postsurgery depression scores were associated with poorer recovery in functional status.

Many patients will, of course, be disheartened by the pain and disability of an acute admission for trauma. The diagnosis should be suspected, however, in postacute patients who are unduly despondent or making disappointing progress in relation to their objectively determined problems. A number of useful screening questionnaires exist. The GDS-15 (Yesavage, 1988) is widely used. Many patients respond to treatment with such relatively non-toxic drugs as lofepramine.

Immediate rehabilitation

Whatever the locus of later rehabilitation efforts (whether at home, in a designated rehabilitation unit or (least preferably) in the acute orthopaedic ward itself) the acute orthopaedic unit can and should offer immediate rehabilitation opportunities to elderly orthopaedic patients. From the 1950s to the 1970s there was a progressive diminution in the duration of non-weight-bearing prescribed after hip fixation (Ceder *et al.*, 1987). Now, with almost universal enthusiasm for immediate weight-bearing, hip fracture patients are encouraged to take at least a few steps on the first postoperative day. Many will need the help of two simply to stand, but will benefit from the demonstration that it can be done. More will be accomplished soon.

While expertise in mobilisation is traditionally the province of the physiotherapist, it is no monopoly. If patients are to walk 'little and often' and a little further each time, they are, in most orthopaedic units, likely to be dependent on nurses for help when they do so. Physiotherapists, fewer and more expensive than nurses, can continue to contribute by assessment, goal setting and review and are normally willing (systems of reimbursement permitting) to collaborate with nursing staff in the common goal of early mobilisation. With adequate pain control and regular encouragement, many patients will make progress towards a target – getting to and from a toilet is one that makes immediate sense to most – and feel an appropriate sense of achievement.

Other activities of daily living should be encouraged in the first few postoperative days in the acute ward. (Here the patient's relatives can usefully be involved. A few days after surgery most patients should have clothes and shoes brought in. Relatives should also be made aware of the patient's progress and prognosis: their cooperation in future plans may be vital.) Patients should be encouraged to dress themselves, minimum necessary help being provided by ward staff. The effectiveness of the occupational therapist, like that of the physiotherapist, can be greatly extended by maximising the nursing contribution in day-to-day activities of daily living rehabilitation and reserving more specialist therapist input for assessment, goal-setting and review.

Rehabilitation-oriented nursing offers a means of bringing to the acute ward a key component of the more specialised care offered in geriatric orthopaedic units. Dependent more on attitudes and education than on additional resources, it is probably underutilised. The key elements of successful nursing in the early rehabilitation of elderly orthopaedic patients are skill in the management of confusion, the early promotion of the patient's own efforts in mobility and self-care, and a positive and sensitive approach to carers. Such an approach will produce gratifying results. In a recent study (Currie *et al.*, 1994) of elderly trauma patients admitted from home to a unit in which such nursing attitudes prevailed, perioperative dependency (measured by the Barthel Index) was shown to be generally brief. A policy of vigorous early mobilisation and the promotion of self-care resulted in 45% of the patients, including some with femoral neck fractures, proceeding straight home (in most instances with additional community support) with a mean length of stay of 8.3 days.

In contrast, much damage can be done by a passive approach in the early postoperative phase. Patients who are viewed as 'waiting for a rehabilitation bed' and hence regarded as 'blocking a bed' are unlikely to be subjected to the active interest, regular rehabilitation and review that might benefit them. A minimal approach to nursing, addressing dependency needs and failing to address early rehabilitation opportunities, will unnecessarily prolong the stay of many elderly patients.

Good pain control is essential for effective early postoperative rehabilitation of elderly trauma patients. For a number of reasons it is difficult. Confused patients may not report pain unless questioned sympathetically. Inexperienced staff may overestimate the risks of inadequate analgesia. A recent study (Currie *et al.*, 1993) showed that in a prospective series of 100 elderly trauma patients the majority experienced significant pain, yet in the 48–hour period following surgery none of the patients received more than half of the maximum recommended number of doses of opioid analgesics. Adequate, regular and regularly reviewed doses of opioids will control postoperative pain safely. Within a few days a switch to simpler analgesia will usually be possible. Codeine, dihydrocodeine and coproxamol are useful. Paracetamol may occasionally be adequate. Non-steroidal anti-inflammatory drugs are dangerous in elderly trauma patients because they are frequently hypotensive and dehydrated and the risk of renal damage is very high.

Geriatrician involvement

It has been stressed already that a fracture, often a proximal femoral fracture, is commonly merely an incident in a long career of chronic illness and disability in an elderly patient. The involvement of geriatricians in the care of elderly orthopaedic patients has been one of the notable developments of the past 30 years or so. In the early stages of the development of cooperation such involvement was often fairly minimal, with geriatricians being asked simply to provide placement for patients who, weeks or months after surgery, had stabilised without prospects of further rehabilitation. With the growing realisation of the potential of collaborative rehabilitation schemes, geriatricians have tended to become involved earlier and earlier. A common form of such collaboration is the orthogeriatric unit (see below).

As in many units around half of the acute orthopaedic beds are occupied by elderly patients, many of them with pre-existing and/or perioperative medical problems, there are grounds for geriatrician involvement in the earliest stages of the management of elderly trauma patients. Prompt and expert assessment of the non-surgical problems by a specialist in the care of the elderly will in many cases minimise preoperative delay. A geriatrician, by definition an expert in the rehabilitation of frail elderly patients, is well placed to assess rehabilitation needs and potential in the light of locally available facilities. As a provider of 'general medicine' for elderly patients, a geriatrician will also serve to minimise delay-inducing referrals to single organ specialists of elderly patients many of whom will have multiple medical problems. Daily specialist geriatrician input is not generally available, but is much appreciated by orthopaedic surgeons (Whittaker & Currie, 1988).

A recent Australian report (Cameron *et al.*, 1993) of a randomised controlled trial of 'accelerated rehabilitation' after proximal femoral fracture provides encouraging evidence in support of geriatrician involvement in the orthopaedic ward. Intervention patients underwent multidisciplinary rehabilitation led by an experienced physician with training in geriatric and rehabilitation medicine. A 20% reduction in length of hospital stay was achieved, together with improved physical independence and an increased likelihood of patients from home returning to their homes.

Orthogeriatric unit

This is now a fairly common and well-established form of orthopaedic–geriatric collaboration (Newman, 1992). Such units vary considerably in facilities, selection procedure, organisation and performance. Most rely heavily on the organisational skills of the geriatrician and the efforts of a multidisciplinary team (nursing, physiotherapy, occupational therapy, social work). While the patients remain 'orthopaedic' by reason of their injuries and previous management, their need for close surgical supervision is not great. The opening of an orthogeriatric unit is not likely to result in a time consuming commitment for orthopaedic surgeons. A brief regular review is all that is required for most patients. Surgical complications requiring urgent assessment will be recognised by medical staff and referred or transferred appropriately.

The principal duty of the orthogeriatric unit is to promote mobilisation, self-care and, in most cases, eventual discharge of frail and often confused elderly patients. This is a complex task requiring patience, sensitivity and an awareness of the problems of the confused elderly patient. As rehabilitation is a matter of learning and because learning is impaired by dementia (the commonest barrier to rehabilitation in the elderly orthopaedic patient) a gently repetitive approach is often required. Perioperative confusional states may clear only slowly. It is not uncommon for a further confusional state to be precipitated by the move from the acute unit to the orthogeriatric unit. The usual principles of management of confusion, namely the identification and treatment of treatable underlying causes, minimal disturbance and minimal sedative medication, apply.

The organisation of nursing is key to the success of an orthogeriatric unit. Nursing must be rehabilitation oriented. Nurses function in effect as extenders of the efforts of more specialist rehabilitation professionals such as physiotherapists and occupational therapists. While the latter make assessments, set targets and review progress, much of the day-to-day and hour-to-hour work of rehabilitation is in practice carried out by nurses. Brief regular periods of mobilisation with an appropriate walking aid, if only to and from the toilet, is an excellent use of nursing resources. Likewise, supervision and encouragement of other activities of daily living such as washing and dressing can be carried out by nurses.

It is important that patients are briefed on admission about the purpose of their stay in an orthogeriatric unit. Many old people take the view that hospitals 'look after you' and require to be persuaded that it is in their interests to do as much as possible for themselves. If this is established and the ward is run in such a way as to encourage a return to normal life in terms of walking, dressing, self-toileting, and less obvious measures such as eating in groups round a table rather than seated alone or, worse, in bed, the message becomes clear. Patients see other patients progressing towards independence, a pre-discharge home visit and eventual successful discharge home and are encouraged to follow their example.

Most patients will go home. Typical outcomes are those reported from a London orthogeriatric unit showing that, following transfer from an orthopaedic unit, the median length of stay was 17 days (Murphy *et al.*, 1987). Including the time spent in the orthopaedic unit, this gave a total median hospital stay of 36 days. The eventual outcome of patients admitted to the unit was that 75% were discharged home, 4% were transferred for other forms of specialist treatment, 15% died and only 6% required admission to a continuing care unit.

A number of barriers to rehabilitation have been identified in patients transferred to an orthogeriatric unit, in that those remaining for more than 6 weeks are likely to be older, female, have had poor premorbid mobility, have had impaired mental function, and have concurrent medical problems rather than just a hip fracture (Whitaker & Currie, 1989) (Table 21.3). These are similar to those identified earlier in the chapter as factors associated with an adverse prognosis in elderly patients on admission to an orthopaedic unit. They are of some value in deciding upon the appropriateness or otherwise of transfer to a rehabilitation ward.

As considerable resources are involved in setting up and running orthogeriatric units, it is not surprising that a number of studies have been set up to evaluate their efficacy. On the basis of a historical comparison, the establishment of a ten bedded orthogeriatric assessment ward in Islington Health District was associated with an increase in the number of patients over 60 years admitted to the orthopaedic unit from 642 in 1980 to 888 in 1985, despite the fact that the number of beds allocated to orthopaedics had been reduced from 103 to 84 (Murphy *et al.*, 1987). Over the same period of time the median duration of stay for patients over the same age in the orthopaedic unit fell from 29 to 20 days, and the proportion spending more than 2 months in the unit fell from 30.8 to 12.9%.

A comparison also has been made between patients who remained in an orthopaedic unit and those transferred to an orthogeriatric ward (Whitaker & Currie, 1988). Those transferred to the orthogeriatric ward were older, had a lower mean mental test score, had a greater number of concurrent medical problems, and were less likely to have had independent mobility prior to the fracture. Despite this a comparable number were discharged to their own homes 6 weeks after admission, suggesting that the orthogeriatric ward provided a more effective rehabilitation programme.

Since then, there have been a number of prospective studies. The first of these randomised patients with fractured proximal femurs to transfer to an orthogeriatric unit or to continued management in orthopaedic wards (Gilchrist *et al.*, 1988). There was no difference in outcome for the two groups in terms of mortality, length of stay or placement, although more medical conditions were recognised and treated in the orthogeriatric unit.

Another study investigated the effectiveness of increased geriatric input into an orthopaedic unit (Kennie *et al.*, 1988). Patients were divided into two groups both of which received support from a physiotherapist and other rehabilitation service, but only the treatment group received thrice weekly visits and supervision of rehabilitation from a geriatrician. It emerged that a higher proportion of subjects in the treatment group regained independence in activities of daily living and were eventually discharged to their own homes, and that their median length of stay was shorter (Table 21.4).

Several factors could account for the disparity in the results of the last two studies

Table 21.3. *Factors associated with proportions of patients still in orthogeriatric unit six weeks after admission*

Factor	Percentage still in hospital at 6 weeks
Aged under 80 years	25.6
Aged 80 years and over	35.0
Male	19.5
Female	32.5
Unrestricted premorbid mobility	17.3
Poor premorbid mobility	38.1
No mental impairment	22.9
Mental impairment	38.7
Surgery within 24 hours	24.8
Surgery between 25 and 48 hours	42.3
Surgery between 49 and 72 hours	56.3
No intercurrent medical problems	17.3
More than four intercurrent medical problems	50.0

Source: Whitaker & Currie (1989).

Table 21.4. *Comparison between patients with proximal femur fracture receiving input from a geriatrician and a control group*

Outcome	Treatment group	Control group
Median stay in days	24(8–197)	41(9–365)*
Percentage independent in activities of daily living	41	25
Percentage discharged home	63	38
Percentage discharged to institution	10	32

Note: * Values in parentheses are ranges.
Source: Source: Kennie *et al.* (1988).

(Currie, 1989). One was that patients in the first of these were transferred to the orthogeriatric unit at a relatively late stage in their convalescence, by which time some of the potential for rehabilitation might have been lost. Again the second used more sensitive measures of outcome, which may have made it easier to detect differences between the treatment and control groups; however, this trial has been seriously criticised. The randomisation process resulted in the intervention group being on average substantially younger and mentally more alert than the control group, which may have accounted for some or much of the difference in outcome (Simpson & Whitaker, 1988).

A later study has compared the outcome of patients with fractured proximal femurs treated in Health Authority sectors, one with access to an orthogeriatric unit, the other without this (Hempshall *et al.*, 1990). The characteristics of the two groups on admission were similar in terms of age, sex ratio, dependency, proportion with significant medical problems and fracture type. The main difference in outcome was that, excluding initial mortality, the median length of stay among patients with access to the orthogeriatric unit was 29.5 as opposed to 38.0 days among patients from the other sector.

The above and a number of other evaluations of orthogeriatric units have been summarised (Newman, 1992). The overall impression is that orthogeriatric units produce a useful impact on length of stay, the most commonly used measure of outcome. Controversy about their usefulness continues, however, and doubts persist about both methodology and the implications of the findings of individual evaluations.

If collaborative care as provided in orthogeriatric units were a simple and uniform intervention, easily defined and readily exportable to another setting, evaluation would, of course, be a more straightforward matter. Orthogeriatric units vary greatly. Their effectiveness depends on a complex and locally determined combination of enthusiasm, resources and competence. Single inputs, such as physiotherapy, skills in geriatric medicine and orthopaedic supervision, to name only three, are probably quite important but impossible to evaluate separately. Length of stay is a crude measure of outcome. Dependency measures such as Barthel are more sensitive. The proportion of patients returning to their previous setting (i.e. avoiding progression to more expensive forms of care) may well be the outcome of the most economic consequence. Other evaluations of orthogeriatric rehabilitation are in progress but it does not seem likely that any dramatic revelations are in store. Progress will be made locally, and progress will become generalised as the overall concept of combined care, necessarily complex and dependent on local factors, for frail elderly trauma patients is more widely accepted. No single evaluation will demonstrate how best to do it everywhere.

Rehabilitation at home

The stimulus for early discharge from hospital was provided by a report from Australia of patients with a fractured proximal femur who were operated on under spinal anaesthesia, mobilised within hours of surgery and sent home as soon as they could walk, with continuing supervision being provided by a physiotherapist and community nurse (Sikorski *et al.*, 1985). Nineteen of 69 patients initially evaluated were considered unsuitable for rapid transit. These included 13 individuals with serious intercurrent medical or surgical conditions, three whose carers refused to have them back, one who lived in poor social circumstances, one who lived too far from the hospital and one with a complicated fracture. The scheme was unsuccessful in another four, one of whom died of advanced cancer, and three of whom were too disabled after surgery to consider discharge home. Despite this the mean length of stay of patients accepted into the scheme was three nights. The incidence of medical, urinary and surgical complications was 26% compared with one of 52% in patients treated conventionally in the same unit prior to introduction of the scheme.

A somewhat similar service has been developed in Peterborough (Pryor *et al.*, 1988), where a previously existing 'hospital at home' service provided opportunities for the intensive support and rehabilitation of elderly trauma patients discharged home. Within the orthopaedic unit, an attempt is made to operate on all patients within 24 hours of admission, and a spinal anaesthetic is used whenever practicable. Patients under 70 years of age normally are treated with internal fixation, while older ones are usually given an Austin–Moore hemiarthroplasty.

At the time of admission, patients are assessed by a doctor and an occupational therapist as to their suitability for early discharge. Factors of particular importance are a history of independence and mobility prior to the injury, and an absence of a serious intercurrent medical disorder.

Once a patient is identified, an occupational therapist performs a home visit to plan any equipment or adaptations necessary for the discharge. A liaison community nursing sister plans with the patient, relatives and community nursing service the amount of nursing help required, and the general practitioner is consulted and involved. After discharge a physiotherapist visits two to three times per week, and follow-up by the surgeon and occupational therapist is provided where necessary.

Analysis of 56 cases revealed that the average hospital stay was 8.2 days ranging from 2 to 21 days, and that the cost of home nursing per patient was £262, an amount far less than the cost of keeping the patient for a comparable period in hospital. The readmission rate was only 3.6% which suggests that few of the accelerated discharges had been inappropriate.

The Community Orthopaedic Project in Essex (1988) makes use of a hospital-based multidisciplinary team in the early discharge and rehabilitation at home of elderly orthopaedic patients including many with hip fractures. As with other comparable schemes, serious confusion appears to exclude patients. Although the scheme has had very considerable local impact in terms of reducing boarding out and feeding resources for elective orthopaedic surgery, no detailed economic or outcome analysis is yet available.

Ideally, all orthopaedic services admitting large numbers of elderly patients should have available, as resources permit, arrangements for early rehabilitation in the acute ward, early discharge and home rehabilitation arrangements for previously fitter patients, and inpatient combined rehabilitation facilities (orthogeriatric units) for patients whose rehabilitation needs are recognised as more complex and needing more time and effort.

Summary and conclusion

Elderly trauma patients, steadily increasing in numbers with the aging of populations and the age-specific increase in osteoporotic fractures, pose complex and urgent challenges for orthopaedic and geriatric services. A variety of collaborative schemes have evolved in different settings. Ideally, elderly trauma patients would have access to rehabilitation according to their needs and geared to maximising early independence and a return to their previous circumstances with appropriate continuing support comprising both rehabilitation and monitoring.

Rehabilitation schemes have evolved that vary considerably in outline and in detail. No ideal arrangements can be prescribed or need be sought. Local variations in process will continue.

Standardisation of outcome measurements is a much more useful and practical goal than standardisation of process. As hip fractures are common and costly, and because rehabilitation services that deal adequately with hip fracture patients can deal also with the wide range of lesser injuries, standardised audit procedures looking at mortality and functional and placement outcomes in hip fracture patients should be evolved and adopted.

References

Astrom, J., Almqvist, S., Berteema, J. & Jonsson, B. (1987). Physical activity in women sustaining a fracture of the neck of femur. *J Bone Joint Surg*, **69**, 381–3.

Barnes, B. & Dunovan, K. (1987). Functional outcomes after hip fracture. *Physical Ther*, **69**, 1675–9.

Bastow, M. D., Rawlings, J. & Allison, S. P. (1983). Benefits of supplementary tube feeding after fractured neck of femur: a randomised controlled trial. *Br Med J*, **287**, 1589–92.

Berggen, D., Gustafson, Y., Eriksson, B., Bucht, G., Hansson, L. I. *et al.* (1987). Post-operative confusion after anaesthesia in elderly patients with femoral neck fractures. *Anesth Analg*, **66**, 497–504.

Broos, P. L. O., Stappaerts, K. H., Luiten, M. D. & Gruwez, J. A. (1988). Home-going: prognostic factors concerning the major goal in treatment of elderly hip fracture patients. *Int Surg*, **73**, 148–50.

Campbell, A. J. (1976). Femoral neck fractures in elderly women: a prospective study. *Age Ageing*, **5**, 102–9.

Cameron, I. D., Lyle, D. M. & Quine, S. (1993). Accelerated rehabilitation after proximal femoral fracture: a randomised controlled trial. *Disabil Rehab*, **15**, 29–34.

Ceder, L., Stormqvist, B. & Hansson, L. I. (1987). Effects of strategy changes in the treatment of femoral neck fractures during a 17 year period. *Clin Orthop*, **218**, 53–7.

Cheng, C. L., Lau, S., Hui, P. W., Chow, S. P., Pun, W. K., Ng, J. & Leong, J. C. Y. (1989). Prognostic factors and progress for ambulation in elderly patients after hip fracture. *Am J Phys Med*, **68**, 230–3.

Clayer, M. T. & Bauze, R. J. (1989). Morbidity and mortality following fractures of the femoral neck and trochanteric region: analysis of risk factors. *J Trauma*, **29**, 1674–8.

Collins, R., Scrimgeour, A., Yusuf, S. & Peto, R. (1988). Reduction in fatal pulmonary embolism and venous thrombosis by perioperative administration of subcutaneous heparin. *New Engl J Med*, **318**, 1162–73.

Community Orthopaedic Project in Essex. (1988). Report to the King's Fund. London.

Cummings, S. R., Black, D. M. & Rubin, S. M. (1989). Lifetime risks of hip, Colles' or vertebral fracture and coronary heart disease among white post-menopausal women. *Arch Intern Med*, **149**, 2445–8.

Currie, C. T. (1989). Hip fractures in the elderly: beyond the metalwork. *Br Med J*, **298**, 473–4.

Currie, C. T., Tierney, A. J., Closs, S. J. & Fairtlough, H. L. (1993). Pain in elderly orthopaedic patients. *J Clin Nursing*, **2**, 41–6.

Currie, C. T., Tierney, A. J., Closs, S. J. & Fairtlough, H. L. (1994). Early supported discharge for elderly trauma patients, a report on a preliminary study. *Clin Rehab*, **8**, 207–12.

Day, J. J., Bayer, A. J., McMahon, M., Pathy, M. S. J., Spragg, B. P. & Rowlands, R. C. (1988). Thiamine status, vitamin supplements and post-operative confusion. *Age Ageing*, **17**, 29–34.

Delmi, M., Repin, C. H., Bengoa, J. M., Delmas, P. D., Vasey, H. & Bonjour, J. P. (1990). Dietary supplementation in elderly patients with fractured neck of the femur. *Lancet*, **335**, 1013–16.

Dolk, T. (1989). Influence of treatment factors on the outcome after hip fractures. *Upsala J Med Sci*, **94**, 209–11.

Eastwood, H. D. H. (1987). Delayed diagnosis of femoral neck fractures in the elderly. *Age Ageing*, **16**, 378–82.

Finsen, V. (1988). Improvements in general health among the elderly: a factor in the rising incidence of hip fractures? *J Epidemiol Commun Health*, **42**, 200–3.

Gilchrist, W. J., Newman, R. J., Hamblen, D. L. & Williams, B. O. (1988). Prospective randomised study of an orthopaedic geriatric inpatient service. *Br Med J*, **297**, 1116–18.

Gustafson, Y., Breggren, D., Brannstrom, B., Bucht, G., Norberg, A., Hanson, L. J. & Winblad, B. (1988). Acute confusional states in elderly patients treated for femoral neck fractures. *J Am Geriatr Soc*, **36**, 525–30.

Gustafson, Y., Brannstrom, B., Norberg, A., Bucht, G. & Winblad, B. (1991a). Underdiagnosis and poor documentation of acute confusional states in elderly hip fracture patients. *J Am Geriatr Soc*, **39**, 760–5.

Gustafson, Y., Brannstrom, B., Breggren, D., Ragnarsson, J. I. & Siggard, J. (1991b). A geriatric-anaesthesiologic program to reduce acute confusional states in elderly patients treated for femoral neck fractures. *J Am Geriatr Soc*, **39**, 655–62.

Hempshall, V. J., Robertson, D. R., Campbell, M. J. & Briggs, R. S. (1990). Orthopaedic geriatric care: is it effective? A prospective population-based comparison of outcome in fractured neck of femur. *J R Coll Phys Lond*, **24**, 47–50.

Hughes, A. V. (1986). Prevention of pressure sores in patients with fractures of the femoral neck. *Injury*, **17**, 19–22.

Ions, G. I. & Stevens, J. (1987). Prediction of survival in patients with femoral neck fractures. *J Bone Joint Surg (B)*, **69**, 384–7.

Kennie, D. C., Reid, J., Richardson, I. R., Kiamari, A. A. & Kelt, C. (1988). Effectiveness of geriatric rehabilitation care after fractures of the proximal femur in elderly women: a randomised clinical trial. *Br Med J*, **297**, 1083–5.

Lord, S. R. & Sinnett, P. F. (1986). Femoral neck fractures: admissions, bed use, outcome and projections. *Med J Aust*, **145**, 492–3.

McQueen, M. M., Littlejohn, M. A., Miles, R. S. & Hughes, S. P. (1990). Antibiotic prophylaxis in proximal femur fracture. *Injury*, **21**, 104–6.

Manninger, J., Kazar, G., Fekete, G., Fekete, K., Frenyo, S., Gyarfas, F., Salacz, T. & Varga, A. (1989). Significance of urgent (within six hours) internal fixation in the management of fractures of the neck of the femur. *Injury*, **20**, 101–5.

Mossey, J. M., Mutran, E., Knott, K. & Craik, R. (1989). Determinants of recovery twelve months after hip fracture: the importance of psychosocial factors. *Am J Pub Health*, **79/3**, 279–86.

Murphy, P. J., Rai, G. S., Lowy, M. & Bielawska, C. (1987). The beneficial effects of joint orthopaedic-geriatric rehabilitation. *Age Ageing*, **16**, 273–8.

Newman, R. J. (1992). Special collaborative rehabilitation schemes following femoral neck fracture. In *Orthogeriatrics*. Oxford: Butterworth-Heinemann.

Pryor, G. A., Williams, D. R. R., Myles, J. W. & Anand, J. K. (1988). Team management of the elderly patient with hip fracture. *Lancet*, **1**, 401–3.

Robbins, J. A. & Donaldson, L. J. (1984). Analysing stages of care in hospital stay for fractured neck of femur. *Lancet*, **2**, 1028–9.

Sexson, S. B. & Lehner, J. T. (1987). Factors affecting hip fracture mortality. *J Orthop Trauma*, **1**, 298–305.

Sikorski, J. M., Davis, N. J. & Senior, J. (1985). The rapid transit system for patients with fractures of proximal femur. *Br Med J*, **290**, 439–43.

Simpson, R. J., Whitaker, N. H. (1988). Hope for broken hips? *Br Med J*, **297**, 1543–4.

Stableforth, P. G. (1986). Supplement feeds and nitrogen and calorie balance following femoral neck fracture. *Br J Surg*, **73**, 651–5.

Taberner, D. A., Poller, L., Thomson, J. M., Lemon, G. & Weighill, F. J. (1989). Randomised study of adjusted versus fixed low dose heparin in prophylaxis of deep vein thrombosis in hip surgery. *Br J Surg*, **76**, 933–5.

Villar, R. N., Allen, S. M. & Barnes, S. J. (1986). Hip fractures in healthy patients: operative delay vs prognosis. *Br Med J*, **297**, 1543–4.

Whitaker, J. J. & Currie, C. T. (1988). An evaluation of the role of geriatric orthopaedic rehabilitation units in Edinburgh. *Health Bull*, **46**, 273–6.

Whitaker, J. J. & Currie, C. T. (1989). Non-orthopaedic problems in the elderly on an acute orthopaedic unit: the case for geriatrician input. *Health Bull*, **47**, 72–7.

Yesavage, J. A. (1988). Geriatric Depression Scale. *Psychopharmacol Bull*, **24**, 709–11.

22

Confusion and injury in old age

J. WATTIS

Confusion may be related to injury in old age in three ways: it may be a cause of injury, it may be a consequence of injury or it may be merely coincidental. Whatever the relation to any specific injury, confusion will, if present, have an impact – often a major impact – on management. The injury associated with confusion may be accidental or, in the case of surgical operations, planned. Surgical operation may be an urgent response to some other trauma or may be elective.

The term 'confusion' is insufficiently precise for medical use. Colloquially, it can refer to anything from a reaction to an embarrassing situation to profound dementia. For discussion here we will deal principally with the syndromes of dementia and delirium. Dementia may predispose to delirium so the two syndromes are not entirely unconnected.

Dementia

Dementia is briefly defined as 'an acquired, global impairment of intellect, memory and personality' (Lishman, 1978). More complicated definitions have been proposed (ICD–10, 1992), but Lishman captures the essence of a decline from previous function that affects more than just memory or cognition. Dementia is a term for a group of conditions of diverse aetiology that are generally age-related. Prevalence, extremely low in those under 65 years of age, rises to 2–3% in the 65–74 year age group, to around 5% in the 75–79 year group, to around 20% in those aged over 80 years (Brayne & Ames, 1988). The brain pathology of Alzheimer's disease is found in many cases, sometimes associated with multi-infarct brain disease and sometimes with less gross radiological signs of vascular damage, especially in very old people (Wallin *et al.*, 1989). The exact proportion of different types of dementia at post-mortem varies from study to study (Brayne & Ames, 1988). Alzheimer's disease has been split into various subtypes (Rossor *et al.*, 1984) and, recently, diffuse Lewy body disease has been shown to account for some cases of dementia (Gibb *et al.*, 1989), possibly as many as 20% of the demented elderly dying in hospital (Perry *et al.*, 1990). Knowledge about the pathology and aetiology of dementia continues to grow rapidly and the diagnosis of senile dementia of the Lewy body type and its implications was reviewed by Harrison & McKeith (1995).

One possible aetiological factor for Alzheimer's disease is head injury. A case-control study of 78 male Alzheimer cases found that the only major difference between patients and controls was a greater occurrence of antecedent head trauma in the patients (French *et al.*, 1985). A later mixed-sex study (Graves *et al.*, 1990) confirmed this finding although another larger study which relied on medical records rather than informant report failed to find an association (Chandra *et al.*, 1989). Although the first two studies may have been subject to reporting bias, the last may have under-recorded cases of head injury because of the stricter criteria used. A possible mechanism for post-traumatic dementia and a possible link with Alzheimer's disease was found by Roberts *et al.* (1991) who found βA4 amyloid at post-mortem in six of 16 head injury patients who survived to 18 days.

There is a possible link with dementia pugilistica. Although originally described as characterised by neurofibrillary tangles without plaque formation, reinvestigation using modern immunocytochemical methods has shown that the brains of patients who suffered from dementia pugilistica did show diffuse deposits of beta amyloid protein identical to that found in Alzheimer's disease (Roberts *et al.*, 1990). This reinforces theories that Alzheimer pathology may be the common result of a variety of insults, including head trauma.

While dementia may be a consequence of trauma, it may also be a cause. The prevalence of falls increases with increasing age but even so, the prevalence of falls resulting in fractures in patients with dementia ('chronic brain syndrome') was about two to three times higher than for non-demented controls (Weisenberg & Gaines, 1989; Buchner & Larson, 1987). Although previously identified with Alzheimer's disease (Wolfson *et al.*, 1990), there is increasing evidence for a possible link with Lewy body dementia, possibly through extrapyramidal mechanisms (McKeith *et al.*, 1994).

Delirium

The concept

The concept of delirium has a long and interesting history ably summarised by Berrios (1981). It was rooted in Greek medicine as early as the fifth century BC when its relation to physical disease was already understood. After some variations in the use of the term in the mid-nineteenth century, delirium returned to its meaning of a cluster of mental and behavioural symptoms occurring in the wake of physical disease. Lipowski (1987) reviewed the definition, frequency and clinical features of delirium. He proposed a definition of delirium as a transient disorder of cognition and attention, accompanied by disturbances of the sleep–wake cycle and of psychomotor behaviour. The International Classification of Diseases (ICD-9) used the term 'acute confusional state' as synonymous with delirium for a short-lived state characterised by clouded consciousness, confusion, disorientation, illusions and often vivid hallucinations, but ICD-10 (1992) returned to the use of the term 'delirium' as a major diagnostic category.

Clinical features

ICD-10 specifies that there must be some disturbance in each of five categories (consciousness, cognition, psychomotor function, the sleep–wake cycle and emotion) for a diagnosis of delirium.

Consciousness

Some patients with delirium show signs of autonomic over-arousal, others are drowsy, perhaps eventually lapsing into coma. The sleep–wake cycle is often disrupted with over-arousal at night and drowsiness by day. Variations in consciousness may be reflected in variations in orientation and cognitive test performance from hour to hour or from minute to minute. Hyper- or hypoactivity may result from the disturbance of consciousness. Lipowski (1987) warns that hypoactive delirium is less likely to be noticed than the hyperactive variety!

Cognition

There is a global disorder of cognition, affecting memory, thinking and the interpretation of percepts. The memory impairment affects registration, retention and recall. This is partly due to a failure of attention and it may be that disturbances of semantic memory (the meaningful way that memories are associated and organised) lie behind problems of disturbed thinking and misperception. Thinking is incoherent with reduced ability to direct and maintain a train of thought, deal with abstract concepts and solve problems. This causes impaired judgement and erratic behaviour. Misperceptions (illusions) occur when a normal perception is distorted or misinterpreted: a running tap appears as an overwhelming cataract or a nurse trying to restrain the patient from leaving hospital is seen as a criminal detaining the patient in wrongful imprisonment. Sometimes there are false perceptions (hallucinations) in the visual or auditory modalities varying from simple unformed shapes to complicated scenes. Visual hallucinations predominate, with some auditory hallucinations, and olfactory and other hallucinations much rarer. False beliefs, incompatible with the patient's cultural background (delusions), are often fragmentary and appear to be based on a disordered attempt to give meaning to the patient's abnormal experience.

Psychomotor disturbances

As well as the more expected overactivity, underactivity and rapid shifts from one to the other also occur.

Disturbance of the sleep–wake cycle

Sleeplessness or complete distintegration or reversal of the normal sleep–wake cycle is often found. Terrifying dreams, merging with hallucinations, are not uncommon.

Emotion

These experiences are often frightening and the patient may react with anxiety, anger, perplexity or withdrawal. Fear may account for the unpredictable and sometimes violent behaviour of patients with delirium.

Vulnerability to delirium in old age

Prevalence

Delirium has been reported in 12–50% elderly general medical inpatients at some time during their stay (Bergmann & Eastham, 1974; Warshaw *et al.*, 1982; Bowler *et al.*, 1994). In surgical patients the rates vary from 9 to 14% (Seymour & Vaz, 1989; Millar, 1981). These differences in prevalence reflect different methodologies, the transitory nature of delirium and difficulties in deciding the 'cut-off' point for such a diagnosis. Nevertheless, even at a conservative estimate, delirium is a significant problem among elderly patients on medical and surgical wards. It may also be wrongly diagnosed as dementia (Bowler *et al.*, 1994). In the community there are no reliable prevalence figures (MacDonald *et al.*, 1989), although future research may be helped by the development of standardised rating scales (O'Keefe, 1994).

Aetiology

As with most medical conditions, the cause of delirium is best understood multifactorially. A model which starts with the brain and considers the internal environment provided by other body systems, the interface provided by the sensory systems and the physical and social environment is useful for understanding not only causation but also management (Figure 22.1).

The brain

Children and old people appear to be specially susceptible to delirium. In children the immaturity of the central nervous system and of the cognitive and memory 'contents' of the system is presumably responsible. In older people, it is hard to separate the effects of aging from those of disease. Most of the changes, neuro-pathological, neurochemical, neurophysiological and neuropsychological, that are found in Alzheimer's disease are found (to a much lesser degree) in the brains of normal aged people.

Of particular interest is the role of acetylcholine as choline acetyl transferase activity in demented patients is inversely related to memory performance (Perry *et al.*, 1978) and because a single 2 mg dose of the anticholinergic drug benzhexol can produce measurable memory impairment, 90 minutes after administration, in cognitively well-preserved old people (Potamianos & Kellett, 1982). Pharmacological agents that interfere with cholinergic function or that produce sedation may contribute to delirium. They may also contribute directly to injury through falls due to postural hypotension (the tricyclic antidepressants) or due to extrapyramidal side-effects (the neuroleptics).

Alcohol is a special example of a drug that can lead to confusion and to injury through a variety of mechanisms. Confusion is produced in acute intoxication and

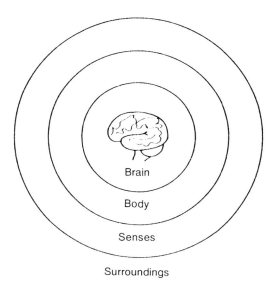

Figure 22.1. An interactive model of 'confusion'. Reproduced from Wattis & Martin (1994, Chapter 5) by permission of Chapman & Hall).

withdrawal states. The *delirium tremens* of alcohol withdrawal can be life-threatening. Thiamine deficiency can lead to the acute confusional state of Wernicke's encephalopathy and to the long-term selective memory deficit of Korsakoff's psychosis. Brain damage as a direct result of alcohol damage, and mediated indirectly through the mechanism of hypertension, can lead to dementia which may be at least partly reversible on stopping alcohol consumption. It is particularly important to include *delirium tremens* and Wernicke's encephalopathy in the differential diagnosis of any patient who becomes confused in the week after admission to hospital for whatever cause (Perkin & Hondler, 1983). Alcohol histories are rarely recorded adequately by admitting doctors (Awad & Wattis, 1990) and treatable conditions are therefore easily overlooked. Thiamine deficiency may also be responsible for postoperative confusion in some poorly nourished old people, independently of alcohol abuse (Older & Dickerson, 1982).

The senses

Since the 1950s it has been known that severe sensory deprivation can produce visual hallucinations, disorientation and cognitive impairment even in healthy young adults (Heron *et al.*, 1956). In a mixed diagnostic group of 150 elderly psychiatric patients, Berrios & Brook (1984) found a significant correlation between visual hallucinations and eye pathology, irrespective of diagnosis. There is also an association between long-standing deafness and paranoid psychosis in old people (Cooper *et al.*, 1974). Although it has not been demonstrated, it seems likely that relative sensory deprivation caused by defective sight and hearing may be a factor in the causation and phenomenology of many cases of delirium.

The environment

Change of environment can contribute to increased confusion, especially if it is rapid and inadequately explained as sometimes happens in emergency hospital admission following injury. Some environments are better than others at providing clues to enable a patient who is already disoriented to improve his/her orientation. Hospitals are notoriously bad at this. The design of the environment and consideration for the patient's experience in planning admission procedures can help reduce confusion. Most importantly, the patient should if possible be accompanied by someone familiar to them who will explain, repeatedly if necessary, what is going on. Staff need to spend time explaining procedures and nursing procedures should allow the patient to get to know a small group of core staff who are looking after him/her.

Postoperative delirium and dementia

Incidence

Nine to 14% of elderly surgical patients experience delirium in the postoperative period (Millar, 1981; Smith *et al.*, 1986; Seymour & Pringle, 1983). For hip fracture patients, the rate rises to over a third (Whittaker, 1989).

Permanent dementia after operation is much rarer. One early study found that 7% of surgical patients, mentally normal before operation, developed 'severe dementia' after operation, possibly linked to sustained hypotension during the operation. Later studies (Simpson *et al.*, 1961; Blundell, 1967) found either no postoperative dementia or much lower rates of sustained impairment. It may be that improvements in anaesthetic technique or the exclusion of 'high risk' emergency operations account for these differences. Nevertheless, anecdotally, relatives often date the onset of cognitive decline to the time of a major operation.

Predisposing factors

These can be divided according to time (preoperative, operative, postoperative) or type (e.g. intrinsic, anaesthetic, environmental). Dementia is known to be manifested according to a 'threshold effect'. A certain amount of neuropathological damage is necessary before dementia manifests itself clinically. It may be that patients who have 'subthreshold' damage are particularly vulnerable to damage at or around the time of operation. For delirium, Whittaker (1989) reviewed the literature and identified the following factors:

> *Preoperative*: increasing age, associated medical problems, pre-existing psychiatric problem (cognitive impairment or depression).
> *Operative*: type of surgery; heart surgery, prolonged surgery and emergency surgery were particularly implicated. Anaesthetic factors included general versus regional anaesthesia, hypoxaemia and hypotension.
> *Postoperative*: haemodynamic problems, infections, respiratory problems, drugs, metabolic problems and sensory deprivation.

To these we would add, at all phases, the effects of drugs (including alcohol/alcohol withdrawal). Bigler *et al.* (1985) demonstrated that not only depressive illness but also the use of antidepressant drugs predicted postoperative confusion. Although they were unable to separate out the effects of depression and its treatment, the more general finding of an association between postoperative delirium and serum levels of anticholinergic drugs (Tune *et al.*, 1981) suggests a probable mechanism. Similarly, sedatives and hypnotics may play an important part in generating postoperative confusion. Occasionally the problem may be a delirium due to benzodiazepine or alcohol withdrawal. Especially in emergency admissions, staff may be unaware of previous long-term benzodiazepine or alcohol use and its cessation on admission may provoke a withdrawal syndrome.

Management of the delirious patient

Prevention

A knowledge of predisposing factors should enable the risk of postoperative delirium to be minimised. The patient's medication should be reviewed and previous alcohol intake noted, appropriate steps being taken to avoid withdrawal states. Nutritional status and vitamin deficiencies should be considered. If there is any doubt, and there is no time for investigation, it is worth considering the use of a high dose thiamine-containing preparation in view of the possible association between thiamine status and postoperative confusion.

Management of the acute phase

This first involves diagnosis and treatment of medical problems. A review of the history (including drugs and alcohol) and a thorough physical assessment should be made looking for evidence of infection, cardiovascular and respiratory problems, fluid and electrolyte imbalance and medication which might be causing problems. In old people it is well to remember that multiple pathology is the rule rather than the exception. The role of pain, urinary retention, constipation and sensory deprivation should also be considered.

Second, management involves good interpersonal care, mainly nursing care. Mac-Donald *et al.* (1989) have pointed out that most of the advice given on this matter is not based on scientific findings and is often quite impracticable in the modern hospital setting. Nevertheless, one nursing study (Williams *et al.*, 1985) showed that interpersonal and environmental nursing interventions reduced the incidence of postoperative confusion from 51.5% in the control group to 43.9% in the treatment group for elderly patients with hip fractures. (After controlling for risk factors, this was statistically significant: $P < 0.02$.) The most effective interventions appeared to be those that provided orientation and clarification, corrected sensory deficit and increased continuity of care. Kitwood (1990) argues that the disability of dementia is partly caused by what he terms the 'malignant social psychology' of dementia. He argues that approaches which diminish respect for the patient as a person, such as 'talking across' the demented patient, increase confusion. His ideas are based on detailed observational studies of the quality of care for people with dementia and can be extended to care of the delirious patient.

Finally, management involves the judicious use of drugs. Despite the risk of extrapyramidal side-effects, short-term use of the antipsychotic butyrophenone, haloperidol, is to be preferred to those drugs with a strong anticholinergic profile such as thioridazine or chlorpromazine. The highly sedative, short-acting droperidol can also be useful. These medications should only be considered when other measures are not working and they are necessary to enable other necessary management or to prevent danger to the patient or others.

Legal aspects

In English statute law nobody has a specific right to give consent to medical treatment for an incapacitated adult. When the patient is incapable of giving a valid consent, any treatment not permitted under the doctrine of necessity is a technical assault. Under the doctrine of necessity 'a doctor is entitled, and probably has a duty, to carry out such emergency treatment as is necessary to preserve the life and health of an *unconscious* (my emphasis) patient' (The Law Commission, 1991). Unfortunately, the position for a conscious but incapacitated patient and the degree of threat to health or life are not defined; nor does the Mental Health Act (1983) help in respect for treatment of physical illness, although its provisions for compulsory admission do allow treatment for psychiatric disorder. Despite the lack of specific legal provision most doctors and nursing staff take the view that they have a duty of care to their patients which obliges them to treat serious illness in a patient who is incapable of consenting to such treatment because of delirium or dementia. The whole area of consent and the incapacitated adult is considered in detail in the Law Commission report referred to above which summarises approaches in a variety of jurisdictions.

Conclusion

Confusion may be related to injury in many ways. It may cause, complicate or be caused by injury and may be short-lived (delirium) or permanent (dementia). The tendency that doctors and other professional carers have to distance themselves from patients who are confused, can militate against quality care which must be based on sound scientific and humane principles. Accurate diagnosis and treatment and good interpersonal care, supplemented when needed by the judicious use of drugs, are essential. The pressure to reduce the length of inpatient stay and move patients on can mean that final decisions are made about placing a patient in a residential or nursing home before adequate time has been allowed for optimal recovery. Older patients with delirium often take a considerable time to regain mental equilibrium, especially if there is underlying demen-tia or continuing physical ill-health. Prolonged invalidism may be due to depressive illness which may masquerade as confusion. The newer antidepressant drugs with minimal anticholinergic action are to be preferred in these circumstances.

Confusion associated with injury provides a challenge to the diagnostic abilities and caring skills of all professionals involved. It is a challenge to be accepted, not avoided.

References

Awad, I. & Wattis, J. P. (1990). Alcohol histories in hospital: does the age and sex of the patient make a difference? *Br J Addict*, **85**, 149–51.

Bergmann, K. & Eastham, E. J. (1974). Psychogeriatric ascertainment and assessment in an acute medical ward. *Age Ageing*, **3**, 174–88.

Berrios, G. E. (1981). Delirium and confusion in the 19th century: a conceptual history. *Br J Psychiatry*, **139**, 439–49.

Berrios, G. E. & Brook, P. (1984). Visual hallucinations and sensory delusions in the elderly. *Br J Psychiatry*, **144**, 662–4.

Bigler, D., Adelhoj, B., Petring, O. U., Pederson, N. O., Busch, P. & Kalhke, P. (1985). Mental function and morbidity after acute hip surgery during spinal and general anaesthesia. *Anaethesia*, **40**, 672–6.

Blundell, E. (1967). A psychological study of the effects of surgery on eighty-six elderly patients. *Br J Social Clin Psychol*, **6**, 297–303.

Bowler, C., Boyle, A., Branford, M., Cooper, S. A., Harper, R. & Lindesay, J. (1994). Detection of psychiatric disorders in elderly medical inpatients. *Age Ageing*, **23**, 307–11.

Brayne, C. & Ames, D. (1988). The epidemiology of mental disorders in old age. In *Mental Health Problems in Old Age*, ed. B. Gearing, M. Johnson & T. Heller. Chichester: John Wiley & Sons/Open University.

Buchner, D. M. & Larson, E. B. (1987). Falls and fractures in patients with Alzheimer-type dementia. *J Am Med Assoc*, **257**, 1492–5.

Chandra, V., Kokmen, E., Schoenberg, B. S. & Beard, C. M. (1989). Head trauma with loss of consciousness as a risk factor for Alzheimer's disease. *Neurology*, **39**, 1576–8.

Cooper, A. F., Curry, A. R., Kay, D. W. K., Garside, R. F. & Roth, M. (1974). Hearing loss in paranoid and affective psychoses of the elderly. *Lancet*, **2**, 851–4.

French, L. R., Schuman, L. M., Mortimer, J. A., Hutton, J. T., Boatman, R. A. & Christians, B. (1985). A case-control study of dementia of the Alzheimer type. *Am J Epidemiol*, **121**, 414–21.

Gibb, W. R. G., Luthert, P. G., Janota, I. & Lantos, P. L. (1989). Cortical Lewy body dementia: clinical features and classification. *J Neurol Neurosurg Psychiatry*, **52**, 185–92.

Graves, A. B., White, E., Koepsell, T. D., Reifler, B. V., van Belle, G., Larson, E. B. & Raskind, M. (1990). The association between head trauma and Alzheimer's disease. *Am J Epidemiol*, **131**, 491–501.

Harrison, R. W. & McKeith, I. G. (1995). Senile dementia of the Lewy body type: a review of clinical and pathological features and implications for treatment. *Int J Geriatr Psychiatry*, **10**, 919–26.

Heron, W., Doane, B. K. & Scott, T. H. (1956). Visual hallucinations after prolonged perceptual isolation. *Can J Psychol*, **10**, 13–16.

ICD-10 Classification of Mental and Behavioral Diseases: clinical descriptions and diagnostic guidelines (1992). Geneva: World Health Organization.

Kitwood, T. (1990). The dialectics of dementia: with particular reference to Alzheimer's disease. *Ageing Society*, **10**, 177–96.

Lipowski, Z. J. (1987). Delirium (acute confusional states). *J Am Med Assoc*, **258**, 1789–92.

Lishman, W. A. (1978). *Organic Psychiatry*, 1st edn. Oxford: Blackwell.

MacDonald, A. J. D., Simpson, A. & Jenkins, D. (1989). Delirium in the elderly: a review and suggestion for a research programme. *Int J Geriatric Psychiatry*, **4**, 311–20.

McKeith, I. G., Fairburn, A. F., Perry, R. H. & Thompson, P. (1994). The clinical diagnosis and misdiagnosis of senile dementia of Lewy body type (SDLT). *Br J Psychiatry*, **165**, 324–32.

Millar, H. R. (1981). Psychiatric morbidity in elderly surgical patients. *Br J Psychiatry*, **138**, 17–20.

O'Keefe, S. T. (1994). Rating the severity of delirium: the delirium assessment scale. *Int J Geriatr Psychiatry*, **9**, 551–6.

Older, M. W. & Dickerson, J. W. (1982). Thiamine and the elderly orthopaedic patient. *Age Ageing*, **11**, 101–7.

Perkin, G. D. & Hondler, C. E. (1983). Injury and confusion, final draft. Wernicke–Korsakoff syndrome. *J Hosp Med*, **30**, 331–4.

Perry, R. H., Irving, D., Blessed, G. *et al.* (1990). Senile dementia of Lewy body type: clinically and neuropathologically distinct type of Lewy body dementia in the elderly. *Neurol Sci*, **95**, 119–39.

Perry, E. K., Tomlinson, B. E., Blessed, G., Bergmann, K., Gibson, P. H. & Perry, R. H. (1978). Correlations of cholinergic abnormalities and mental test scores in senile dementia. *Br Med J*, **2**, 1457–9.

Potamianos, G. & Kellett, J. M. (1982). Anticholinergic drugs and memory: the effects of Benzhexol on memory in a group of geriatric patients. *Br J Psychiatry*, **140**, 470–2.

Roberts, G. W., Allsop, D. & Bruton, C. (1990). The occult aftermath of boxing. *J Neurol Neurosurg Psychiatry*, **53**, 373–8.

Roberts, G. W., Gentleman, S. M., Lynch, A. & Graham, D. I. (1991). βA4 amyloid protein deposition in brain after head trauma. *Lancet*, **338**, 1422–3.

Rossor, M. N., Iversen, L. L., Reynolds, G. P., Mountjoy, C. Q. & Roth, M. (1984). Neurochemical characteristics of early and late onset types of Alzheimer's disease. *Br Med J*, **288**, 961–4.

Seymour, D. G. & Pringle, R. (1983). Postoperative complications in the elderly surgical patient. *Gerontology*, **29**, 262–70.

Seymour, D. G. & Vaz, F. G. (1989). A prospective study of elderly general surgical patients. II. Postoperative complications. *Age Ageing*, **18**, 316–26.

Simpson, B. R., Williams, M., Scott, J. F. & Crompton Smith, A. (1961). The effects of elective surgery and anaesthesia on old people. *Lancet*, **2**, 887–93.

Smith, R. J., Roberts, N. M., Rodgers, R. J. & Bennet, S. (1986). Adverse cognitive effects of general anaesthesia in young and elderly patients. *Int Clin Psychopharmacol*, **1**, 253–9.

The Law Commission. (1991). *Mentally Incapacitated Adults and Decision-Making: An Overview*. London: HMSO.

Tune, L., Holland, A., Folstein, M., Damlouji, N., Gardner, T. & Coyle, J. (1981). Association of postoperative delirium with raised serum levels of anticholinergic drugs. *Lancet*, **2**, 651–3.

Wallin, A., Blennow, K., Gottfries, C. G., Langstrom, G. & Uhlemann, C. (1989). White matter low attenuation on computed tomography in Alzheimer's disease and vascular dementia. *Acta Neurol Scand*, **80**, 518–23.

Warshaw, G. A., Moore, J. T., Friedman, S. W. *et al.* (1982). Functional disability in the hospitalised elderly. *J Am Med Assoc*, **248**, 847–50.

Wattis, J. P. & Martin, C. (1994). *Practical Psychiatry of Old Age*, 2nd edn. London: Chapman & Hall.

Weisenberg, L. B. & Gaines, J. (1989). The increased rate of fractures of the hip and spine in Alzheimer's patients. *West J Med*, **151**, 206.

Whittaker, J. J. (1989). Postoperative confusion in the elderly. *Int J Geriatr Psychiatry*, **4**, 321–6.

Williams, M. A., Campbell, E. B., Raynor, W. J., Mlynarczyk, S. M. & Ward, S. E. (1985). Reducing acute confusional states in elderly patients with hip fractures. *Res Nursing Health*, **8**, 329–37.

Wolfson, L., Whipple, R., Amerman, P. & Tobin, J. N. (1990). Gait assessment in the elderly: a gait abnormality rating scale and its relation to falls. *J Gerontol*, **45**, 12–19.

23
Some ethical issues

L. GORMALLY

Introduction

Only a limited selection of the ethical issues that arise in relation to management of injury in the aging will be discussed here. Limitations of space require the discussion to be in somewhat general terms. The issues for consideration concern:

- rationing decisions,
- decisions about the appropriateness and inappropriateness of treatment options,
- decisions about the conduct of research with the elderly.

Rationing decisions

If we think of rationing as essentially involving decisions establishing priorities between different claims on limited resources, we can usefully distinguish five levels at which such decisions are made (Klein, 1993):

1. the level at which the total National Health Service budget is determined,
2. the level at which resources are allocated to broad sectors or client groups, such as, for example, the elderly or renal patients,
3. the level at which resources are allocated to types of organisational provision (e.g. hospital or community care) and treatment (e.g. the development of renal transplantation),
4. the level at which it is decided which types of patients shall have access to available services and facilities, and
5. the level at which it is decided exactly which forms of investigation, treatment and care are to be provided to a patient who has been granted some access to services.

351

Decisions at levels 4 and 5 are traditionally regarded as the preserve of the clinician. There can hardly be much doubt that they should remain so at level 5. There is some doubt as to whether it should continue to be the case at level 4. It is suggested that the value of types of treatment for specific patient groups can be specified in terms of some cost-utility formula (such as Quality Adjusted Life Year (QALY) measures are used to supply). If that were possible there might be no distinctive role for the clinician at level 4. Even if one ignores, however, the highly contestable character of cost-utility formulae (Banner, 1992), it is clear from the phenomenon of patient heterogeneity that there can be no mechanical solution to decision-making at level 4. Since within any group of patients, whose responses to a given type of intervention will differ significantly, it is not reasonable to ration by reference to a standard outcome of that treatment in such a group.

Even if it is clear that a technical device such as a cost-utility formula cannot displace the role of clinical judgement at level 4, clinicians who have the responsibility of deciding which types of patient should have access to available services and facilities may be influenced by one line of argument about the health care entitlements of the elderly. This rests on the claim that age correlates with some factor which is morally relevant to fair rationing of medical services. Thus some maintain that age correlates with the capacity to benefit from treatment; others maintain that achievement of old age means one has had one's reasonable share of the benefits of the health care system. But old age as such is a poor predictor of an individual's capacity to benefit from medical interventions (Jahnigen & Binstock, 1991; Knaus *et al.*, 1991; see Chapter 19), and people vary enormously in the use they make of health care services over the course of a life. It is certainly morally relevant to take into account a person's capacity to benefit from treatment when one is obliged to ration scarce medical services, as one has an obligation to make the best use of those services. The basis of one's judgement should be assessment of the individual patient's capacity to benefit from some possible course of treatment and not the patient's age. In general, age is not as such a basis for fair rationing of scarce medical services (Boyle, 1992).

The above considerations suggest that level 4 rationing decisions have a problematic status. They cannot be reasonably made on the basis of cost-utility formulae, nor is it clear that they can be made except by reference to individualised clinical assessment of patients. If that is so, then the distinction between level 4 and level 5 rationing decisions is a distinction between deciding whether to treat a patient at all and deciding how much to investigate and treat a patient. If such decisions have to be made because demand exceeds the medical services available then the obvious basis for selection is the extent to which a patient can benefit from investigation and treatment.

Clinicians may have to make such decisions because of the constraints imposed upon them by decisions made at levels 1–3. Those decisions may be very unwise, particularly because of the consequences they have for a society's treatment of the elderly. Macroallocation decisions may have consequences subversive of recognition of the fundamental values of human dignity and human solidarity (Gormally, 1992).

Decisions about the appropriateness and inappropriateness of treatment

The classical idea of justice comprehends more than just fairness in the allocation of distributable goods, such as health care services. It embraces whatever is owing to others in the way of action and restraint. For individuals to possess the virtue of justice in this sense is for them to possess the fundamental disposition required in human relationships. For a society to exhibit justice in this sense is for it to have laws and institutional arrangements conducive to right relationships between individuals.

The 'others' to whom we have obligations of justice are human beings, and not some subclass of human beings identified by reference to possession of some range of exercisable psychological abilities (of understanding, choice and communication). Those who restrict entitlement to just treatment to some subclass of human beings are frequently somewhat arbitrary in specifying the precise psychological abilities they deem required if one is to have a claim to justice (i.e. if one is to be a subject of justice). Furthermore, and this is more crucial, they are unavoidably arbitrary in determining at what point in the development of the 'relevant' abilities a human being is entitled to just treatment. This arbitrariness is sufficient to invalidate the proposal to restrict the subjects of justice to some subclass of human beings. For it is part of our basic understanding of the notion of justice that it excludes arbitrariness about whom we should treat justly. If we allow that to be determined in an arbitrary fashion then our legal and social arrangements are precisely the contrary of justice. Membership of the fundamental community of those entitled to be treated justly has to be determined in a way which avoids any of the arbitrariness which may occur in determining the membership of less fundamental communities, such as the community of doctors or the community of a chess club. One can avoid arbitrariness in determining membership of the fundamental community of those entitled to be treated justly only by recognising that all human beings are subjects of justice (Gormally, 1993, 1995).

This recognition is expressed positively when we say that all human beings, simply in virtue of being human, possess an ineliminable dignity and value and basic human rights. The most fundamental of these rights is the right not to be unjustly killed. One may aim to bring about a person's death either by positive acts or by deliberately omitting to provide what is owing to that person (Gormally, 1994).

Ordinary care in the way of shelter, warmth, food and fluids is owing to vulnerable human beings on the part of those who have undertaken their care. The provision of ordinary care is directed to sustaining an individual's existence. By contrast, specifically medical care is directed to the restoration of health or of some approximation to health or to the palliation of symptoms. Health is a condition of bodily well-functioning (Kass, 1985). The distinction between ordinary care and medical care in terms of their different purposes is important to understanding when it is reasonable to abandon ordinary care and when it is reasonable to abandon medical treatment.

In a disaster situation involving scarcity of basic resources one may not be able to provide one or other form of basic nursing care. Otherwise such care should be provided. To deny it to a human being for whom one has responsibility, when it is possible to provide it, generally amounts to saying that the very existence of that human being is not worthwhile. That view of another human being's existence is incompatible with the recognition of his or her dignity. Indeed it makes the death of that human being appear to be a 'benefit' which doctors might aim to secure (Gormally, 1993).

Withholding of ordinary care, and especially of food and fluids, would not have a homicidal character if what motivates it is either knowledge that the patient is in the terminal phase of dying, and needs to be allowed to die, or knowledge that the method of delivering the food and fluids is itself proving a truly grave burden to the patient.

Judgement about the appropriateness or inappropriateness of medical care and treatment should be based on two kinds of consideration: (1) the achievability of the specific purpose (therapeutic or palliative) of the treatment, and (2) the degree to which it may prove burdensome to the patient, in other words excessively painful, or psychologically taxing, or disruptive of lifestyle, or in other ways unacceptably costly (Gormally, 1987).

In determining whether treatment is burdensome in one or another respect one must rely at least in part on what the competent patient thinks. And since whether treatment proves burdensome depends to some extent on an individual patient's disposition and sensibility, clinicians need to consult those who have been close to incompetent patients in order to make a sensitive judgement about whether some treatment is likely to prove burdensome.

Clinical judgement on which treatment is appropriate is primarily influenced by considering which is most likely to secure the therapeutic (or palliative) goal that presents itself for achievement. This is clear enough, for example, from consideration of approaches to fracture management in the aged. Thus in the case of proximal femoral fractures conservative management is not generally indicated because the long bed rest it requires is associated with a high complication rate 'and the end result may well be poor due to shortening and deformity' (Chapter 19).

Inevitably, in treating the elderly, questions arise about the worthwhileness of certain interventions. In addressing them it is important to ensure that the focus remains on the question of whether the treatment is sufficiently beneficial to the patient, and not to allow this question to be replaced by a question about whether a patient is worth benefiting. The discussion in Chapter 19 on the management of fractures in cases of metastatic bone tumours is instructive in relation to this issue. Clift

& Rowley are quite clear that such fractures should be treated 'with internal fixation even if the patient has only a short time to live' because the fractures cause considerable pain and disability and 'fixation greatly helps with pain relief'. Even though the benefit to be secured is perhaps relatively short-term, operative management is indicated because it clearly contributes to good palliative care. The fact that a benefit is short-term does not mean that it is inconsiderable.

Consideration of benefit to the patient seems to yield a negative answer, however, to the question whether to treat by operation femur fractures in those with advanced dementias. The issue of benefit is resolved by looking at the consequences of such treatment. If the most important factors in explaining death as an outcome of operative management are 'the (patient's) degree of independence before injury and . . . mental ability score' (Clift & Rowley, referring to Ions & Stevens, 1987), then there must be serious grounds for doubting the benefit of operative management of femur fracture in a patient with advanced dementia.

As we have already noted, an important error in evaluating the prospective benefits of treatment to elderly injured patients is that of allowing age itself to play a large part in that evaluation. Age as such is a poor predictor in the individual case of the outcome of treatment. Co-morbidity and the underlying physiological condition of the patient (such as his cardiovascular function) offer a much more reliable basis for predicting the outcome of treatment (Knaus *et al.*, 1991.)

Research on the elderly

When an experimental therapy or procedure is straightforwardly for the benefit of the experimental subject, then the moral issue is relatively simple. Providing what is undertaken offers some prospect of needed benefit which is not otherwise available, then one may run the risk of harms which are proportionate to the possible benefits. (One would not be reasonable by this criterion if, for example, one ran a significant risk of being killed in order to secure the benefit of mobility.)

The moral issues are more complex in cases of randomised clinical trials in which, typically, one group receives experimental therapy, another the standard therapy, and a third group a placebo. First, it is clear that patients should not be entered for such trials without their adequately informed consent, and specifically their consent to the possibility that they may be receiving no therapy. Second, it should also be clear that the option of no therapy should not involve the risk of significant disadvantage to the patients earmarked for it. Third, however, even if these conditions are satisfied there remains a problem about the responsibility of doctors. A doctor's primary responsibility is to heal the sick persons who are his patients here and now; how can he be said to honour such a commitment if he gives them placebos?

Whether one proceeds with clinical research in many situations depends on whether patients are competent to participate in it, so something ought to be said about competence to consent. 'Competence in the medical setting is the capacity for conscious and reasoned choices about one's own health and medical care' (Pellegrino, 1991). Competence is not an 'all or nothing' concept: incompetence to make investment decisions does not imply incompetence to decide whether one wants fried onions with one's sausage and mash. A person is capable of giving valid consent to participation in clinical research if he understands what is being proposed, and specifically what the short-term and long-term consequences of participation are for his health and well-being. One has reason to believe a person capable of the requisite understanding if he has shown himself capable of assimilating and assessing the significance of information of similar complexity. A person needs to be provided with information 'adequate for the choice to be made' (Kennedy, 1992); in the case of clinical research, information which accurately identifies the possible impact of the research on the research subject, and the consequences of the alternatives to participation.

In cases of non-therapeutic research the direct purpose is not medical benefit to the subjects of research but the advancement of knowledge.

Non-therapeutic research should never involve risk of serious harm to the research subject, not even to the consenting research subject. For it is wrong for persons to allow their bodies to be reduced to the status of instruments for securing scientific knowledge, and they would so reduce them if their bodily well-being were placed seriously at risk. The situation is, of course, different with risky therapeutic research when the justification for it is the possibility of improving the bodily well-being of the experimental subject; if one genuinely envisages serving someone's bodily well-being then one is not simply instrumentalising that person's body.

Research on the elderly who are incompetent, as on the incompetent in general, raises distinct issues. The duty of those charged with the responsibility of proxy (or vicarious) consent is to act for the good of the incompetent person. This is fundamental to understanding the duties of a proxy.

In cases of therapeutic research it is reasonable to consent to such research on an incompetent patient if the risks incurred are in proportion to the potential benefit to the patient.

In the case of non-therapeutic research a proxy cannot justifiably consent to research which might involve any risk of harm to an incompetent patient. There are two reasons for this. The first (already mentioned) is that the responsibility of the proxy is to act strictly for the good of the incompetent patient whose interests he represents. The second, that it belongs to the general justification of risk-taking in relation to research that it relies on the fact that it is freely undertaken. Hence, where it cannot be, subjection to risks is not justified.

This general position on the ethics of research may seem to be damagingly restrict-
ive, but the largely unrecognised danger in clinical research is a tendency to the
idolatry of scientific method. Single-minded preoccupation with the pursuit of truth by
the experimental method (and particularly preoccupation with an ideal of 'proof'; see
Anscombe, 1983) very easily leads to subversion of respect for other fundamental
values and specifically to the instrumentalising of human life, i.e. treating human
beings as though they were subordinate to the achievement of the scientist's goals. We
need to get scientific research in general, and clinical research in particular, into
perspective. Two observations are to the point. The first is that it is possible to think
that on balance the consequences of scientific research have been more harmful than
beneficial. Just that thought was indeed expressed some 15 years ago by a distin-
guished English philosopher when he wrote: '. . . it seems to me indisputable, with
hindsight, that we should be on balance far better off than we are if, in 1900 or in 1920,
all scientific research had come to a permanent stop. With the experience of what (has)
happened (since), we have little reason to doubt that the net practical result of future
research will be increasingly disastrous' (Dummett, 1981). One does not need to go all
the way with this contention in order to recognise that the tendency of scientists to give
over-riding weight to the advancement of knowledge is a serious threat to human
dignity and other values. A society which accommodates and rationalises this tendency is certainly an undesirable society.

The second point to note about clinical research in particular is the tendency greatly
to exaggerate the extent to which improvements in longevity and health are owing to
specifically medical interventions. We had come close to the present level of public
health before the pharmacological revolution started, thanks largely to improved diet
and public health measures (Nicholson, 1986). If we bear in mind the limited contribution to human health of medical interventions we will be less inclined to chafe at strict
ethical controls on medical research.

References

Anscombe, G. E. M. (1983). Sins of Omission? The non-treatment of controls in clinical trials.
In *Proceedings of the Aristotelian Society*, Suppl. **57**, 223–7.

Banner, M. (1992). Economic devices and ethical pitfalls: quality of life, the distribution of
resources and the needs of the elderly. In *The Dependent Elderly. Autonomy, Justice and
Quality of Care*, ed. L. Gormally, pp. 158–80. Cambridge: Cambridge University Press.

Boyle, J. (1992). Should age make a difference in health care entitlement? In *The Dependent
Elderly. Autonomy, Justice and Quality of Care*, ed. L. Gormally, pp. 147–57. Cambridge:
Cambridge University Press.

Dummett, M. A. E. (1981). Ought research to be unrestricted? *Gräzer Philosophische Studien.
Internationale Zeitschrift für Analytische Philosophie*, **12/13**, 281–98.

Gormally, L. (1987). A response (to Roy Fox. Palliative care and aggressive therapy). In

Medical Ethics and Elderly People, ed. R. J. Elford, pp. 177–98. Edinburgh: Churchill Livingstone.

Gormally, L. (1992). The aged: non-persons, human dignity and justice. In *The Dependent Elderly. Autonomy, Justice and Quality of Care*, ed. L. Gormally, pp. 181–8. Cambridge: Cambridge University Press.

Gormally, L. (1993). Against voluntary euthanasia. In *Principles of Health Care Ethics*, ed. R. Gillon, pp. 763–74. Chichester: John Wiley.

Gormally, L. ed. (1994). *Euthanasia, Clinical Practice and the Law*. London: The Linacre Centre.

Gormally, L. (1995). Walton, Davies, Boyd and the legalization of euthanasia. In *Euthanasia Examined. Ethical, Clinical and Legal Perspectives*, ed. J. Keown, pp. 113–40. Cambridge: Cambridge University Press.

Ions, G. K. & Stevens, L. (1987). Prediction of survival in patients with femoral neck fractures. *J Bone Joint Surg*, **69B**, 384–7.

Jahnigen, D. W. & Binstock, R. H. (1991). Economic and clinical realities: health care for elderly people. In *Too Old for Health Care? Controversies in Medicine, Law, Economics and Ethics*, ed. R. H. Binstock & S. G. Post, pp. 13–43. Baltimore and London: The Johns Hopkins University Press.

Kass, L. (1985). *Toward a More Natural Science. Biology and Human Affairs*. New York: The Free Press.

Kennedy, I. (1992). Consent to treatment: the capable person. In *Doctors, Patients and the Law*, ed. C. Dyer, pp. 44–71. Oxford: Blackwell Scientific Publications.

Klein, R. (1993). Rationality and rationing: diffused or concentrated decision-making? In *Rationing of Health Care in Medicine*, ed. M. Tunbridge, pp. 73–81. London: Royal College of Physicians.

Knaus, W. A. Wagner, D. P. & Draper, E. A. (1991). The APACHE III prognostic system: risk prediction of hospital mortality for critically ill hospitalized adults. *Chest*, **100**, 1619–36.

Nicholson, R. H. ed. (1986). *Medical Research with Children: Ethics, Law and Practice*. Oxford: Oxford University Press.

Pellegrino, E. D. (1991). Informal judgements of competence and incompetence. In *Competency. A Study of Informal Competency Determinations in Primary Care* (*Philosophy and Medicine*, vol. 39), ed. M. A. G. Cutter & E. E. Shelp, pp. 29–45. Dordrecht: Kluwer Academic Publishers.

Index

Page references to tables and figures appear in italics.